T0259977

Cannabis as Medicine

Cannabis as Medicine

Edited by
Betty Wedman-St Louis

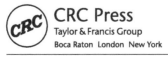

CRC Press
Taylor & Francis Group
Boca Raton London New York

CRC Press is an imprint of the
Taylor & Francis Group, an **informa** business

CRC Press
Taylor & Francis Group
6000 Broken Sound Parkway NW, Suite 300
Boca Raton, FL 33487-2742

© 2020 by Taylor & Francis Group, LLC
CRC Press is an imprint of Taylor & Francis Group, an Informa business

International Standard Book Number-13: 978-0-367-15054-9 (Paperback)
International Standard Book Number-13: 978-0-367-15055-6 (Hardback)

Library of Congress Cataloging-in-Publication Data

Names: Wedman-St Louis, Betty, author.
Title: Cannabis as medicine / Betty Wedman-St Louis.
Description: Boca Raton : Taylor & Francis, 2019. | "A CRC title, part of the
Taylor & Francis imprint, a member of the Taylor & Francis Group, the
academic division of T&F Informa plc." | Includes bibliographical references.
Identifiers: LCCN 2019017494| ISBN 9780367150549 (pbk. : alk. paper) |
ISBN 9780367150556 (hardback : alk. paper)
Subjects: LCSH: Cannabis—Therapeutic use.
Classification: LCC RM666.C266 W43 2019 | DDC 615.7/827—dc23
LC record available at https://lccn.loc.gov/2019017494

Visit the Taylor & Francis Web site at
http://www.taylorandfrancis.com

and the CRC Press Web site at
http://www.crcpress.com

Dedication

To Connor and so many others who have learned that cannabis can greatly improve their quality of life

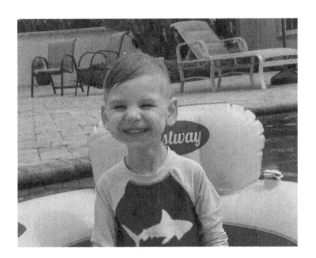

Contents

Acknowledgments

My deepest gratitude to all the contributors for making *Cannabis as Medicine* a reality. So many individuals have asked me how to get started in understanding how to use cannabis and now they have an excellent guide with many research studies reviewed all in one book. Everyone who reads this book will understand the benefits of using cannabis as a nutraceutical supplement and/or medicinal therapy.

A special thank you goes to Randy Brehm for believing that *Cannabis as Medicine* was needed as a CRC Press/Taylor & Francis Group reference for healthcare professionals.

Betty Wedman-St Louis, PhD
Clinical Nutritionist in Private Practice, St. Petersburg, Florida

Editor

Betty Wedman-St Louis, Ph.D., is a licensed nutritionist specializing in digestive diseases, diabetes, cancer, and environmental health issues who has been a practicing nutrition counselor for over 40 years. Her BS in foods and business from the University of Minnesota introduced her to how the food industry influences eating habits. Dr. Wedman-St Louis completed her MS in nutrition at Northern Illinois University where she studied the relationship between prolonged bed rest and space flight weightlessness nutrient requirements. She had a private practice at the Hinsdale Medical Center before completing her Ph.D. in nutrition and environmental health from The Union Institute in Cincinnati. Dr. Wedman-St Louis completed her doctorate internship at WUSF-Tampa in multimedia production for distance learning and online course development. Dr. Wedman-St Louis is the author of numerous published articles on current nutrition topics including phosphates in food, folate, vitamin B12, seafood nutrition, alpha lipoic acid, and diabetes. She has authored columns for "The Hinsdale Doings," "Chicago Sun-Times," and "Columbia Missourian" and has taught undergraduate and graduate courses on nutrition. She currently writes a personal health column for the "Tampa Bay Times" and maintains a private practice in Pinellas Park, Florida.

Contributors

Will Bankert
Shimadzu Scientific Instruments
Columbia, Maryland

Uwe Blesching

Kenneth Blum
Substance Abuse Disorder Institute
Philadelphia, Pennsylvania

Natascia Bruni
Istituto Farmaceutico Candioli Srl
Bernasco, Italy

Alline C. de Campos
University of Sao Paulo
Sao Paulo, Brazil

Robert Clifford
Shimadzu Scientific Instruments
Columbia, Maryland

Franco Dosio
University of Torino
Torino, Italy

Alexander Fossi
Thomas Jefferson University
Philadelphia, Pennsylvania

Daniela Gastaldi
University of Torino
Torino, Italy

Felipe V. Gomes
University of Sao Paulo
Sao Paulo, Brazil

Francisco S. Guimarães
Department of Pharmacology, Ribeirão
   Preto Medical School
University of Sao Paulo
Sao Paulo, Brazil

Robert T. Hoban
Hoban Law Group
Denver, Colorado

Samia R. Joca
University of Sao Paulo
Sao Paulo, Brazil

Joshua S. Kaplan
Western Washington University
Bellingham, Washington

Scott Kuzdzal
Shimadzu Scientific Instruments
Columbia, Maryland

Kaylee Martig
Western Washington University
Bellingham, Washington

Chris D. Meletis
Naturopathic Physician
Beaverton, Oregon

Joseph J. Morgan
Substance Abuse Disorders Institute
Philadelphia, Pennsylvania

Simonetta Oliaro-Bosso
University of Torino
Torino, Italy

Carlo Della Pepa
University of Torino
Torino, Italy

Enrica Pessione
University of Torino
Torino, Italy

Charles V. Pollack, Jr.
Thomas Jefferson University
Philadelphia, Pennsylvania

Keelee Reid
Western Washington University
Bellingham, Washington

Miles Sarill
CV Sciences
Watertown, Massachusetts

Judith Spahr
Thomas Jefferson University
Philadelphia, Pennsylvania

Betty Wedman-St Louis
Clinical Nutritionist in Private Practice
St. Petersburg, Florida

Paul Winkler
Shimadzu Scientific Instruments
Columbia, Maryland

Introduction

COMMEMORATING RAPHAEL MECHOULAM, PH.D.

In 2018 the International Association for Cannabinoid Medicine (IACM) thanked Professor Raphael Mechoulam for his extraordinary lifework in cannabis research.

Professor Mechoulam was born in Sofia, Bulgaria, on November 5, 1930, and moved to Israel in 1949 with his family where he studied chemistry and went on to receive his Ph.D. at the Weizmann Institute, Rehovoth, Israel, in 1958. After post-doctoral studies at the Rockefeller Institute in New York (1959–1960), he joined the scientific staff of the Weizmann Institute (1960–1965) before moving to the Hebrew University of Jerusalem where he became professor and Lionel Jacobson Professor of Medicinal Chemistry. Professor Mechoulam was chairman of IACM from 2003 to 2005 and continues contributing to cannabis research in helping millions of people suffering from endocannabinoid deficiency disorders.

In Zach Klein's documentary film *The Scientist*, Dr. Mechoulam states that cannabinoid medicine "is not being used as much as it should be in the clinic" referring to the treatment of patients with numerous conditions. He further states that as a scientist "in a small country like Israel with a limited budget, he chose to work on cannabinoid chemistry and approached the U.S. National Institutes of Health (NIH) for a grant in 1962." As Klein's film indicates, Mechoulam states NIH told him "the topic you're interested in, the constituents of cannabis sativa, is not a relevant topic for the U.S. It's not used in the U.S. When you have something more relevant, ask us for a grant."

Undeterred, Mechoulam started his cannabinoid research and he answers questions about that research.*

Question: **Where did you get cannabis for your research?**
Reply: I got hashish for research from the Israeli police. I even thanked the police for the supply in my original papers.

The hashish from which Mechoulam isolated THC and CBD had been obtained from the police in Jerusalem and he brought it to his laboratory on a bus despite the inquisitive looks and remarks from fellow passengers unfamiliar with the smell.

As the film *The Scientist* identifies, a year later Mechoulam got a phone call from a NIH pharmacologist. Mechoulam's reply in the film was "all of a sudden they had a change of mind so I asked them what happened. Well, apparently someone high up—an important person, maybe a senator—had called NIH and asked 'what does cannabis do?' According to Mechoulam, this person's son had been caught smoking

---

* Editor Note: Zach Klein's documentary film, "Raphael Mechoulam is *The Scientist*" (highlighted by Fred Gardner in *O'Shaughnessy's*, Winter 2015/16, https://beyondthc.com/oshaughnessys-winterspring-201516/), provided content and quotations for this review. Professor Mechoulam provided endorsement of the review and addressed questions from the editor. (*The Scientist* (2015). Directed by Zach Klein. Y.Klinik Productions. Retrieved from: http://mechoulamthescientist.com/.)

pot and he wanted to know if marijuana destroyed his mind and NIH knew nothing about marijuana." So the NIH pharmacologist went to Mechoulam's laboratory to learn about cannabis.

Question: **How did your 1964 science article on the structure of delta-9-tetrahydrocannabinol happen?**
Reply: As the psychoactive component of cannabis apparently had never been isolated in pure form and its exact structure had not been established, these were the aims of our research.

The NIH pharmacologist learned that we had discovered the active compound and had a large amount—about 10 grams THC—which he took back to the United States. As Mechoulam states, "so he got the world's supply of THC, took it to the U.S.—actually he probably smuggled it because I don't think he had a license to take it to the U.S. But then, of course, nobody was looking for THC. It was not a known compound."

Question: **How was your research in cannabis funded?**
Reply: As of 1965, for about 45 years, by the NIH.

Safety data was limited although the medical literature had reported cannabis use for centuries, so human experiment was needed. As Klein reported in *The Scientist,* Mechoulam and his wife, Dahlia, invited some friends to "take 10 milligrams of pure THC on a piece of cake while five took only the cake without THC." "None of us had ever used cannabis before. All those that took the THC were affected, but surprisingly, they were affected differently." Some said, "Well, we just feel kind of strange, in a different world. We want to sit back and enjoy." Another one said, "Nothing happens"—but he didn't stop talking all the time. A third one said, "Well, nothing's happened"—but every 15–20 seconds he would burst out laughing, Mechoulam observed. According to Mechoulam, "these effects are well-known today. People are differently affected."

Question: **When researching THC affect in the body, you have been quoted as indicating individuals are affected differently. From your years of research, do you have any clues as to why and what makes this difference?**
Reply: Most drugs have somewhat different actions in different individuals—particularly those drugs that act on the central nervous system. All of us somewhat differ—biochemically and physiologically—from each other, hence drug actions differ.

RESEARCH

1964: Structure of delta-9-THC described in a paper by R. Mechoulam & Y. Gaoni
1992: Mechoulam & Devane working at Hebrew University identified an endogenous cannabinoid—arachidonoyl ethanolamide or AEA which they named "anandamide" after the Sanskrit word for "bliss."

Question: **What led to your research for using cannabis in epilepsy?**

Reply: For centuries cannabis had been used in epilepsy, hence it seemed reasonable to test (first in animals) CBD for anti-epileptic effects. Then we tested it in patients.

A Brazilian study of CBD as a treatment for epilepsy sparked Mechoulam's interest when he heard "an Arab story of the 15th century and it says that one of the Arab leaders had epilepsy. A physician came over and gave him cannabis and it cured him. But he had to take it for his entire life." The Brazilian trials took place in San Paulo with 10 people who were not affected by known drugs for epilepsy. High doses of cannabidiol—200 mg per day—were used and no seizures occurred during the use of cannabidiol.

In 1986, your **Cannabinoids as Therapeutic Agents** concluded with the last sentence "Are we missing something?" Klein asked you to explain what you were asking and you replied, "Plant cannabinoids have been evaluated in the test tube. They had been evaluated in animals and to a certain extent in human patients. But nothing was known at that time about the mechanism."

Mechoulam rated the discovery of a cannabinoid receptor in rat brain by Allyn C. Howlett, Ph.D., pharmacologist at St Louis University School of Medicine in 1988 as a major key to the further understanding of cannabis mechanisms. He pointed out that receptors are made for compounds that we produce, "not because there is a plant that produces cannabinoids." This led to the discovery of the human endocannabinoid system and endogenous cannabinoids.

According to Klein's interview with Mechoulam for *The Scientist,* "we initially worked on brains of pigs" in search for the endogenous cannabinoid. "It is generally accepted that the organs of pigs and the organs of humans are somewhat closely related, so we wanted to work on pig brains but they were not easy to find in Jerusalem." The pig brains were supplied by a butcher in Tel Aviv but the price kept increasing as research advanced. Finally in 1992 a small amount of compound was identified as arachidonoyl ethanolamide. "It was only like a few droplets in the end of a little test tube" but pharmacologist Roger Pertwee, Ph.D., defined the compound as a cannabinoid.

CANNABIS FUTURE

Question: **What do you see as future research needs in cannabis?**

Reply: We badly need clinical trials. At the moment most medical use is based on individual reports.

Question: **In your opinion, why is cannabis as medicine not available to all who can benefit from it?**

Reply: In Israel we have at present about 35,000 patients who get medical cannabis— by approval of the Ministry of Health. Presumably all patients that need it. In some countries (or states) apparently the ruling bodies have not yet decided, presumably due to old laws.

1 What is Hemp?

Miles Sarill
CV Sciences

CONTENT

The passage of the Agricultural Improvement Act of 2018 establishes a marked shift in United States federal policy toward the cultivation and utilization of hemp, while distinguishing it from the drug varieties of cannabis [1]. As farmers begin to cultivate hemp, as herbalists begin extracting its constituents, and as patients and consumers begin ingesting these extracts, we must ask: "What is hemp?" The distinctions between true agricultural hemp and drug-type cannabis plants (i.e., marijuana) extend beyond legal importance. In this chapter, the botanical, genetic, agricultural, and phytopharmacological characteristics of this plant will be discussed.

Hemp is a cultivar of the plant Cannabis sativa L. and is defined by the US federal government as containing less than 0.3% Δ-9-tetrahydrocannabinol (THC) or its carboxylic acid form THCA by dry weight. THC is converted from THCA upon heat exposure in a process known as decarboxylation and is a principal constituent mediating the psychoactive, euphoric and sometimes psychotoxic effects of consumption of drug-type cannabis plants [2]. It is important to note that THC is but one of many phytocannabinoids found in cannabis, with as many as 120 being reported [3]. The dominant phytocannabinoid in agricultural hemp is cannabidiol (CBD), which is presently being researched for its antioxidant, immunomodulatory, anticonvulsant, and cytoprotective properties without any abuse potential or psychotoxicity [4,5]. Hence, although THC-rich cannabis strains are most popular for adult recreational use and show clinical efficacy in various medicinal applications, hemp-derived CBD preparations are becoming increasingly popular for both legal and practical reasons (Figure 1.1).

Hemp has been incorporated into various civilizations' agricultural practices globally for at least 10,000 years [6]. Hemp is a major crop in the production of fiber, food, and fuels and has been used in antiquity across many cultures to produce textiles, rope, and paper [7]. Evidence for the use of fiber hemp to produce food and medicinal extracts can be found in ancient Chinese texts extending back to at least 2,000 years [8]. Modern industrial uses of hemp fiber include the production of plastic-like composite materials and concrete alternatives [9,10]. Hemp seeds are edible and rich in amino acids, minerals, and essential fatty acids including the ω-3 polyunsaturated fatty acid alpha-linolenic acid [11]. Hemp is a bio-accumulator and has been examined as an important crop in soil restoration and regenerative agriculture [12,13]. Given that hemp may be useful for restoring soil from toxins including

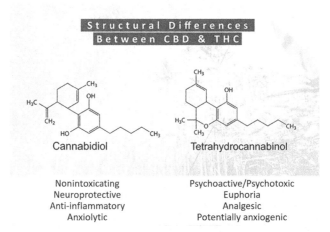

Nonintoxicating
Neuroprotective
Anti-inflammatory
Anxiolytic

Psychoactive/Psychotoxic
Euphoria
Analgesic
Potentially anxiogenic

FIGURE 1.1 The two molecules may appear similar, but the ring closure in Δ-9-tetrahydrocannabinol distinguishes a completely different pharmacodynamic quality in comparison to cannabidiol.

heavy metals, dioxins, etc., medicinal-grade hemp cultivated for phytocannabinoid extraction must be grown in low-pollution environments.

It has been suggested that cannabis genus plants can be further characterized into sativa, indica, and ruderalis species [14]. Other botanists prefer to categorize indica varieties as a subspecies of cannabis sativa [15]. The botanical differences between these species include their morphology, with C. sativa plants generally being taller and having narrower leaves than the smaller, bushier C. indica cultivars [16]. A common notion that is propagated among dispensaries and patient communities are that C. indica species have more relaxing and sleep-inducing properties compared to the uplifting and energizing properties of C. sativa drug-type strains [17]. Terpenoids, the scent molecules present in the cannabis plant, exert their own biological activity and may account for some of the pharmacological differences between C. sativa and C. indica strains [17–19].

Dividing the cannabis genus into sativa, indica, and ruderalis varieties may not be the most appropriate designation. Agricultural hemp is a cultivar of C. sativa but recent genetic research, however, illustrates that hemp shares some characteristics more in common with C. indica drug-type cultivars [20]. Researchers genotyped 81 marijuana and 43 hemp samples, analyzing single-nucleotide polymorphisms (SNPs) to establish and associate differences between C. sativa and C. indica ancestry, at a genome-wide level. In addition to the fact that many drug-type cannabis strain names did not reflect their associated genetic identity, true agricultural food and fiber hemp was found to have significant genomic differences from drug varieties of cannabis sativa, and more closely resemble some C. indica strains.

An important genetic distinction between agricultural food and fiber hemp in comparison to drug-type cannabis plants may be SNPs in the gene THCA synthase [21]. This gene codes for the enzyme that is responsible for the final step in the production of THCA in plants. THCA and other cannabinoids are produced by the plant in response to light exposure, to prevent damage to the leaves. Often medicinal and recreational cannabis growers will incorporate bright indoor lighting to encourage the highest expression of THCA, which may be a strain on the energy grid. True agricultural hemp can be grown outdoors, supporting the putative environmental benefits of cultivation, without leading to heightened THCA expression due to the aforementioned SNP.

Perhaps rather than trying to fit hemp into any specific cannabis subspecies, defining the chemical composition of the plant in terms of its cannabinoid expression is a more useful distinction. Cannabis varieties can be divided into five different chemical phenotypes (chemotypes). Type I chemotype plants are most often considered drug-type plants with a lowCBD/THC content ratio, due to the high expression of THCA or THC. An intermediate chemotype II displays roughly 1:1 CBD/THC ratios. Type III chemotype plants are the category that most agricultural hemp fit into, with a dominant expression of CBD with concentrations exceeding 0.5% dry weight and THC less than 0.3% dry weight. An additional type IV chemotype exists with cannabigerol (CBG) as the dominant cannabinoid, and type V with no significant detectable cannabinoids present in the plant [22,23].

Ratios of cannabinoids are not the only factor to consider when examining a hemp or cannabis plant. It is imperative to remember that cannabis is a plant of at least 400 different molecules including as many as 120 cannabinoids, terpenoids, alkaloids, polyphenols including flavonoids and stilbenoids, lignamides, tocopherols, and tocotrienols [3,19,24–28]. Different parts of the plant contain different constituents, with the highest percentage of cannabinoids present in trichromes located primarily in the flowering tops, but also present in other aerial parts [28]. Extraction of the seeds provides highly unsaturated fatty acids along with the novel anti-neuroinflammatory phenylpropanamide family of compounds including cannabisin B and N-trans-caffeoyltyramine [25]. Roots of the cannabis plant have an herbal history of being recommended for inflammation associated with arthritis and gout. Interestingly, however, cannabis and hemp roots contain virtually no CBD, THC, or other cannabinoids. Instead, extracting the root provides bitter alkaloids cannabisativine and triterpenoids friedelin and epifriedelanol exerting an anti-inflammatory effect [26,29].

A dominant terpenoid present in agricultural hemp is β-caryophyllene (BCP), a sesquiterpene present in many pungent herbs including *Nigella sativa* seed oil and oregano [30,31]. BCP is being studied as a powerful anti-inflammatory and antinociceptive. The effects of BCP in inflammation and immunomodulation extend to its role as an agonist of the cannabinoid receptor type 2 (for an in-depth discussion on the endocannabinoid system and cannabinoid receptors, please read further chapters) [32]. In contrast, strains dominant in the monoterpene β-myrcene are known to promote a sedative effect. β-myrcene is a $GABA_A$ receptor agonist at the benzodiazepine site and is known to cause "couch-lock," which may account for the sedative properties of β-myrcene dominant C. indica strains [17,33].

Beyond botanical morphology or classifying cannabis plant chemotypes based on cannabinoid levels, assessing content of terpenoids represents a novel chemotaxonomic approach. Researchers assessed 2,237 individual cannabis flower samples for cannabinoid and terpenoid content. It was found that CBD-dominant hemp-like type III cannabis plants display a unique profile of terpenes statistically different from drug-type cannabis varieties. Type III samples contained higher content of BCP relative to other terpenes such as β-myrcene, whereas the content of BCP was lower in most other varieties tested [19].

Because of the wide biological diversity of phytonutrients present in the hemp plant, extraction of a broad-spectrum of constituents is necessary to achieve the greatest bioactivity. Allopathic medicinal and pharmacological paradigm focuses on utilizing one compound to regulate one receptor to treat one disease. As a result, much of the present focus is on preparing isolated or purified cannabinoids. Doing so, ignores new research on the synergistic properties of phytocannabinoid-terpenoid interactions in pharmacological activity and that there is synergy among broad-spectrum cannabis extracts known as the entourage effect.

Epidiolex is 99% isolated CBD prepared by G.W. Pharmaceuticals and approved by the FDA in 2018 for the treatment of severe epilepsy associated with Lennox-Gastaut and Dravet syndromes [34,35]. A standard dose for this CBD preparation is 20 mg/kg/body weight daily, much higher than commercial preparations of CBD-rich hemp extracts typically consumed. A recent meta-analysis has shown, however, that there are potential clinical benefits of CBD-rich cannabis extracts over isolated CBD preparations such as Epidiolex in treatment resistant epilepsy [36]. CBD-rich cannabis extracts presented a better therapeutic profile, requiring significantly lower doses to be clinically effective than isolated CBD while causing less adverse reactions. Authors concluded that differences in clinical outcomes between isolated CBD and the broad-spectrum CBD-rich cannabis extracts arise from potential synergy among CBD, the many phytocannabinoids, and other cofactors within the cannabis plant: the entourage effect. *In vitro* evidence corroborates these findings by demonstrating that cannabinoids combined with a botanical drug cannabis extract containing minor cannabinoids and cofactors display significantly more biological diversity in their affinity for molecular targets than isolated cannabinoids [37].

With the immense popularity of CBD products available for consumers, it is imperative to choose a brand that captures a broad-spectrum of constituents from the aerial parts of hemp, operates an audited GMP (Good Manufacturing Practice) laboratory, and uses certified hemp seeds or strains. Because the legal status of CBD-containing dietary supplements is still under consideration in the United States, seeking out companies that have conducted formal safety research and attained generally recognized as safe (GRAS) self-affirmation on a hemp extract further supports their use [38]. Ultimately, within the United States, we suspect that there will be three main channels of distribution for cannabis products. Isolated drugs such as Epidiolex will be available through the pharmaceutical channel, preparations of drug-type THC dominant or mixed CBD:THC cannabis plants sold in medicinal and recreational dispensaries, and CBD-dominant agricultural hemp extracts sold through natural health retailers and mainstream distribution channels. Hence, with its broad range of constituents and multitude of cultivars, cannabis offers something for everyone.

REFERENCES

1. Pal L, Lucia L. Renaissance of industrial hemp: A miracle crop for a multitude of products. *BioResources.* 2019;14(2):2460–4.
2. Mechoulam R, Gaoni Y. The absolute configuration of delta-1-tetrahydrocannabinol, the major active constituent of hashish. *Tetrahedron Lett* [Internet]. 1967 Mar;12:1109–11. Available from: www.ncbi.nlm.nih.gov/pubmed/6039537.
3. Morales P, Hurst DP, Reggio PH. Molecular targets of the phytocannabinoids: A complex picture. In: Kinghorn AD, Falk H, Gibbons S, Kobayashi J, editors, *Progress in the Chemistry of Organic Natural Products.* Cham: Springer International Publishing, 2017, vol. 103, pp. 103–31. Available from: http://link.springer.com/10.1007/978-3-319-45541-9.
4. Machado Bergamaschi M, Helena Costa Queiroz R, Waldo Zuardi A, Crippa JAS. Safety and side effects of cannabidiol, a Cannabis sativa constituent. *Curr Drug Saf* [Internet]. 2011;6(4):237–49. Available from: www.eurekaselect.com/openurl/content.php?genre=article&issn=1574-8863&volume=6&issue=4&spage=237.
5. Schoedel KA, Szeto I, Setnik B, Sellers EM, Levy-Cooperman N, Mills C, et al. Abuse potential assessment of cannabidiol (CBD) in recreational polydrug users: A randomized, double-blind, controlled trial. *Epilepsy Behav* [Internet]. 2018;88:162–71. Available from: doi:10.1016/j.yebeh.2018.07.027.
6. Schultes RE, Klein WM, Plowman T, Lockwood TE. Cannabis: An example of taxonomic neglect. In: *Cannabis and Culture* [Internet]. Berlin, New York: De Gruyter Mouton. Available from: www.jstor.org/stable/41762285%0A.
7. Touw M. The religious and medicinal uses of Cannabis in China, India and Tibet. *J Psychoactive Drugs.* 1981;13(1):23–34.
8. Brand EJ, Zhao Z. Cannabis in Chinese medicine: Are some traditional indications referenced in ancient literature related to cannabinoids? *Front Pharmacol.* 2017 Mar;8:1–11.
9. Holbery J, Houston D. Natural-fiber-reinforced polymer composites in automotive applications. JOM [Internet]. 2006 Nov;58(11):80–6. Available from: http://link.springer.com/10.1007/s11837-006-0234-2.
10. Arnaud L, Gourlay E. Experimental study of parameters influencing mechanical properties of hemp concretes. *Constr Build Mater* [Internet]. 2012 Mar;28(1):50–6. Available from: https://linkinghub.elsevier.com/retrieve/pii/S0950061811004065.
11. Callaway JC. Hempseed as a nutritional resource: An overview. *Euphytica* [Internet]. 2004 Jan;140(1–2):65–72. Available from: http://link.springer.com/10.1007/s10681-004-4811-6.
12. Campbell S, Paquin D, Awaya JD, Li QX. Remediation of benzo[a]pyrene and chrysene-contaminated soil with industrial hemp (Cannabis sativa). *Int J Phytoremediation* [Internet]. 2002 Apr;4(2):157–68. Available from: www.tandfonline.com/doi/abs/10.1080/15226510208500080.
13. Ahmad R, Tehsin Z, Malik ST, Asad SA, Shahzad M, Bilal M, et al. Phytoremediation potential of hemp (Cannabis sativa L.): Identification and characterization of heavy metals responsive genes. *Clean - Soil, Air, Water* [Internet]. 2016 Feb;44(2):195–201. Available from: doi:10.1002/clen.201500117.
14. Hillig KW. Genetic evidence for speciation in cannabis (cannabaceae). *Genet Resour Crop Evol* [Internet]. 2005 Mar;52(2):161–80. Available from: http://link.springer.com/10.1007/s10722-003-4452-y.
15. Pollio A. The name of cannabis: A short guide for nonbotanists. *Cannabis Cannabinoid Res* [Internet]. 2016;1(1):234–8. Available from: www.ncbi.nlm.nih.gov/pubmed/28861494.

16. Anderson LC. Leaf variation among Cannabis species from a controlled garden. *Bot Mus Lealf Harv Univ* [Internet]. 1980;28(1):61–9. Available from: www.jstor.org/stable/41762825.

17. Piomelli D, Russo EB. The Cannabis sativa versus Cannabis indica debate: An Interview with Ethan Russo, MD. *Cannabis cannabinoid Cannabinoid Res* [Internet]. 2016;1(1):44–6. Available from: www.ncbi.nlm.nih.gov/pubmed/28861479.

18. Russo EB. Cannabidiol claims and misconceptions. *Trends Pharmacol Sci* [Internet]. 2017;38(3):198–201. Available from: doi:10.1016/j.tips.2016.12.004.

19. Orser C, Johnson S, Speck M, Hilyard A, Afia I. Terpenoid chemoprofiles distinguish drug-type *Cannabis sativa* L. Cultivars in Nevada. *Nat Prod Chem Res* [Internet]. 2018;6(1):1–7. Available from: www.omicsonline.org/open-access/terpenoid-chemoprofiles-distinguish-drugtype-cannabis-sativa-l-cultivars-in-nevada-2475-7675-1000304-98201.html.

20. Sawler J, Stout JM, Gardner KM, Hudson D, Vidmar J, Butler L, et al. The genetic structure of marijuana and hemp. Tinker NA, editor. *PLoS One* [Internet]. 2015 Aug 26;10(8):e0133292. Available from: http://dx.plos.org/10.1371/journal.pone.0133292.

21. Kojoma M, Seki H, Yoshida S, Muranaka T. DNA polymorphisms in the tetrahydro-cannabinolic acid (THCA) synthase gene in "drug-type" and "fiber-type" Cannabis sativa L. *Forensic Sci Int* [Internet]. 2006 Jun;159(2–3):132–40. Available from: https://linkinghub.elsevier.com/retrieve/pii/S037907380500407X.

22. Mandolino G, Carboni A. Potential of marker-assisted selection in hemp genetic improvement. *Euphytica*. 2004;140(1–2):107–20.

23. Pacifico D, Miselli F, Micheler M, Carboni A, Ranalli P, Mandolino G. Genetics and marker-assisted selection of the chemotype in Cannabis sativa L. *Mol Breed* [Internet]. 2006 Apr;17(3):257–68. Available from: http://link.springer.com/10.1007/s11032-005-5681-x.

24. Liu Q, Guo T, Hou P, Li F, Guo S, Song W, et al. Stilbenoids and cannabinoids from the leaves of Cannabis sativa f. sativa with potential reverse cholesterol transport activity. *Food Funct*. 2018 Dec 13;9(12):6608–17.

25. Zhou Y, Wang S, Ji J, Lou H, Fan P. Hemp (*Cannabis sativa* L.) seed phenylpropionamides composition and effects on memory dysfunction and biomarkers of neuroinflammation induced by lipopolysaccharide in mice. *ACS Omega* [Internet]. 2018 Nov 30;3(11):15988–95. Available from: http://pubs.acs.org/doi/10.1021/acsomega.8b02250.

26. Ryz NR, Remillard DJ, Russo EB. Cannabis roots: A traditional therapy with future potential for treating inflammation and pain. *Cannabis Cannabinoid Res*. 2017;2(1):210–6.

27. Falk J, Munné-Bosch S. Tocochromanol functions in plants: Antioxidation and beyond. *J Exp Bot* [Internet]. 2010 Jun;61(6):1549–66. Available from: www.ncbi.nlm.nih.gov/pubmed/20385544.

28. Andre CM, Hausman J-F, Guerriero G. *Cannabis sativa*: The plant of the thousand and one molecules. *Front Plant Sci* [Internet]. 2016;7(February):19. Available from: www.ncbi.nlm.nih.gov/pubmed/26870049.

29. Latter HL, Abraham DJ, Turner CE, Knapp JE, Schiff PL, Slatkin DJ. Cannabisativine, a new alkaloid from *Cannabis sativa* L. root. *Tetrahedron Lett* [Internet]. 1975 Jan;16(33):2815–8. Available from: http://linkinghub.elsevier.com/retrieve/pii/S0040403900750039.

30. Venkatachallam SKT, Pattekhan H, Divakar S, Kadimi US. Chemical composition of *Nigella sativa* L. seed extracts obtained by supercritical carbon dioxide. *J Food Sci Technol*. 2010;47(6):598–605.

31. Leyva-López N, Gutiérrez-Grijalva EP, Vazquez-Olivo G, Heredia JB. Essential oils of oregano: Biological activity beyond their antimicrobial properties. *Molecules.* 2017;22(6).

32. Pradier B, Zimmer A, Racz I, Klauke A-L, Markert A, Gertsch J, et al. The cannabinoid CB2 receptor-selective phytocannabinoid beta-caryophyllene exerts analgesic effects in mouse models of inflammatory and neuropathic pain. *Eur Neuropsychopharmacol* [Internet]. 2013;24(4):608–20. Available from: doi:10.1016/j.euroneuro.2013.10.008.

33. Costa CA, Kohn DO, De Lima VM, Gargano AC, Flório JC, Costa M. The GABAergic system contributes to the anxiolytic-like effect of essential oil from Cymbopogon citratus (lemongrass). *J Ethnopharmacol* [Internet]. 2011;137(1):828–36. Available from: doi:10.1016/j.jep.2011.07.003.

34. Mellis C. Cannabidiol for drug-resistant seizures in the Dravet syndrome. *J Paediatr Child Health.* 2018;54(1):101–2.

35. Thiele EA, Marsh ED, French JA, Mazurkiewicz-Beldzinska M, Benbadis SR, Joshi C, et al. Cannabidiol in patients with seizures associated with Lennox-Gastaut syndrome (GWPCARE4): A randomised, double-blind, placebo-controlled phase 3 trial. *Lancet* [Internet]. 2018 Mar;391(10125):1085–96. Available from: https://linkinghub.elsevier.com/retrieve/pii/S0140673618301363.

36. Pamplona FA, Da Silva LR, Coan AC. Potential clinical benefits of CBD-Rich cannabis extracts over purified CBD in treatment-resistant epilepsy: Observational data meta-analysis. *Front Neurol.* 2018 Sep;9:1–9.

37. De Petrocellis L, Ligresti A, Moriello AS, Allarà M, Bisogno T, Petrosino S, et al. Effects of cannabinoids and cannabinoid-enriched cannabis extracts on TRP channels and endocannabinoid metabolic enzymes. *Br J Pharmacol.* 2011;163(7):1479–94.

38. Marx TK, Reddeman R, Clewell AE, Endres JR, Béres E, Vértesi A, et al. An assessment of the genotoxicity and subchronic toxicity of a supercritical fluid extract of the aerial parts of hemp. *J Toxicol.* 2018;2018.

2 Endocannabinoid System & Cannabinoid Receptors

Betty Wedman-St Louis
Clinical Nutritionist

CONTENTS

The endocannabinoid system (ECS) is the most widely distributed receptor system in the human body that needs to adjust to constant change within the body and the external environment. The ECS regulates our biology through a homeostasis balance found in all vertebrate species. The system is maintained through endocannabinoids activating cannabinoid receptors CB_1 and CB_2 found throughout the body. The discovery of the endocannabinoid system stemmed from the 1992 Mechoulam and Devane research identifying the endogenous cannabinoid AEA (arachidonoyl ethanolamide) which was named "anandamide" after the Sanskrit word for bliss [1].

Cannabis has been important as a botanical herb for millenia, but it has only been in the past 25 years that medical science has unlocked its benefits. The discovery of cannabinoid receptors in the ECS—brain, skin, digestive tract, liver, cardiovascular system, bone, and genitourinary tract—provided a better understanding of this unexplained regulatory system [2].

Four kinds of cannabinoids can influence the endocannabinoid system regulation:

- **Endocannabinoids** are fatty acid cannabinoids produced naturally in the body (anandaminde [AEA] and 2-arachidonoylglycerol [2-AG])
- **Phytocannabinoids** are concentrated in the resin of cannabis buds and leaves with over 100 identified in the cannabis plant
- **Pharmaceutical cannabinoids** are manufactured in a laboratory that may or may not contain cannabis and sold as drugs
- **Synthetic cannabinoids** are manufactured artificially to mimic the effects of natural cannabinoids

The CB_1 endocannabinoid receptors were found to be more abundant in the central nervous system and brain, while the CB_2 receptors are predominately in the immune system. Endocannabinoid receptors are produced as needed by cells in the body from fatty acid molecules in the cell membrane. Both innate endocannabinoids and phytocannabinoids found in cannabis can activate CB_1 and CB_2 receptors [3].

The ECS initiates the production of new nerve cells to replace damaged cells and enhance memory along with improving neuroplasticity or new learning. Neurons communicate by electrochemical signaling, but when over-activity occurs, endocannabinoids are released to quiet the neuronal activity whether this occurs in the brain (e.g. multiple sclerosis), the immune system (e.g. cancer), or the gastrointestinal tract (e.g. Crohn's disease, IBS).

Inflammation is a protective response to infection (HIV/AIDS) or physical damage (brain trauma) whereby endocannabinoid regulation is critical to return the body to homeostasis. Chronic inflammation and autoimmune diseases create over-activated responses that result in constant endocannabinoid intervention. If homeostasis is not achieved, a chronic pathological condition evolves and the ECS can lose its effectiveness which results in disease progression [4].

Endocannabinoids are lipophilic, so transport processes—intestinal absorption, membrane permeability, protein-binding and distribution to tissues and organs, including the brain—need fatty acids for functioning. As a lipophilic compound, endocannabinoids linger in the system longer than hydrophilic substances and its beneficial effects last longer and wear off slowly. Lipophilic molecules generally diffuse across cell membranes and enter the blood stream for absorption [5].

Both CB_1 and CB_2 receptors are present in the gastrointestinal tract which can cause intestinal motility issues in an inflamed gut [6]. Endocannabinoids and their receptors are also involved in gastric secretions, ion transport, and cell proliferation in the gut. Since food is our primary source of essential fats, the human body has recognized the need for regulating homeostasis via fatty acid uptake in the gut [7].

The endocannabinoid system has significant implications in mammalian reproduction when it signals implantation of a fertilized egg onto the uterine wall. Inadequate anandamide (AEA) could lead to miscarriage or an ectopic pregnancy [8]. High levels of endocannabinoids in maternal milk are critical in developing suckling in a newborn and offsetting infant colic. As John Hick, M.D. states in *The Medicinal Power of Cannabis* [9]

> most people have not had their cannabinoid system supplemented since they were breast-fed. If they were not breast-fed, this system has not been supported since birth.

BEYOND CB_1 AND CB_2

In recent years, research on endocannabinoid receptors has moved beyond CB_1 and CB_2 to include the ionotropic cannabinoid receptor—transient receptor potential vanilloid 1 ($TRPV_1$)—and the regulatory metabolic and catabolic enzymes—FAAH (fatty acid amide hydrolase) and MAGL (monoacylglycerol lipase).

The primary functions of $TRPV_1$ in the body are to detect and regulate body temperature in addition to responding to pain, especially in the treatment of neuropathic pain. $TRPV_1$ is predominately expressed in peripheral sensory neurons and is widespread in the cardiovascular system. These sensors are also involved in nociception, taste perception, osmolarity sensing, as well as thermosensation.

Chronic inflammation such as in rheumatoid arthritis (RA) causes an activation of the sympathetic nervous system signaling the peripheral norepinephrine release to activate both AEA and 2-AG endocannabinoids. These endocannabinoids modulate transient receptor potential channels (TRPs) located on the sensory nerve fibers and induce pain signals along with secreting pro-inflammatory neuropeptides. Transit receptor potential vanilloid 1 can mediate chronic inflammation through interaction between the endocannabinoids and the sympathetic nervous system [10].

Fatty acid amide hydrolase (FAAH) is a main gatekeeper in cardiac functions, substance abuse disorders, and regulation of nociception [11–14]. Cell culture and animal studies have shown inhibiting FAAH may be a treatment option in anxiety disorders [15]. Certain flavonoids have been found to inhibit FAAH in its effort to break down the endocannabinoid anandamide [16]. Anandamide is responsible for maintaining basic endocannabinoid signaling. FAAH inhibition increases endocannabinoid concentrations and decreases pro-inflammatory cytokines while increasing the production of anti-inflammatory cytokines [10].

Monoacylglycerol lipase (MAGL) is a key enzyme that converts monoacylglycerol to the free fatty acid and glycerol which results in the degradation of lipoprotein triglycerides. This may be a possible therapeutic target to regulate the homeostatic action of endocannabinoids for pain, anxiety, and inflammatory bowel disease [17]. MAGL inhibition has also been shown to reduce cancer cell growth and brain inflammation [18]. Blocking MAGL, which controls levels of a pain-reducing metabolite in the brain and regulates neuroinflammation, could provide a therapeutic benefit in neurodegenerative disorders like Parkinson's disease and Alzheimer's disease.

CLINICAL CHALLENGES

Cannabis plants vary significantly based on species, cultivation, and processing. A cannabis plant can have more than 700 different chemical compounds including about 120 phytocannabinoids and more than 200 terpenes [19]. Terpenes have been shown to be synergistic with phytocannabinoids in producing therapeutic results for lowering inflammation, reducing pain, and protecting neurons. Full spectrum cannabis tinctures and extracts are recommended for improved therapeutic effect.

PHARMACEUTICAL & SYNTHETIC CANNABINOIDS

The U.S. Food & Drug Administration has approved several cannabinoid-based medicines with Epidiolex being the first cannabis-derived drug allowed. The active ingredient in Epidiolex is cannabidiol.

Dronabinol, a sticky man-made resin formulated from sesame oil, is sold as Marinol for treating anorexia. It is sold as a capsule in various strengths and may cause drowsiness and confusion in some patients.

Nabilone sold as Cesamet claims to activate CB_1 cannabinoid receptors to reduce nausea and vomiting. A capsule of Cesamet is used to reduce nausea and vomiting in chemotherapy patients and contains 1 mg nabilone plus povidone and corn starch. Povidone (polyvinylpyrrolidone) is used in the pharmaceutical industry as a synthetic polymer for aiding absorption in the human gastrointestinal tract [20].

Synthetic cannabinoids are products that are sold as K2, spice, "fake weed," or synthetic marijuana. They are made from various chemicals that can cause serious side effects. Synthetic cannabinoid products can be toxic in addition to causing psychoactive effects. They are designed to be similar to natural THC from the cannabis plant but often have greater binding effects to CB_1 receptors that can cause paranoia, anxiety, and seizures [21].

FULL SPECTRUM CANNABIS

Cannabis is much more than phytocannabinoids. As the graphic illustrates, cannabinoids make up a small percentage of the plant's potential as a botanical medicine. Terpenes, sesquiterpenes, and flavonoids are important considerations as synergy between these components is identified. Only from full spectrum cannabis oils and tinctures and raw juicing will the full benefit of this plant be recognized.

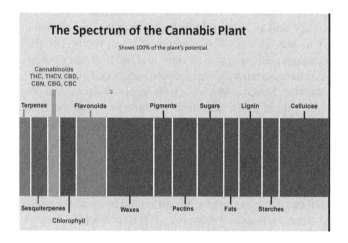

REFERENCES

1. Pacher P, Batkai S, Kunos G. The endocannabinoid system as an emerging target of pharmacotherapy. *Pharmacol Rev* 2006;58(3):389–462.
2. Russo EB. Beyond cannabis: Plants and the endocannabinoid system. *Trends Pharmacol Sci* doi:10.1016/j.tips.2016.04.005.
3. Ligresti A, De Petrocellis L, Di Marzo V. From phytocannabinoids to cannabinoid receptors and endocannabinoids: Pleiotropic physiological and pathological roles through complex pharmacology. *Physiol Rev* 2016;96(4):1593–1659.
4. Nagarkatti P, Pandey R, Rieder SA, et al. Cannabinoids as novel anti-inflammatory drugs. *Future Med Chem* 2009;1(7):1333–49.
5. Lipophilic foreign compounds. www.springer.com/cda/content/document/cda/9781461410485.

6. Mathison R, et al. Effects of cannabinoid receptor-2 activation on accelerated gastrointestinal transit in lipopolysaccharide-treated rats. *Br J Pharmacol* 2004;142:1247–54.

7. DiPatrizio NV, et al. Endocannabinoid signal in the gut controls dietary fat intake. *PNAS* 2011; 108:12904–8.

8. Maccarrone M. Endocannabinoids: Friends and foes in reproduction. *Prog Lipid Res* 2009;48(6):344–54.

9. Hichs J. *The Medicinal Power of Cannabis*. Skyhorse Publishing, New York, 2015.

10. Lowin T, Straub RH. Cannabinoid-based drugs targeting CB1 and TRPV1, the sympathetic nervous system, and arthritis. *Arthritis Res Ther* 2015;17(1):226.

11. Alfulaij N, Meiners F, Michalek J, et al. Cannabinoids, the heart of the matter. *J Am Heart Assoc* 2018;7:e009099.

12. Schacht JP, Selling RE, Hutchison KE. Intermediate cannabis dependence phenotypes and the FAAH C385A variant: An exploratory analysis. *Psychopharmacology (Berl)* 2009;203(3):511–17.

13. Cravatt BF, Lichtman AH. The endogenous cannabinoid system and its role in nociceptive behavior. *J Neurobiology* 2004;61(1):149–60.

14. Panlilio LV, Justinova Z, Goldberg SR. Inhibition of FAAH and activation of PPAR: New approaches to the treatment of cognitive dysfunction and drug addiction. *Pharmacol Ther* 2013;138(1):84–102.

15. Berardi A, Schelling G, Campolongo P. The endocannabinoid system and Post Traumatic Stress Disorder (PTSD): From preclinical findings to innovative therapeutic approaches in clinical settings. *Pharmacol Res* 2016;111:668–78.

16. Thors L, Belghiti M, Fowler CJ. Inhibition of fatty acid amide hydrolase by kaempferol and related naturally occurring flavonoids. *Br J Pharmacol* 2008;155:S244–S252.

17. Petrosino S, Di Marzo V. FAAH and MAGL inhibitors: Therapeutic opportunity from regulating endocannabinoid levels. PMID:20047159.

18. Nomura DK, Morrison BE, Blankman JL, et al. Endocannabinoid hydrolysis generates brain prostaglandins that promote neuroinflammation. *Science* 2011;334(6057):809–13.

19. Hendriks H, et al. Mono-and sesqui-terpene hydrocarbons of the essential oil of Cannabis sativa. *Phytochem* 1975;14:814–15.

20. Davis MP. Oral nabilone capsules in the treatment of chemotherapy-induced nausea and vomiting and pain. *Expert Opin Investig Drugs* 2008;17(1):85–95.

21. Centers for Disease Control and Prevention. Marijuana and public health. https://www.cdc.gov/marijuana/faqs.htm

3 Why Terpenes Matter— The Entourage Effect

Betty Wedman-St Louis
Clinical Nutritionist

CONTENTS

There is a lot more to cannabis than its cannabinoid content. Other therapeutic compounds in cannabis contribute to its smell and aromatic diversity. Terpenes have garnered increased attention as a result of the "entourage effect" which emphasizes that the therapeutic benefits of cannabis are improved when full spectrum compounds—multiple cannabinoids + terpenoids + flavonoids—are used instead of single cannabinoids. The terms terpene and terpenoid are frequently used interchangeably, but they have different meanings. Terpenes are hydrocarbons (the only elements present are hydrogen and carbon), whereas terpenoids have been denatured by oxidation—drying and curing the flowers or chemically modified.

Terpenes form the largest group of plant products and are the most common ingredient in volatile oils. They are sometimes referred to as isoprenoids due to the fact that all terpenes are derived from a 5-carbon precursor isoprene. Terpenoids are identified as monoterpenoids and monoterpenoid lactones, sesquiterpenoids and sesquiterpenoid lactones, diterpenoids, and triterpenoids. The triterpenoids form the largest group and are broken down into saponins, steroid saponins, cardenolides, bufadienolides, phytosterols, cucurbitacins, nortriterpenoids, and carotenoids [1]. Pharmacological interest in terpenoids is at an all time high as a plant-based diet takes on new meaning for health and well-being.

- Monoterpenoids are the simplest class of isoprenoids with more than 1,000 identified in algae, marine organisms, and insects. It is now realized that they have a considerable range of properties and are receiving increasing attention from the pharmaceutical industry [2]. They have a strong smell such as spearmint or lavender and vary in pharmacological properties as expectorants, insecticides, and antiseptics.
- Monoterpenoid lactones have been used to stimulate mucosal and gastric secretions within the human body.
- Sesquiterpenoids occur with monoterpenoids in plant essential oils and can be used as antifungals, insecticides, or as an antibiotic in treatment of staphylococcus aureus and candida albicans [3].
- Sesquiterpenoid lactones have cytotoxicity properties with ongoing anti-tumor research.
- Diterpenoids are usually toxic, but some have antibiotic, antiviral, anti-inflammatory properties with the Ginkgo biloba plant being the most prized phytochemical for treatment of memory loss [4].
- Triterpenoid saponins are plant glycosides that have medicinal implications as antifungals, antimicrobials, and adaptogens. Glycyrrhizin from licorice root is the most widely used anti-inflammatory triterpenoid saponin today.
- Steroid saponins are used therapeutically as expectorants, cell wall enhancers, cholesterol-lowering agents, and anti-inflammatory stimulants. Diosgenin from wild yam was used in the development of the first oral contraceptive [5].
- Cardenolides and bufadienolides are highly poisonous but provide cardiac glycosides to perform a specific action on myocardial muscle and calm myocardial infarction. Digitalis from the foxglove plant is an example of this function.
- Phytosterols are needed for plant membranes and cell growth. Sitosterol, stigmasterol, and campesterol are the most common phytosterols. Beta-sitosterol lowers plasma concentrations of LDL cholesterol [6].
- Cucurbitacins have cytotoxic, anti-tumor, and antileukemic properties.
- Nortriterpenoids are terpenoids that have been oxidized and degraded whereby they demonstrate antibacterial properties.
- Carotenoids are 40-carbon tetraterpenoids with lipid soluble terpenes found in all plants. The value to animals comes from splitting the C-40 molecule into a 20-carbon isoprenoid alcohol known as Vitamin K—a process that occurs after ingestion [7].

MAJOR TERPENOIDS IN CANNABIS

The essential oil or volatile oil found in cannabis is a mixture of about 200 terpenoids. No terpenoids are unique to cannabis, and the qualitative and quantitative profiles of terpenoids vary between batches of the same seed source [8]. Terpenoids along with cannabinoids and other compounds are synthesized inside the plant trichomes (cannabis flowers) and usually represent no more than 10% of the trichome content with subsequent losses based on storage, drying, and growing conditions [9].

The U.S. Food and Drug Administration (FDA) regard terpenes as food additives with GRAS (generally recognized as safe) status, despite their activity on receptors and neurotransmitters. But more research is needed to improve the accuracy of how they function medicinally and synergistically. A brief description of the major terpenoids found in cannabis follows:

MONOTERPENOIDS

β-Myrcene usually is the dominant monoterpenoid in all cannabis plants. It is also found in bay leaves, mango, lemon grass, thyme, hops.

- Sedative, muscle relaxant, anti-inflammatory, analgesic
- Anti-tumor, antioxidant
- Increases CB_1 receptor saturation allowing increased psychoactive effect

Limonene is also found in rosemary, juniper, peppermint, fruit rinds and is the second most common terpene in nature.

- Anxiolytic, anti-carcinogenic, treatment for GERD & gallstones
- Mood, stress relief

Terpinolene is one of the least common terpenes but is also found in nutmeg, tea tree, cumin.

- Sedative, antispasmodic
- Antioxidant, anti-tumor, antifungal, antibacterial

α-Pinene is also found in pine needles, rosemary, basil, parsley, dill.

- Anti-inflammatory, bronchodilatory, antiMRSA, AChE inhibitor
- Alertness, memory

β-Pinene

- Anti-tumor

Cis-O-Cimene is also found in parsley, basil, mangos, kumquats.

- Antiviral, antifungal, decongestant, antibacterial
- Anti-inflammatory, antioxidative

Linalool is also found in mint, cinnamon, coriander, and lavender

- A study of 12 hospitalized depressed patients indicated nine reduced their need for antidepressant medication through inhalation of linalool vapor which increased serotonin and dopamine in the brain [10].

- Anxiolytic, local anesthetic, analgesic, anticonvulsant
- Used topically as burn treatment
- Relaxation, stress relief, elevates mood, sedative
- Can restore cognitive function, useful in neurodegenerative disorders

SESQUITERPENOIDS

Levels of sesquiterpenoids may increase after drying in storage due to a reduction of monoterpenoids. This was particularly noted by Ross and ElSohly where β-caryophyllene increased from 1.33% to 5.45% after three months storage [11].

β-Caryophyllene is the primary sesquiterpenoid in cannabis, but it is also found in black pepper, oregano, cloves, and cinnamon. It is found in all cannabis chemovars and is the volatile compound used in drug detection.

- Anti-inflammatory, gastro-protective, analgesic, antimalarial, antifungal, antibacterial, anti-tumor
- CB_2 agonist for treatment of inflammation, pain, seizures
- Only terpenoid known to directly activate a cannabinoid receptor and frequently referred to as a "dietary cannabinoid"

α-Humulene is also found in hops, coriander, cloves, basil, sage.

- Anti-inflammatory, antibacterial, antifungal
- Anorectic/suppresses appetite
- Anti-tumor

To provide a perspective on how much monoterpenoid and sesquiterpenoid can be found in a cannabis sample, a GC-MS analysis of major terpenoids in volatile oil freshly extracted from cannabis inflorescences is given as follows [12]:

Compound	% Oil
α-Pinene	1.11–31.0
β-Pinene	0.6–7.95
β-Myrcene	8.23–67.11
Limonene	0.2–16.38
Linalool	0.09–2.8
O-Cimene	0.04–10.28
β-Caryophyllene	1.33–28.02
α-Humulene	0.28–12.61

DITERPENOIDS & TRITERPENOIDS

Diterpenoid paclitaxel and the semi-synthetic analogue docetaxel have been used in breast and prostate cancers [13,14]. Triptolide is a diterpenoid which has been reported to have antineoplastic activity through inhibiting cell growth at low concentrations and inducing apoptosis at high concentrations [15]. Triterpenoids are close to steroids in structure and are also extensively studied in hormone-related cancers and other types of cancer [16].

Plant derived terpenoids provide a broad spectrum of medicinal benefits, but limited research on the terpenoids found in cannabis and their synergistic properties has limited their use in therapeutic treatment options. As Yang and Dou declare, these compounds exhibit multiple properties including antioxidant, anti-inflammatory and anti-tumor benefits [17].

MINOR TERPENOIDS IN CANNABIS

Some minor cannabis terpenoids enhance the benefits of major terpenoids, but research is limited on their therapeutic use [18]. A number of them listed below are acetylcholinesterase (AChE) inhibitors. Acetylcholine in the brain is used to facilitate communications between nerve cells.

- Pulegone
  - AChE inhibitor
  - Sedative

- 1,8-Cineole
  - Increases cerebral blood flow
  - Stimulant
  - Antibiotic, antiviral, anti-inflammatory

- Terpineol
  - AChE inhibitor
  - Antibiotic, antioxidant
  - Sedative, relaxing effect

- Δ-3-Carene
  - Anti-inflammatory
  - Used to dry out excess tears, mucus, sweat

- Geraniol
  - Anti-tumor, antibacterial, antifungal
  - Antioxidant
  - Neuroprotectant

- Bisabolol
  - Anti-inflammatory, antimicrobial
  - Antioxidant

- Nerolidol
  - Sedative
  - Potent antimalarial

LINALOOL AND BRAIN FUNCTION

Neuroscience has long been reporting on how the sense of smell induces powerful affective experiences due to the intricate neuro-anatomy of olfactory processing [19]. Terpenes and flavonoids are the aromatic compounds in cannabis that the brain translates into individualized mechanisms that are still not fully elucidated [20]. These essential oils of cannabis act synergistically and may increase glutathione production in the liver [21,22].

Using the monoterpenoid linalool as an example, a rat study has shown that linalool blocks the excitatory brain chemical glutamate resulting in anti-convulsant and sedative properties. The brain chemical acetylcholine is reduced by linalool which reduced muscle contractions and rigidity. Linalool has anesthetic-like-effects to reduce excitability of the cells in the spinal cord which transmits pain signals to the brain [23]. In a mouse study, linalool reduced brain plaques and tangles which are characteristic of Alzheimer's disease and reversed behavioral and cognitive impairments [24].

Ota et al. [25] reported that 15 healthy male adults (mean age 31 ± 6 years) with no history of psychiatric illness or contact with psychiatric services were enrolled in a study to assess the effect of linalool on brain function. Linalool inhalation for 10 minutes in a quiet room resulted in CBF reductions in the right superior temporal gyrus to insula anterior cingulate cortex, which indicated the linalool influence on glutamatergic transmission to cause sedative and anxiolytic activity. The psycho-neurological effects of linalool impact its role in the gut-brain connection, stress, pain, and overall discomfort using a small dose of three to six drops of oil [26].

As the European Pharmacopeia, Sixth Edition (2007) states, terpenoids are pharmacologically versatile because of their lipophilic nature, whereby they interact with cell membranes, neurological signaling systems, neurotransmitter receptors, and G-protein coupled receptors [27].

TERPENE PRODUCTION IN CANNABIS

Many factors influence a plant's terpene content: climate, weather, age, fertilizers, and time of day harvested. As Russo elaborates, terpenes increase with light exposure but decrease with soil fertility [28]. According to Franz and Novak [29], the essential oil composition of the chemovar is more genetic than environmentally determined, but controlled environmental conditions of light, heat, and humidity have proven to provide good consistency for plant-based pharmaceutical quality [30,31].

BIOLOGICAL ACTIVITY OF TERPENES

Many terpenes in nature function as a defense mechanism and are used as commercial insecticides which disrupt the insect nervous system. These compounds target the cell membranes and can facilitate other toxins passing into the membranes [32]. A similar effect is seen against microorganisms, and pharmacologists can use this phenomenon to achieve drug delivery through the skin [33].

As Gershenson and Dudareva point out, terpenes may play roles as a conveyor of information over distances because of their low molecular weight in a lipophilic package. Most of the terpene cell-mediated communication research has been reviewed in plant-insect interactions [34], but the role of terpenes in the natural world has provided a glimpse into why full spectrum cannabis products offer synergistic benefits over single cannabinoids.

TERPENE EXTRACTION

Terpene extraction is a well-established industry within the fragrance world, and isolation of cannabis-derived terpenoids has become a specialized industry. Steam distillation is effective, but the heat and oxygen in the process can compromise the content of the terpenoids isolated. Processing with a vacuum pump using nitrogen gas and distilled water reduces the temperature of extraction, so volatile compounds are not lost [35].

The beneficial qualities of terpenoids can be seriously damaged if heated past their boiling point as identified by the Steep Hill analysis [36].

Terpenoid	Vaporizes Temperature
Pinene	311°F (155°C)
Myrcene	334°F (168°C)
Limonene	349°F (176°C)
Linalool	388°F (198°C)
O-Cimene	122°F (50°C)
Terpinolene	365°F (185°C)
Caryophyllene	320°F (160°C)
Humulene	388°F (198°C)

TERPENOID ANALYSIS

Cannabis Science and Technology [37] reported that most states are now starting to require cannabis products to be tested for terpenes listed in the American Herbal Monograph [8]. Only by understanding the terpene composition of different chemovars can research lead to more personalized medicinal choices. Patients and healthcare professionals need terpene profiles on cannabis products, so they can better manage symptoms.

The primary cannabinoids in cannabis are: delta-9-THC, CBD, CBG, and CBC. Delta-9-THC is the most psychoactive compound with terpenes modifying its effects. THCV (tetrahydrocannabivarin) is a variant of THC found in some chemovars of cannabis with somewhat reduced psychoactivity. CBD occurs in almost all cannabis plants, is not psychoactive, and has many of the same therapeutic effects of THC. CBG (cannabigerol) is non-psychoactive and is a powerful analgesic. CBC (cannabichromene) is found mostly in immature plants and is similar to CBD. [The "A" cannabinoids are raw plant; those no "A" are decarboxylated plant compounds.]

Therapeutic synergistic benefits of cannabis cannabinoids and terpenes can best be summarized in this manner:

- THCA (non-psychoactive)
  - *Anti-cancer*—caryophyllene, humulene, limonene, myrcene
  - *Anti-inflammatory*—pinene, caryophyllene, cineol, myrcene
  - *Anti-spasmodic*—myrcene

- THCVA
  - *Anti-inflammatory*—pinene, caryophyllene, cineol, humulene, myrcene

- CBDA
  - *Anti-inflammatory*—pinene, caryophyllene, cineol, humulene, myrcene
  - *Anti-cancer*—caryophyllene, humulene, limonene, myrcene

- CBGA
  - *Anti-inflammatory*—pinene, caryophyllene, cineol, humulene, myrcene
  - *Analgesic*—myrcene

- CBGVA
  - *Anti-inflammatory*—pinene, caryophyllene, cineol, humulene, myrcene

- CBCA
  - *Antifungal*—pinene, caryophyllene, limonene, terpinolene
  - *Anti-inflammatory*—pinene, caryophyllene, cineol, humulene, myrcene

- CBCVA
  - *Anti-inflammatory*—pinene, caryophyllene, cineol, humulene, myrcene

- THC (psychoactive)
  - *Anti-cancer*—caryophyllene, humulene, limonene, myrcene
  - *Anti-inflammatory*—pinene, caryophyllene, cineol, humulene, myrcene
  - *Anti-spasmodic*—myrcene
  - *Analgesic*—myrcene
  - *Bronchodilator*—pinene, cineol

- THCV
  - *Anti-inflammatory*—pinene, caryophyllene, cineol, humulene, myrcene
  - *Anti-convulsive*—linalool

- CBD
  - *Anti-inflammatory*—pinene, caryophyllene, cineol, humulene, myrcene
  - *Anti-cancer*—caryophyllene, humulene, limonene, myrcene
  - *Anti-depressant*—cineol, limonene, linalool
  - *Analgesic*—myrcene
  - *Anti-spasmodic*—myrcene
  - *Sedative*—linalool, myrcene. terpinolene

- CBDV
  - *Anti-convulsive*—linalool

- CBC
  - *Anti-inflammatory*—pinene, caryophyllene, cineol, humulene, myrcene
  - *Antifungal*—pinene, caryophyllene, limonene, terpinolene
  - *Anti-cancer*—caryophyllene, humulene, limonene, linalool
  - *Analgesic*—myrcene
  - *Antibacterial*—pinene, caryophyllene, cineol, humulene, limonene, linalool, terpinolene
  - *Sedative*—linalool, myrcene, terpinolene

- CBG
  - *Anti-cancer*—caryophyllene, humulene, limonene, myrcene
  - *Antifungal*—pinene, caryophyllene, limonene, terpinolene
  - *Antibacterial*—pinene, caryophyllene, cineol, humulene, limonene, linalool, terpinolene
  - *Analgesic*—myrcene
  - *Anti-depressant*—limonene, linalool

CANNABIS VS. MARINOL®

Marinol® is a brand name for dronabinol which is an FDA approved medicine used to treat nausea and vomiting from cancer chemotherapy. Dronabinol has also been used to improve appetite and reduce weight loss in HIV patients. But Marinol® consists of only synthetic delta-9-THC suspended in a sesame oil base and contains no terpenes. At such an expensive price, Marinol® misses out on the "entourage effect" of other cannabinoids, terpenoids, and flavonoids. Selecting full spectrum cannabinoid products offers increased therapeutic benefits.

JUICING CANNABIS FOR HEALTH BENEFITS

Juicing fresh buds and leaves allows an individual the opportunity to consume large amounts of THCA (non-psychoactive form of THC) and CBDA for anti-inflammatory, antioxidant, and cancer fighting properties. Cannabis juice has stimulatory properties for the immune system. The terpenes in raw cannabis juice have mood-altering and therapeutic benefits which need more clinical studies. Cannabis juice can be made by combining fresh-from-the-plant bud and leaves, and trim into a blender or juicer. If a blender is used, sieve or squeeze the juice through cheesecloth to eliminate the plant material. The juice tastes bitter, so it can be mixed into other liquids to modify the taste. Preserve large quantities by freezing it in ice cube trays to use as desired. Be sure to use ONLY fresh, organic plant material and check for mold and mildew before juicing.

Growing your own freshly harvested cannabis allows control of the cultivation of the plants. Maintaining a perpetual harvest ensures an adequate supply of raw cannabis. Every cultivar grows differently, so environmental factors (temperature, humidity, light intensity) need to be managed along with pest control to insure a healthy crop. Growing a home cannabis garden can be an investment of $100 to $1,000 with harvesting guidelines available on websites like Leafly.com [38].

TERPENOID FUTURE RESEARCH

Terpenes are lipophilic compounds that easily cross cell membranes and the blood-brain barrier to provide a wide array of pharmacological properties [39]. The future hopefully will provide increased research into how cannabis-derived terpenoid products offer specific therapeutic benefits. As laws prohibiting research in cannabis continues to evolve, terpenoids will be at the forefront for further development.

A dispensary owner in San Francisco described terpenes in this manner:

> Terpenes are the driving force behind the diverse effects of cannabis. If **THC** is the engine, **terpenes** are the steering wheel and tires!

REFERENCES

1. Harborne JB, Baxter H. *Phytochemical Dictionary: A Handbook of Bioactive Compounds from Plants.* Taylor and Francis, Washington, DC, 1993.
2. Charlwood BV, Charlwood KA. Monoterpenoids. In: Charlwood BV, Banthorpe DV (eds). *Terpenoids - Methods in Plant Biochemistry.* Academic Press, San Diego, CA, 1991.
3. Duke JA. *Handbook of Medicinal Herbs.* CRC Press, Boca Raton, 1985.
4. De Feudis FV. *Ginkgo Biloba Extract (EGb 761): Pharmacological Activities and Clinical Applications.* Editions Scientifiques Elsevier, New York, 1991.
5. Harborne JB, Baxter H. *Phytochemical Dictionary: A Handbook of Bioactive Compounds from Plants.* Taylor and Francis, Washington, DC, 1993.
6. Lehninger AL. *Principals of Biochemistry.* Worth Publishers, New York, 1982.
7. Flores-Perez U, Rodriguez-Concepcion M. Carotenoids. In: Saltar A, Wiseman H, Tucker G, ed. *Phytonutrients.* Wiley & Sons, 2012, pp. 89–93.
8. Cannabis Inflorescence Cannabis spp. Standards of Identity, Analysis and Quality Control. American Herbal Pharmacopoeia 2014.
9. Hazekamp A. *Medicinal Use of Cannabis: A Review.* Leidan, Netherlands, 2008–2009.
10. Guzman-Gutierrez SL, Gomez-Cansino R, Garcia-Zebadua JC, et al. *J Ethnopharmacol* 2012;143(2):673–9.
11. Ross SA, Elsohly MA. The volatile oil composition of fresh and air-dried buds of Cannabis sativa L. *J Nat Prod* 1996;59:49–51.
12. Cannabis Inflorescence Cannabis spp. Standards of Identity, Analysis and Quality Control. American Herbal Pharmacopoeia 2014.
13. Saloustros E, Mavroudis D, Georgoulias V. Paclitaxel and docetaxel in the treatment of breast cancer. *Expert Opin Pharmacother* 2008;9:2603–16.
14. Mancuso A, Oudard S, Sternberg CN. Effective chemotherapy for hormone-refractory prostate cancer (HRPC): present status and perspectives with taxane-based treatments. *Crit Rev Oncol Hematol* 2007;61:176–85.
15. Kiviharju TM, Lecane PS, Sellers R, et al. Antiproliferative and proapoptotic activities of triptolide (PG490), a natural product entering clinical trials, on primary cultures of human prostatic epithelial cells. *Clin Cancer Res* 2002;8:2666–74.
16. Rzeski W, Stepulak A, Szymanski M, et al. Betulinic acid decreases expression of bcl-2 and cyclin D1, inhibits proliferation, migration and induces apoptosis in cancer cells. *Naunyn Schmiedebergs Arch Pharmacol* 2006;3374:11–20.
17. Yang H, Dou QP. Targeting apoptosis pathway with natural terpenoids: implications for treatment of breast and prostate cancer. *Curr Drug Targets* 2010 Jun;11(6):733–44.

18. McPartland JM, Russo EB. Cannabis and cannabis extracts: greater than the sum of their parts? *J Cannabis Therap* 2001;1:103–32.
19. Krusemark EA, Novak LR, Gitelman DR, et al. When the sense of smell meets emotion: anxiety-state-dependent olfactory processing and neural circuitry adaptation. *J Neuroscience* 2013;33(39):15324–32.
20. Matsunaga M, Isowa T, Yamakawa K, et al. Psychological and physiological responses to odor-evoked autobiographic memory. *Neuro Endocrinol Lett* 2001;32(6):774–80.
21. Sultan MT, Butt MS, Karim R, et al. Nigella sativa fixed and essential oil modulates glutathione redox enzymes in potassium bromate induced oxidative stress. *BMC Complementary Altern Med* 2015;15:330.
22. Amorati R, Foti MC, Valgimigli L. Antioxidant activity of essential oils. *J Agric Food Chem* 2013;61(46):10835–47.
23. Elisabetssky E, Marschner J, Onofre Souza D. Effects of linalool on glutamatergic system in the rat cerebral cortex. *Neurochem Res* 1995;20(4):461–5.
24. Sabogal-Guaqueta AM, Osorio E, Cardona-Gomez GP. Linalool reverses neuropathological and behavioral impairment in old triple transgenic Alzheimer's mice. *Neuropharmacology* 2016;102:111–20.
25. Ota M, Sato N, Sone D, et al. (-)-Linalool influence on the cerebral blood flow in healthy male volunteers revealed by three-dimensional pseudo-continuous arterial spin labeling. *Indian J Psychiatry* 2017;59(2):225–7.
26. Mayer LA. The neurobiology of stress and gastrointestinal disease. *Gut* 2000;47:861–9.
27. Buchbauer G. Biological activities of essential oils. In: Baser KHC, Buchbauer G, eds. *Handbook of Essential Oils: Science, Technology, and Applications*. CRC Press, 2010, pp. 235–280.
28. Russo, EB. Taming THC: the potential cannabis synergy and phytocannabinoid-terpenoid entourage effects. *Br J Pharmacol*. 2011 Aug;163(7):1344–64.
29. Franz C, Novak J. Sources of essential oils. In: Baser KHC, Buchbauer G, eds. *Handbook of Essential Oils: Science, Technology, and Applications*. CRC Press, 2010, pp. 39–82.
30. Potter DJ. The propagation, characterisation and optimisation of Cannabis sativa L. as a phytopharmaceutical. 2009 PhD. King's College, London, 2009.
31. Fischedick JT, Hazekamp A, Erkelens T, et al. Metabolic fingerprinting of Cannabis sativa L., cannabinoids and terpenoids for chemotaxonomic and drug standardization purposes. *Phytochem* 2010;71:2058–73.
32. Gershenzon J, Dudareva N. The function of terpene natural products in the natural world. *Nat Chem Biol* 2007;3(7):408–14.
33. Kanikkannan N, Kandimalla K, Lamba SS, et al. Structure-activity relationship of chemical penetration enhancers in transdermal drug delivery. *Curr Med Chem* 2000;7:593–608.
34. Dudareva N, Negre F, Nagegowda DA, et al. Plant volatiles: recent advances and future perspectives. *Crit Rev Plant Sci* 2006;25:417–40.
35. Zuodong J, Kempinski C, Chappell J. Extraction and analysis of terpenes/terpenoids. *Curr Protoc Plant Biol* 2016;1:345–58.
36. Terpenes. Steep Hill Global Leader in Cannabis Testing and Analytics. www.steephill.com/science/terpenes.
37. Characterizing Cannabis. Cannabis Science and Technology. Jan 29, 2018. www.canabissciencetech.com/cannabis-strains/characterizing-cannabis.
38. How to harvest cannabis continually throughout the year. www.leafly.com/news/growing/how-to-harvest-cannabis-year-round.
39. Fukumoto S, Sawasaki E, Okuyama S, et al. Flavonoid components of monoterpenes in citrus essential oils enhance the release of monoamines from rat brain slices. *Nutr Neeurosci* 2006;9:73–80.

4 Cannabis Flavonoids— Antioxidant & Anti-Inflammatory Benefits

Betty Wedman-St Louis
Clinical Nutritionist

CONTENTS

A limited number of botanical plants qualify as both a food and a drug—cannabis is one of those botanicals. Another plant that qualifies is garlic which is employed as a flavoring agent in cooking but is also used to control hypertension and blood lipid levels. Psyllium (plantago) seed is another example. Psyllium seeds are incorporated into breakfast cereals and used widely as an OTC (over-the-counter) bulk laxative for purchase without a doctor's prescription [1].

As Elizabeth Pennisi wrote in *Science* "to many, cannabis is a recreational drug; to some it is a medicine. Now it is increasingly seen as a crop, to be grown in quantity and engineered for better traits—not just pharmacological effects, but also fiber content and the rapid, efficient growth needed for biofuels. Science is poised to play a bigger role in improving it" [2].

Recognition of the polyphenols found in cannabis and their potential in health is a big step beyond cannabinoids and their function in the body. Now that the antioxidant benefits of polyphenols have emerged as an important factor in cell signaling and modulation of mitochondrial function, flavonoids in cannabis take on a new therapeutic role [3]. Flavonoids are polyphenolic compounds that are divided into six subclasses: flavonols, flavones, flavanones, catechins, anthocyanidins, and

27

isoflavones. Individual differences within each group arise from variations in the hydroxyl groups, alkylation and/or glycosylation.

- **Flavonols**: quercetin, kaempferol, myricetin, galangin, fisetin (ex- broccoli)
- **Flavones**: apigenin, chrysin, luteolin, balcalin, baicalein (ex- skullcap)
- **Catechins**: epicatechin, epigallocatechin, epicatechin gallate (ex- green tea)
- **Flavanones**: eriodictyol, hesperitin, naringenin (ex- grapefruit)
- **Anthocyanidins**: cyanidin, pelargonidin, delphinidin, peonidin, malvidin (ex- pomegranate)
- **Isoflavonoids**: genistein, daidzein, glycitein, formononetin (ex- soybeans)

Flavonoids are molecules responsible for the color of fruit and flowers and provide powerful antioxidants along with stress modifiers, antiviral compounds, and anti-carcinogens [4]. In nature, they offer a wide range of functions in plants but primarily act as yellow pigments in petals and leaves to attract pollinating insects as well as protection against oxidative stress. Some flavonoids stimulate protein synthesis and others are known as anti-inflammatory agents. Botanicals containing flavonoids are used frequently as therapeutic compounds in diuretics and antispasmodics [5].

U.S. PATENT ON CANNABIS

The U.S. Department of Health and Human Services (HHS) owns the original patent US6630507 B1 on Cannabinoids as Antioxidants and Neuroprotectants filed on 4-21-1999 and granted 10-07-2003. The abstract of the patent reads:

Cannabinoids have been found to have antioxidant properties, unrelated to NMDA receptor antagonism. This new found property makes cannabinoids useful in the treatment and prophylaxis of a wide variety of oxidation associated diseases, such as ischemic, age-related, inflammatory and auto-immune diseases. The cannabinoids are found to have particular application as neuroprotectants, for example in limiting neurological damage following ischemic insults, such as stroke and trauma, or in the treatment of neurological diseases, such as Alzheimer's disease, Parkinson's disease and HIV dementia [6].

U.S. federal law indicates cannabis has "no accepted medical use" and yet the same government owns a patent for the medical use of marijuana. Over the years from 1965 to present, the National Institutes of Health (NIH) in Bethesda, Maryland, funded research in cannabis both as a drug of abuse and for its potential therapeutic properties. So when antioxidant properties were discovered, NIH licensed and patented cannabis production for research inside and outside NIH according to Mark Rohrbaugh who holds a doctorate in biochemistry and law and is a special advisor at NIH. Renate Myle, an NIH spokeswoman, indicated the patent expires on April 21, 2019 [7].

HEALTH BENEFITS OF FLAVONOIDS

Flavonoids are important in both human and animal nutrition [8] and more than 20 have been reported in cannabis [9]. Diets rich in phenolic compounds have been linked to a reduced incidence of chronic diseases—cancer, cardiovascular disease, and neurodegenerative conditions [10]. The flavones and flavonols in cannabis exert a wide range of biological effects along with terpenes and cannabinoids. The anti-inflammatory, anti-cancer, and neuroprotective properties are reviewed by Andre et al. in Current Nutrition Food Science [11] with flavones and flavonols being the primary ones [12]. A brief review of the flavonoids in cannabis has been provided as follows:

- **Cannflavin A,B,C** are methylated isoprenoid flavones with anti-inflammatory activity that inhibits the prostaglandins inflammatory pathway and enhance synergy with terpenoids [13,14].
- **Vitexin and Isovitexin** are used therapeutically for gout and inhibiting thyroid peroxidase [15].
- **Kaempferol** has been reported to have an antidepressant effect [15].
- **Apigenin** has been shown to be capable of stimulating the monoamine transporter, which alters neurotransmitter levels and acts as an anxiolytic and sedative on the GABA receptors along with cannabinoids [16].
- **Quercetin** inhibits viral enzymes and can have antiviral effects along with inhibiting prostaglandin production as an anti-inflammatory agent. It has synergistic benefits with cannabinoids to increase anti-inflammatory effects. Quercetin has also been shown to inhibit MAO (monoamine oxidase enzyme), so it can create possible interactions with some pharmaceuticals [17].
- **Luteolin and Orientin** have been shown to have pharmacological properties of antioxidants, anti-inflammatories, antibiotics, and anti-cancer [16].
- **Liganamides/Lignans** have been found in cannabis fruits and roots [18]. These phenolic amides and liganamides have health-promoting properties such as antioxidants, antivirals, antidiabetic, antitumorigenic and anti-obesity, but human studies are scarce [19]. Sun et al. [20] have shown anti-inflammatory properties in vitro while Cui-Ying et al. [21] have demonstrated cytotoxic activities of lignans that may be confirmed in cannabis.

Just as phenolic compounds in plants act as antioxidants and protect plants from oxidative stress, they have been shown to reduce the incidence of chronic diseases in humans [22]. Flavonoid bioactivity in human health includes regulation of cell signaling, anti-proliferative properties, free radical scavenging, and inhibition of angiogenesis [23].

- **Flavonols**—quercetin, kaempferol, and myricetin—are the most abundant flavonoids in plant foods and are usually present in most leafy vegetables, broccoli, and berries [23].
- **Flavones**—apigenin, luteolin, and anthocyanidins—are found in small amounts in grains, leafy vegetables, and herbs [23].
- **Catechins**—are abundant in tea, apples, grapes, chocolate, and red wine [23].
- **Flavonones**—naringenin and hesperetin—are found in citrus fruits and their juices [23].
- **Isoflavones**—daidzein and genistein—are found primarily in soy foods [23].

Limited human research in flavonoids and cannabis flavonoids is available but one intervention study on the biological activity of flavones provides insight. Fresh and cooked parsley was used as the flavone source. The treatment group had higher blood antioxidant enzyme activity of superoxide dismutase, glutathione peroxidase, glutathione reductase, and catalase [24].

Flavonoids may also be active in the intestinal lumen. Apigenin and luteolin inhibit TNF-induced proinflammatory gene expression in murine intestinal epithelial cells, and a similar effect was demonstrated in human epithelial cells that indicate activity against inflammatory bowel disease (IBD) [25,26].

FLAVONOIDS IN CANNABIS

According to Florez-Sanchez and Verpoorte [27], flavonoid content in cannabis varies from one plant tissue to another with no flavonoids detected in the roots. The orientin content in flowers and leaves did not differ significantly due to gender or cannabis plant chemovars. The orientin contents in seedlings and fruits were 14 times less than the contents in leaves and did not significantly differ among chemovars. Vitexin contents in fruits were similar and the lowest of all plant tissues. The lowest quercetin contents were detected in fruits and the highest in male flowers. The luteolin content in male flowers was significantly different from the leaves. The kaempferol levels did not show significant differences between the three chemovars studied. In leaves, the apigenin contents did not vary significantly by gender, but the flower contents were significantly different by gender.

As reported by Florez-Sanchez and Verpoorte cannabinoid levels accumulate during growth and development of the trichomes, but flavonoids decreased [27]. Accordingly, the isovitexin content did not significantly change during this period.

Another study of flavonoids in cannabis by Raharjo [28] reported apigenin and luteolin in leaves and flowers of Cannabis Four way plants with different results possibly due to plant age.

QUERCETIN

Quercetin is found in all vascular plants including cannabis [29]. Quercetin is a potent antioxidant that is more potent than ascorbic acid, alpha tocopherol, and BHT according to Gadow et al. [30]. McPartland and Russo [31] indicate flavonoids may block free radical formation, whereas Musonda and Chipman [32] describe flavonoids like quercetin as scavenging superoxide anions to catalyze many Fenton reactions.

LUTEOLIN

Luteolin is a common flavonoid found in many types of plants including cannabis. Plants rich in luteolin have been used in Chinese traditional medicine for treatment of hypertension, inflammation, and cancer. Luteolin like other flavonoids is glycosylated in plants and hydrolyzed to free luteolin during digestion [33]. It passes through the intestinal mucosa as glucuronides [34]. The anti-inflammatory effect of luteolin may be linked to its anti-cancer function where it induces apoptosis through redox regulation, DNA damage, and protein kinases for inhibiting proliferation of cancer cells and suppressing angiogenesis [35]. Luteolin is blood-brain barrier permeable, which allows for its therapeutic use in central nervous system diseases including brain cancer [36].

FLAVONOIDS & ANTI-INFLAMMATION

Inflammation is one of the body's defense mechanisms to guard against infection and heal injuries. Chronic inflammation can result in disorders like arthritis, COPD (Chronic Obstructive Pulmonary Disease), IBS (irritable bowel syndrome), and cancer. Macrophages are activated by molecules like cytokines and toxins from pathogens. The activated macrophages produce inflammatory molecules like tumor necrosis factorα (TNFα), interleukins (ILs), and free radicals, which cause neutrophils and lymphocytes to come to the inflammation site. Flavonoids, like luteolin, suppress the production of cytokines and suppress inflammation triggers. Because inflammation and its signaling pathways are associated with carcinogens, flavonoids may contribute to cancer prevention.

Antibiotics are frequently used to treat inflammation but are often accompanied by side effects and the development of resistant strains [37]. The traditional treatment of antibiotic resistant strains of bacteria is administration of vancomycin [38]. Xu and Lee [39] tested 38 flavonoids for activity against strains of methicillin-resistant S. aureus (MRSA) and found growth inhibited by the aglycones of the flavonols and flavones tested.

Flavonoids were also reported effective against viral activity. Quercetin inhibited HIV [40] and was effective in the treatment of AIDS [41] along with kaempferol, quercetin, and myricin. Lin et al. [42] reported bioflavonoids also showed antiviral activity.

ANTIOXIDANT ACTIVITY OF FLAVONOIDS

Flavonoids, in conjunction with other antioxidants—Vitamin C and E—are believed to inhibit lipid peroxidation in the phospholipid bilayer caused by ROS (reactive oxygen species). Flavonoids are likely to be located between the aqueous phase and phospholipid bilayer due to their hydrophilicity, so they can trap radicals at the interface of the membranes [43].

Duthie and Crozier [44] have shown that many flavonoids can be effective antioxidants in a wide range of oxidative systems by their ability to scavenge peroxyl radicals. In addition, some flavonoids can chelate metal ions responsible for the generation of ROS and inhibit the initiation of lipoxygenase reaction [45]. Flavonoids also exert antioxidant abilities through protection or enhancement of endogenous antioxidants through alleviating oxidative stress by inducing glutathione-S-transferase (GST) [46]. Quercetin, myricetin, and fisetin were shown to pay a protective role against cancer by detoxifying xenobiotics [47].

The antioxidant ability of phenolic compounds is based on their structure and the ease with which a hydrogen atom can be donated to a free radical. Studies have shown that aglycones—quercetin, luteolin, myricetin, and kaempferol—have greater antioxidant capacity than other flavonoids [48]. But further studies are needed to explore the bioavailability of flavonoids and their antioxidant effects.

OXIDATIVE STRESS & CELL FUNCTION

It is not known whether the human body's natural antioxidant defense system—superoxide dismutase (SOD), catalases, and selenium-glutathione peroxidase—is sufficient to counteract the increase in free radicals that occur during chronic diseases [49]. The human body attempts to maintain a balance between ROS production and the level of antioxidants to produce homeostasis, but with ROS overproduction, the endogenous defense mechanisms can be overwhelmed.

Body cells and tissues are continually threatened by the damage caused by free radicals and reactive oxygen species produced through normal oxygen metabolism and exogenous factors. In addition, free radicals can attract inflammatory mediators that contribute to a generalized inflammatory process. Flavonoids are powerful antioxidants with the ability to scavenge ROS and inhibit their destruction [50].

OXIDATIVE STRESS & MITOCHONDRIAL DYSFUNCTION

Mitochondria are the center of cellular energy production in the body and the major source of ROS [51]. Mitochondria produce superoxide anions as byproducts of electron leakage [52]. Under normal physiological conditions, mitochondrial ROS is removed by the cellular antioxidant defense system—superoxide dismutases (SOD), catalase, and glutathione peroxidase. However, under pathological conditions, the mitochondrial ROS is over produced leading to excess radicals that damage the mitochondria and cells [53]. The uncontrolled overproduction of ROS overwhelms the cellular antioxidant capacity and impairs the mitochondria.

Mitochondrial dysfunction produces functional losses and structural changes, which disrupt the membrane and causes ATP depletion resulting in low energy metabolism. Associations between mitochondrial dysfunction, aging, and neurodegenerative diseases have been characterized as oxidative stress on the neuronal system, especially due to its high lipid content and metabolic rate [54]. Supplementation with antioxidants can reduce the oxidative load and improve endothelial cell integrity [55].

CANNABIS FLAVONOIDS AS SYNERGY AGENTS

The health benefits of fruits, vegetables, and botanicals are due to synergy or interactions between different bioactive compounds [56]. Cannabis compounds exert their therapeutic effects in humans in a similar manner. Flavonoids modulate the pharmacokinetics of THC via inhibition of the hepatic P450 enzymes-3A11 and 3A4 [57].

As McPartland stated [58], other cannabinoids, terpenoids, and flavonoids can reduce tetrahydrocannabinol-induced anxiety, cholinergic deficits, and immunosuppression. Full spectrum cannabis extracts containing a mixture of all these compounds are needed for the full therapeutic benefits for this precious plant.

REFERENCES

1. Awang DVC, *Tyler's Herbs of Choice - The Therapeutic Use of Phytomedicinals*. CRC Press, 2009, pp. 1–6.
2. Pennisi E. A new neglected crop: cannabis. *Science* 2017;356(6335):232–233.
3. Vauzour D, Vafeiadow K, Spencer JPE. Polyphenols. In: Salter A, Wiseman H, Tucker G, eds. *Phytonutrients*. Wiley-Blackwell, 2012, pp. 110–145.
4. Evans WC. *Trease and Evan's Pharmacognosy*. 13th ed. Philadelphia Bailliere Tindall (The Curtis Center), 1989, p. 420.
5. Batchelder HJ. Pharmacognosy. *Protoc J Bot Med* 1995;1(1):159–163.
6. US 6630507 B1. Cannabinoids as antioxidants and neuroprotectants. http://patents. google.com/patent/US6630507.
7. Wallace A. Patent No. 6,630,507: Why the U.S. government holds a patent on cannabis plant compounds. www.thecannabist.co/2016/08/22/marijuana-patents-6630507-research-dea-nih-fda-kannalife/61255.
8. Manthey JA, Buslig BS. Flavonoids in the living system. *Adv Exp Med Biol* 1998;439:1–7.
9. ElSohly MA, Slade D. Chemical constituents of marijuana: the complex mixture of natural cannabinoids. *Life Sci* 2005;78:539–548.
10. Arts IC, Hollman PC. Polyphenols and disease risk in epidemiologic studies. *Am J Clin Nutr* 2005;81:317–325.
11. Andre CM, Larondelle Y, Evers D. Dietary antioxidants and oxidative stress from a human and plant perspective: a review. *Curr Nutr Food Sci* 2010;6:2–12.
12. Flores-Sanchez IJ, Verpoorte R. Secondary metabolism in cannabis. *Phytochem Rev* 2008;7:615–639.
13. Barron D, Ibrahim RK. Isoprenylated flavonoids-a survey. *Phytochemistry* 1996; 43:921–982.
14. Werz O, Seegers J, Schaible A, et al. Cannaflavins from hemp sprouts, a novel cannabinoid-free hemp food product, target microsomal prostaglandin-E 2 synthase-1 and 5-lipoxygenase. *Pharmanutr* 2014;2:53–60.
15. Murti K, Panchal MA, Gajera V, et al. Pharmacological properties of Matricaria recutita: a review. *Pharmacognosy* 2012;3:348–351.
16. Hostetler GL, Ralston RA, Schwartz SJ. Flavones: food sources, bioavailability, metabolism and bioactivity. *Adv in Nutr* 2017;8(3):423–435.
17. Malavolta M, Costarelli L, Giacconi R, et al. Modulator of cellular senescence: mechanisms, promise, and challenges from in vitro studies with dietary bioactive compounds. *Nutr Res* 2014;34(12):1017–1035.
18. Sakakibara I, Ikeya Y, Hayashi K, et al. Three phenyldihydronaphthalene legnamides from fruits of Cannabis sativa. *Phytochemistry* 1992;31:3219–3223.
19. Andre CM, Hausman J-F, Guerriero G. Cannabis sativa: the plant of the thousand and one molecules. *Front Plant Sci* 2016;7:19.
20. Sun J, Gu Y-F, Su X, et al. Anti-inflammatory lignanamides from the roots of Solanum melongena L. *Fitoterapia* 2014;98:110–116.
21. Cui-Ying M, Wing Keung L, Chun-Tao C. Lignanamides and nonalkaloidal components of Hyoscyamus niger seeds. *J Nat Prod* 2002;65:206–209.
22. Arts IC, Hollman PC. Polyphenols and disease risk in epidemiological studies. *Am J Clin Nutr* 2005;81:317–325.
23. Wang L, Lee I-M, Zang SM, et al. Dietary intake of selected flavonols, flavones and flavonoid-rich foods and risk of cancer in middle-aged and older women. *Am J Clin Nutr* 2009;89:905–912.
24. Nielson SE, Young JF, Daneshvar B, et al. Effect of parsley (Petroselinum crispum) intake on urinary apigenin excretion, blood antioxidant enzymes and biomarker for oxidative stress in human subjects. *Br J Nutr* 1999;81:447–455.

25. Ruiz PA, Haller D. Functional diversity of flavonoids in the inhibition of the proinflammatory Nf-αB, IRF, and Akt signaling pathways in murine intestinal epithelial cells. *J Nutr* 2006;136:664–671.

26. Kim JA, Kim D-K, Kang O-H, et al. Inhibitory effect of luteolin on TNF-alpha-induced IL-8 production in human colon epithelial cells. *Int Immunopharmacol* 2005;5:209–217.

27. Flores-Sanchez IJ, Verpoorte R. PKS activities and biosynthesis of cannabinoids and flavonoids in Cannabis sativa L. plants. *Plant Cell Physiol* 2008;49(12):1767–1782.

28. Raharjo TJ. Studies of cannabinoid biosynthesis in Cannabis sativa L.: the polyketide synthase. PhD thesis, 2004, Leiden University, the Netherlands.

29. Turner CE, ElSohly MA, Boeren EG. Constituents of Cannabis sativa L. XVII. A review of the natural constituents. *J Nat Prod* 1980;43:169–304.

30. von Gadow A, Joubert E, Hansmann CG. Comparison of antioxidant activity of aspalathin with that of other plant phenols of rooibos tes (Aspalathus linearis), αtocpherol, BHT and BHA. *J Agricult Food Chem* 1997;45:632–638.

31. McPartland JM, Russo EB. Cannabis and cannabis extracts: greater than the sum of their parts? *J Cannabis Therap* 2001b;1:103–132.

32. Musonda CA, Chapman JK. Quercetin inhibits hydrogen peroxide (H2O2)-induces NK-kappaB DNA binding activity and DNA damage in HepG 2 cells. *Carcinogenesis* 1998;19(9):1583–1589.

33. Hempel J, Pforte H, Raab B, et al. Flavonols and flavors of parsley cell suspension culture change the antioxidative capacity of plasma in rats. *Nahrung* 1999;43:201–204.

34. Shimor K, Okada H, Furugori M, et al. Intestinal absorption of luteolin and luteolin 7-O-beta-glucoside in rats and humans. *FEBS lett* 1998;438:220–224.

35. Lin Y, Shi R, Wang X, et al. Luteolin, a flavonoid with potential for cancer prevention and therapy. *Curr Cancer Drug Targets* 2008;8(7):634–646.

36. Wruck CJ, Claussen M, Fuhrmann G, et al. Luteolin protects rat PC12 and C6 cells against MPP+ innduced toxicity via an ERK dependent Keapl=Nrf2-ARE pathway. *J Natural Transm.* Suppl 2007;72:57–67.

37. Bylka W, Matlawska I, Pilewski NA. Natural flavonoids as antimicrobial agents. *JANA* 2004;7(2):24–31.

38. Beale JM. Antibacterial antibiotics. In: Block JH, Beale JM, eds. *Wilson and Gisvold's Textbook of Organic Medicinal and Pharmaceutical Chemistry.* 11th ed. Lippincott Williams & Wilkins, New York, 2004, pp. 299–366.

39. Xu H, Lee SF. Activity of plant flavonoids against antibiotic-resistant bacteria. *Phytother Res* 2001;15:39–43.

40. Kim H, Woo ER, Shin CG, et al. A new flavonol glycoside gallate ester from Acer okamotoanum and its inhibitory activity against Human Immunodeficiency Virus-1 (HIV-1) integrase. *J Nat Prod* 1998;61:145–148.

41. Paterson DL, Swindells S, Mohr J, et al. Adherence to protease inhibitor therapy and outcomes in patients with HIV infection. *Ann Intern Med* 2000;133:21–30.

42. Lin YM, Flawin M, Schure R, et al. Antiviral activity of bioflavonoids. *Planta Medica* 1999;5:120–125.

43. Ross JA, Kasum CM. Dietary flavonoids: bioavailability, metabolic effects, and safety. *Annu Rev Nutr* 2002;22:19–35.

44. Duthie G, Crozier A. Plant-derived phenolic antioxidants. *Curr Open Lipidol* 2000;11:43–47.

45. Mc Anlis GT, Mc Eneny J, Pearce J, et al. The effect of various dietary flavonoids on the susceptibility of low density lipoproteins to oxidation in vitro using both metallic and non-metallic oxidizing agents. *Biochem Soc Trans* 1997;25:142S.

46. Hander H, Schneider H. Dietary orthophenols that induce glutathione S transferase and increase the resistance of cells to hydrogen peroxide are potential cancer chemo-preventatives that act by two mechanisms: the alleviation of oxidative stress and the detoxification of mutagenic xenobiotics. *Cancer Lett* 2000;156:17–24.
47. Dirven HAAM, van Omen B, van Bladeren PJ. Involvement of human glutathione S-transferase isoenzymes in the conjugation of cyclophoshamide metabolites with glutathione. *Cancer Res* 1995;54:6215–6220.
48. Noroozi M, Anderson WJ, Lean MEJ. Effect of flavonoids and Vitamin C on oxidative DNA damage to human lymphocytes. *Am J Clin Nutr* 1998;67:1210–1218.
49. Clark SF. The biochemistry of antioxidants revisited. *Nutr in Clin Prac* 2002;17:5–17.
50. Garcia-Lafuente A, Guillamon E, Villares A, et al. Flavonoids as anti-inflammatory agents: implcations in cancer and cardiovascular disease. *Inflamm Res* 2009;58:537–552.
51. Kim SH, Kim H. Inhibitory effect of astaxanthin on oxidative stress-induced mito-chondrial dysfunction- a mini-review. *Nutrients* 2018;10:1137.
52. Nunnari J, Suomalainen A. Mitochondria: in sickness and in health. *Cell* 2012;148:1145–1159.
53. Starkov AA. The role of mitochondria in reactive oxygen species metabolism and signaling. *Ann NY Acad Sci* 2008;1147:37–52.
54. McManus MJ, Murphy MP, Franklin JL. Mitochondria-derived reactive oxygen species mediate capase-dependent and -independent neuronal deaths. *Mol Cell Neurosci* 2014;63:13–23.
55. Kluge MA, Fetterman JL, Vita JA. Mitochondria and endothelial function. *Circ Res* 2013;112:1171–1188.
56. Liu RH. Health-promoting components of fruits and vegetables in the diet. *Adv Nutr Int Rev J* 2013;4:384S–392S.
57. Russo EB. Taming THC: potential cannabis synergy and phytocannabinoid-terpenoid entourage effects. *Br J Pharmacol* 2011;163:1344–1364.
58. McPartland JM, Pruitt PL. Side effects of pharmaceuticals not elicited by comparable herbal medicines: the case of tetrahydrocannabinol and marijuana. *Altern Ther Health Med* 1999;5(4):57–62.

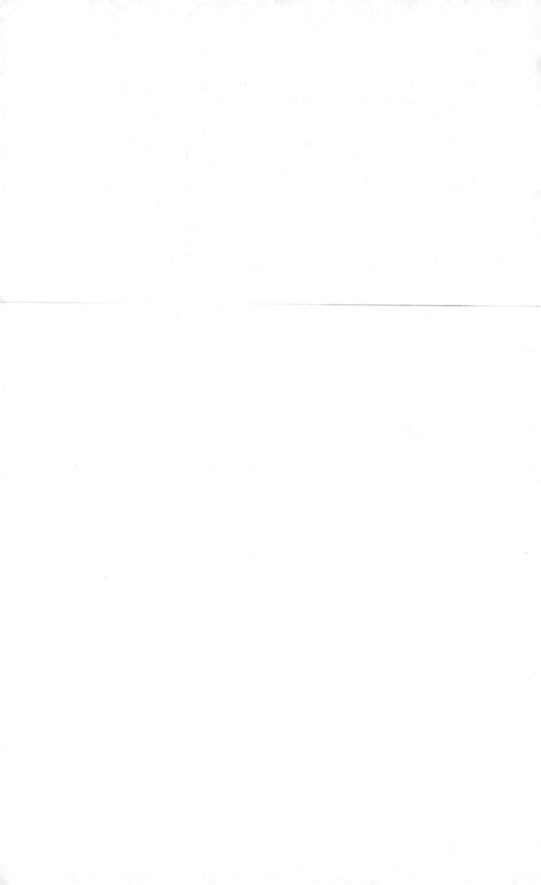

5 Cannabis Pharmacology
An Interview with Ethan B. Russo, M.D.

Betty Wedman-St Louis
Clinical Nutritionist

CONTENTS

In 2011 Ethan B. Russo, M.D. authored *"Taming THC: potential cannabis synergy and phytocannabinoid—terpenoid entourage effects"* and classified cannabis as a medicinal plant based on the research by Mechoulam and his research papers of 1998 [1]. Russo's current focus in "Taming THC…" was to answer the question about whether cannabis was strictly a vehicle for delivery of psychoactive THC.

Once the endocannabinoid system (ECS) and its receptors were identified throughout the human body, it was determined that phytocannabinoids functioned analogously to innate cannabinoids and each phytocannabinoid—THC, CBD, CBC, CBG, THCV, CBDV—was assessed on their function within the ECS. Terpenoid components were reported as responsible for the aroma of cannabis, but few studies on pharmacology were reported until 1999.

Cannabis is one of the oldest known botanical drugs and has a controversial history. Even, today its medicinal value is questioned as legalization is considered. Dr. Russo shares his expertise in an interview about Cannabis As Medicine.

BWS: **If clinicians are going to personalize the cannabinomics, what research needs to be done and how do we educate healthcare professionals about the synergy?**

EBR: Personalized medicine with cannabis will require the presence of safe, effective, and consistent preparations. It is a minimum requirement that every consumer, whether medical or adult use, be provided a certificate of analysis on the material they are purchasing. A good deal of current available literature documents the medical attributes of various cannabinoids and terpenoids, but is rarely addressed in medical school or residency training. The pharmacological effects of cannabis components will need to be confirmed and expanded through additional biomedical research, particularly in the setting of randomized controlled trials, an approach that is severely restricted under current laws in the USA.

BWS: **What do you see as the future of cannabis-based medicines: smoking, vaping, oral capsules, oromucosal spray, and tinctures for use on a daily basis?**

EBR: Smoking is not a defensible delivery approach for medicine. Vaporization is appropriate for situations in which a quick intervention is needed, such as pain paroxysm or impending seizure. More appropriate for chronic conditions are cannabis tinctures and oral preparations that allow prolonged effects, less frequent dosing, and the avoidance of intoxication, reinforcement, and peaks and valleys of activity.

LIMITED CANNABIS RESEARCH

Cannabis has been used for over 500 years in the treatment of pain, inflammation, neuralgia, migraine, and dysmenorrhea, [2] but it was determined to be of "little medical use" and removed from medical formularies. Limited clinical studies have been done on cannabis use especially for pain due to four major obstacles outlined by Notcutt et al. [3]: absence of reliable and standardized preparations, difficulties with delivery methods, political and legal difficulties, and side-effects.

BWS: **Medical and nursing students find it hard to understand how medicinal plants can have analgesic benefits when each batch of cannabis offers a different phytocannabinoid profile. How can this be explained?**

EBR: This limitation is not universal at all. Both Sativex®/nabiximols and Epidiolex®/cannabidiol have been highly standardized sufficiently to allow regulatory approval as pharmaceuticals with the same quality and consistency profiles as New Chemical Entities (NCEs).

BWS: **Any suggestions you could share to help explain phytocannabinoid ability to enhance native systems, especially related to pain.**

EBR: THC and CBD are both anti-inflammatory analgesics, but these properties are also common to many other cannabinoids and terpenoids that are available in specific cannabis chemovars. A good example is that of beta-caryophyllene, a sesquiterpenoid in cannabis that is simultaneously a cannabinoid by virtue of being a potent full agonist at the CB_2 receptor, more potent than THC. As such, it can notably contribute to pain relief in a preparation that contains a significant concentration.

BWS: **Several recent papers on cannabis and pain list the categories of pain as nociceptive (physical injury), inflammation (using THC + CBD) for neuropathic disease [amputation, chemotherapy], and central [affects mood, sense of well-being] dysfunction of nervous system. What is your opinion of cannabis use for pain?**

EBR: In various randomized controlled trials, cannabis-based medicines have proven safe and effective for a wide variety of pain syndromes. Cannabis is less effective in acute settings, such as tooth extraction, but clearly shines in chronic syndromes, especially neuropathic pain and in its ability to produce opioid-sparing effects.

CBD + THC

Cannabidiol (CBD) is a major non-psychotropic cannabinoid that is almost as abundant as THC, especially in hemp. The proportion of CBD:THC is selected for in the cannabis plant-breeding program by the grower. Cannabidiol can inhibit CB_1 and diminish THC's undesirable effects in a dose-related preparation. Cannabidiol by itself is anxiolytic and can reduce inflammation and tachycardia. An oromucosal spray, Sativex® (GW Pharmaceuticals), a botanical extract of cannabis plants, has a CBD:THC ratio of 1:1.

BWS: **Environmental factors have significant influence in modulating cannabinoids present in different parts of the plant at different stages of growth. Can you give me some general guidelines to insure quality cannabis is being used for medicine?**

EBR: Genetics are the primary force affecting the biochemical composition of cannabis, but the plant does respond to environmental changes such as insect attack or other ecological demands that promote certain alterations, particularly in the terpenoid entourage. This biochemical variance can be minimized through the use of vegetative propagation ("cloning") in conjunction with stringent control of growth parameters (heat, light, soil, etc.) along with employment of pooled samples for extraction. This level of standardization has been successful in allowing pharmaceutical development with regulatory approval of Sativex®/ nabiximols in 30 countries and Epidiolex®/cannabidiol in the United States as botanical medicines.

BWS: **More THC + CBD products are available with a 1:1 ratio. Does the use of both cannabinoids offer improved medical benefits?**

EBR: This is absolutely clear at this point. In the Johnson et al. study in opioid-resistant cancer pain, there was no significant difference between a high-THC extract and placebo, whereas the combination of high-THC and high-CBD extract (Sativex®) produced statistically significant improvement in analgesia. THC and CBD synergize pain control, while the latter prolongs the overall effect and improves the therapeutic index by reducing associated adverse effects such as anxiety and tachycardia.

WHOLE PLANT BENEFITS

In *"Taming THC: potential cannabis synergy and phytocannabinoid-terpenoid entourage effects,"* Dr. Russo details how cannabis compounds influence the medicinal effects of this plant even in small amounts.

BWS: **Could the lack of "whole plant" benefits be a factor in poor results of pain management using synthetic cannabinoids?**

EBR: Synthetic cannabinoids are frequently misleading reflections of what cannabis as a botanical whole plant medicine can achieve. Synthetic THC

(Marinol®) is a poorly tolerated and infrequently utilized prescription drug that has a very narrow therapeutic index in comparison to the better tolerated and versatile nature of properly constituted cannabis-based medicines containing a complete entourage that synergizes beneficial properties such as pain control, while minimizing adverse events associated with THC alone.

BWS: **Explain how a small amount of terpenoids can enhance the benefits of THC + CBD and improve symptom management.**

EBR: Caryophyllene is an impressive analgesic and anti-inflammatory that also exerts an anti-addictive effect for opioids and other agents. Alpha-pinene attenuates or even eliminates short-term memory impairment from THC. Limonene is a powerful anti-depressant and immune-stimulator. Linalool is an anti-anxiety and anticonvulsant agent. These are just a few examples.

BWS: **Terpenoids offer pain reduction benefits as well as other benefits, but research lags on their contributions. Why are terpenoids lost in the production of cannabis products?**

EBR: Terpenoids are frequently lost when CO_2 extraction is done with a single pass. This can be rectified in separate runs for cannabinoids and terpenoids with subsequent combination of the two. Ethanol extraction is considered better by many in preserving terpenoid fractions.

BWS: **Does more analytical work for separation and detection need to be added to laboratory certification?**

EBR: Perhaps. There are existing standards for techniques of analysis for cannabis that are accepted by certifying agencies. See American Herbal Products Association, American Herbal Pharmacopoeia, and the Patient-Focused Certification program of Americans for safe access: www.safeaccessnow. org/.

BWS: **Why do testing labs only report six to ten cannabinoids when 70+ have been identified?**

EBR: Labs test for what is most common and components for which laboratory standards are available. Some of the 125 natural cannabinoids in cannabis are trace compounds, or even artifacts of analysis produced by exposure to heat.

CANNABIS PHARMACOGNOSY

"Many physicians fail to recognize that pharmacognosy (the study of medicinal plants) has led directly or indirectly to an estimated 25 percent of modern pharmaceuticals," Dr. Russo writes in "Role of Cannabinoids in Pain Management" [4]. The endocannabinoid system plays a critical role in pain and inflammation through a potent anti-inflammatory antioxidant activity superior to Vitamins C and E. Cannabinoids may enhance the analgesic effects of opioids to permit lower doses and analgesics and minimize incidence or severity of side effects.

REFERENCES

1. Russo EB. Taming THC: potential cannabis synergy and phytocannabinoid-terpenoid entourage effects. *Br J Pharmac* 2011;163:1344–1364.
2. Iversen L, Snyder SH. *The Science of Marijuana.* Oxford University Press, Oxford, 2000.
3. Notcutt W, Price M, Miller R, et al. Initial experiences with medical extracts of cannabis for chronic pain: results from 34 "N of 1" studies. *Anaesthesia* 2004;59:440–452.
4. Russo EB, Hohmann AG. Role of cannabinoids in pain management. Deer TR, et al. (eds). *Comprehensive Treatment of Chronic Pain by Medical Interventional and Integrative Approaches.* doi:10.1007/978-1-4614-1560-2_18.

6 Endocannabinoids & Phytocannabinoids in Pain Management*

Chris D. Meletis
Naturopathic Physician

CONTENTS

Chronic pain is one of the most common complaints affecting modern society with an estimated 25.3 million U.S. adults (11.2%) suffering from this health concern.[1] Furthermore, almost 40 million adults (17.6%) have severe levels of chronic pain.[1] One of the most severe forms of chronic pain is neuropathic pain, which results from damage to the central or peripheral nervous systems.[2] This damage can result from physical trauma such as accidents, surgery, and stroke, diseases such as diabetes, cancer, and immune disorders, and medications such as cancer chemotherapy drugs.[2] Neuropathic pain is also often associated with accompanying mental health disorders such as depression, anxiety, sleep problems, and reduced social interactions.[3]

Standard first-line treatments for neuropathic pain (such as tricyclic antidepressants and selective serotonin norepinephrine reuptake inhibitors) are often not completely effective on all types of neuropathy.[4] In fact, at least 50% of people with neuropathic pain do not notice any clinically meaningful pain relief from their medications.[2] Some medications used for neuropathic pain are accompanied by side effects including dizziness, sedation, depression, and sleep disorders,[2] making them a bad choice for many people.

Another widespread source of chronic pain is osteoarthritis of the knee or hip. Osteoarthritis is the most frequent cause of joint problems in the United States.[5] An estimated 10% of men and 13% of women aged 60 years or older have knee osteoarthritis.[5] In a society where people spend excessive amounts of time staring down at their cell

* Author Note: Reprinted from *Townsend Letter*, November 2018, http://www.townsendletter.com/). Permission to reuse granted by *Townsend Letter, The Examiner of Alternative Medicine.*

phones or looking at their computer, it's not surprising that neck pain is another common disorder that annually affects 30% to 50% of the general population.[6] Furthermore, at any given time, 31 million people in the United States experience low back pain.[7]

Opioids are commonly prescribed to treat chronic pain, either as a first or second line of treatment. Sales of opioid drugs nearly quadrupled from 1999 to 2014.[8] However, opioid drugs are addictive, and overdose of this medication is common. According to Centers for Disease Control and Prevention statistics, drug overdoses killed 63,632 Americans in 2016 and almost two-thirds (66%) of those deaths were the result of a prescription or illicit opioid.[9]

An abundance of research indicates that phytocannabinoids—substances such as cannabidiol (CBD) derived from cannabis and hemp plants—may be effective alternatives. Phytocannabinoids exert much of their actions through the endocannabinoid system, which is involved in pain control. This article will discuss in detail the role of the endocannabinoid system in pain management, how two common phytocannabinoids (THC, the psychoactive component of cannabis and CBD, the non-psychoactive component) differ in their effects on pain, and how a relative newcomer in the realm of natural pain management supplements known as palmitoylethanolamide (PEA) works with the endocannabinoid system to control pain.

THE ENDOCANNABINOID SYSTEM AND PAIN

Endocannabinoids produced within the body including anandamide (arachidonyl ethanolamide) and 2-arachidonylglycerol (2-AG) are able to activate receptors in the endocannabinoid system. Two important receptors in this system that are involved in pain management are CB_1 and CB_2.[10] In the central nervous system, CB_2 receptor mRNA is not present in the neuronal tissue of human or rat brains.[11] However, it *is* found in brain cells known as microglia when they are activated.[11] Microglia can become activated in states of inflammation and activated microglia themselves can produce pro-inflammatory molecules. The presence of CB_2 in activated microglia indicates it may be involved in blocking the effect of painful stimuli in inflammatory processes of the nervous system.[11] Activation of CB_2 receptors blocks the pain response to thermal and mechanical stimuli,[12,13] thermal and tactile hypersensitivity produced by peripheral inflammation,[13-15] and neuropathic pain.[16] The effects of CB_2 receptors on neuropathic pain and inflammation are particularly noteworthy as those conditions are often resistant to treatment, as noted earlier.

An extensive amount of evidence points to the endocannabinoid system's role in pain control. According to preclinical studies in animal models, activation of CB_1 or CB_2 receptors leads to a reduction in chemotherapy-induced allodynia (a pain response from stimuli that don't normally cause pain).[17] Further evidence that the endocannabinoid system is involved in pain regulation is the similarity between endocannabinoids and the pain reliever acetaminophen. The acetaminophen metabolite and endocannabinoid reuptake inhibitor AM 404 indirectly activates CB_1 receptors, which may be responsible for analgesia induced by acetaminophen.[18] Likewise, some non-steroidal anti-inflammatory drugs (NSAIDs) are able to influence the cannabinoid system. The inflammatory enzyme COX-2 breaks down anandamide, an endocannabinoid involved in the regulation of pain perception.[11,19] NSAIDs inhibit the action of the enzyme

COX-2, which in turn prevents anandamide destruction.[11,19] Furthermore, clinical studies revealed altered endocannabinoid signaling in patients with chronic pain.[20]

Endocannabinoids control pain in a way that is much safer compared with opioids, although they can indirectly work through the same receptors. CB_2 receptors indirectly stimulate opioid receptors found in primary afferent pathways.[21] Furthermore, CB_1 expression is weak in the areas of the brain stem that regulate respiration. This suggests that respiratory depression, a potentially fatal adverse effect of opioid drugs, would not occur when using cannabinoids as painkillers.[10] Additionally, CB_1 receptor agonists (substances that enhance the activity of CB_1) work differently on neurotransmission pathways compared with opioids to induce analgesia.[22]

This difference in pathways may explain why in animal models of neuropathic pain cannabinoid receptor agonists last longer compared with morphine.[23]

Researchers are beginning to look beyond the classical CB_1 and CB_2 receptors as potential mediators of some of the beneficial effects of endocannabinoids and phytocannabinoids. For example, type 1 vanilloid receptors ($TRPV_1$) may regulate some cannabinoid effects. The $TRPV_1$ receptor has been identified in neurons that play a role in pain signaling.[17] Other undiscovered cannabinoid receptors may exist, and these receptors may partly mediate some of the analgesic effects associated with cannabinoids.[24,25]

THC VS. CBD IN NEUROPATHIC PAIN

CB_1 receptors inhibit pain signaling pathways.[10] CB_2 receptors, on the other hand, reduce pain via anti-inflammatory effects.[10] THC directly acts on CB_1 receptors of the endocannabinoid system,[26] which are primarily expressed in the brain, and it can also act on CB_2 receptors.[27]

CBD, although it has a low affinity for CB_1 and CB_2 receptors, indirectly acts on the CB_1 receptors by suppressing the enzymatic breakdown of the endogenous cannabinoid anandamide, increasing the duration of time anandamide stays in the system.[28] As noted earlier, anandamide is involved in the regulation of pain perception.

CBD's effects on the CB_1 receptor counteract the psychoactive effects of THC.[29] In most studies, CBD has thus been shown to inhibit adverse effects of THC including intoxication, sedation, and tachycardia.[29] CBD also acts on the CB_2 receptor, and therefore exerts anti-inflammatory effects important for pain control.[10] The ability of THC or CBD to act on CB_2 receptors blocks activation of the brain cells known as microglia, thereby preventing the development of neuropathic pain.[27]

A number of animal studies indicate CBD alone can reduce neuropathic pain. A mouse model of neuropathic pain caused by injury found that CBD alone had beneficial effects on pain reduction.[30] Although CBD's effects were less powerful than THC, CBD administration was not associated with the psychoactive side effects that accompanied THC.[30] In a rat model of sciatic nerve pain and inflammatory pain, oral treatment with CBD (2.5–20 mg/kg for neuropathic sciatic pain and 20 mg/kg for inflammatory pain) or intraplantar injection from a week to 14 days post-injury reduced the sensitization to painful stimuli.[31] Cannabidiol administration also correlated with a lower level of several inflammatory mediators, such as prostaglandin E(2) (PGE(2)), lipid peroxide, and nitric oxide (NO).[31] In this study, CBD's beneficial effects on pain appeared to be due to its actions on the vanilloid receptors rather than

CB_1 or CB_2. The authors concluded, "The results indicate a potential for therapeutic use of cannabidiol in chronic painful states."

CBD has also been shown to be effective in a mouse model of diabetic neuropathy. In diabetic mice, moderate or high doses of cannabidiol administered intranasally beginning at onset of diabetes or high doses of CBD given through an intraperitoneal route were associated with a reduction in the development of two measures of diabetic neuropathy: sensitivity to heat and increased pain after being touched (tactile allodynia).[27] This effect lasted during cannabidiol treatment and for the additional four assessments over two months after CBD was discontinued. CBD had no effect on neuropathic pain that was present prior to CBD treatment. One other benefit of CBD was that mice given either medium or high doses of intranasal/intraperitoneal CBD at diabetes onset had lower densities of microglia in the dorsal spinal cord, an indication of reduced microglia activation.[27]

Rodent models of neuropathy caused by chemotherapy drugs indicate CBD is useful in this instance as well. In a mouse model of neuropathy caused by the chemotherapy drug cisplatin, CBD or THC reduced but did not prevent neuropathy symptoms.[32] In another mouse study, both CBD and THC alone reduced mechanical allodynia caused by the chemotherapy medication paclitaxel.[33] CBD also reduced pain associated with the chemotherapy drug oxaliplatin but not vincristine, while THC significantly reduced vincristine-associated pain but not pain associated with oxaliplatin.[33] Doses of CBD or THC that were too low to be effective when given separately, when given together were effective against pain caused by oxaliplatin but not vincristine.[33]

Although CBD's ability to inhibit neuropathic pain is only half that of THC, CBD can be given in higher doses without the psychoactive effects that occur with THC.[2] Furthermore, long-term use of CBD has been associated with improved efficacy in regard to pain control compared with short-term administration.[2]

With the promising results achieved in animal studies, it is surprising that clinical trials investigating the use of CBD alone on neuropathic pain are lacking. All of the clinical studies have evaluated the use of CBD combined with THC. Many of these studies have found the combination of the two phytocannabinoids to be effective in neuropathic pain.[34-36]

JOINT PAIN AND PHYTOCANNABINOIDS

Endocannabinoids and phytocannabinoids are able to affect pain pathways in the joints. Cannabinoid receptors, including CB_1, CB_2, GPR_{55}, PPARα, and PPARγ, have been found on human articular cartilage from patients with symptomatic osteoarthritis (OA).[37] According to one group of researchers, "Chondrocytes from OA joints were shown to express a wide range of cannabinoid receptors even in degenerate tissues, demonstrating that these cells could respond to cannabinoids."[37] OA leads to a combination of inflammatory, nociceptive, and neuropathic pain. The endocannabinoid system has been shown to reduce all of these types of pain.[38]

CBD was studied for its effects on experimental osteoarthritis in rats. After administration of peripheral CBD (100–300 μg) to rats with end-stage OA, there was a dose-dependent decline in joint afferent firing rate.[39] Furthermore, although 100 or 200 μg of CBD did not produce any benefits, 300 μg CBD was associated with increased withdrawal threshold and weight bearing. Local CBD administration also alleviated acute, transient joint inflammation. Prophylactic administration of CBD blocked the development of subsequent joint pain and nerve damage. The researchers concluded, "These findings suggest that CBD may be a safe, useful therapeutic for treating OA joint neuropathic pain."

In collagen-induced arthritis (CIA), a model for rheumatoid arthritis, CBD at 5 mg/kg per day i.p. or 25 mg/kg per day orally resulted in clinical improvement associated with protection against severe joint damage.[40] CBD led to a reduction in IFN-gamma production and decreased synthesis of tumor necrosis factor by knee synovial cells. In vitro, CBD induced a dose-dependent inhibition of lymphocyte proliferation, both mitogen-stimulated and antigen-specific, and suppression of Zymosan-triggered reactive oxygen burst by peritoneal granulocytes.[40] In mice, CBD blocked the rise in serum tumor necrosis factor caused by lipopolysaccharides.[40] According to the authors, "Taken together, these data show that CBD, through its combined immuno-suppressive and anti-inflammatory actions, has a potent anti-arthritic effect in CIA."

Despite promising preclinical studies and reports from clinical practice as well as a great deal of in vitro justification as to why cannabinoids likely support joint health,[41] there is a paucity of human studies investigating the effects of cannabinoids on joint pain.[41]

PHYTOCANNABINOID USE IN OTHER FORMS OF PAIN

Phytocannabinoids have been studied for their effects on other forms of pain. In a randomized, double-blind, placebo-controlled trial, the semisynthetic THC analog nabilone was shown to reduce pain and improve quality of life and sleep in people with fibromyalgia.[42] In another study, kidney transplant patients experiencing pain were given CBD.[43] The study included seven patients who were given an initial dose of up to 100 mg/day of CBD. Two participants experienced complete improvement of pain, four had a partial response in the first 15 days, and one subject experienced no change.

Furthermore, cannabinoid-rich hemp oil reduced body pain and improved other symptoms in girls who had an adverse reaction to the human papillomavirus (HPV) vaccine.[44] Other evidence indicates the oil of cannabis seeds reduces pain in patients with chronic musculoskeletal inflammation, an effect attributed to the ideal omega-3/omega-6 ratio content.[45]

Treating pain properly involves addressing more than just physical discomfort. Pain is a multidimensional problem that also encompasses impairments in mood, cognition, and function. Cannabidiol has been shown to improve mental health in a number of studies.

THE ROLE OF PALMITOYLETHANOLAMIDE (PEA) IN PAIN MANAGEMENT

A promising new strategy for resolving pain is to use palmitoylethanolamide (PEA) in combination with CBD. When in pain, the body produces PEA, which acts as a natural painkiller.[46] PEA is also found in foods such as egg yolks, peanuts, and soybeans. It is not found in cannabis and is not classified as an endocannabinoid. However, it acts on the endocannabinoid system by helping the body use anandamide more effectively.[46]

Accumulating evidence points to the role of neuroinflammation, characterized by infiltration of immune cells, activation of mast cells and glial cells, and synthesis of inflammatory mediators in the peripheral and central nervous systems, in chronic pain.[46] PEA is an anti-inflammatory and pro-resolving lipid mediator that reduces mast cell activation and regulates glial cell behaviors.[46–48]

A meta-analysis of 12 double-blind, controlled, and open-label clinical trials found that PEA supplementation leads to a progressive decrease in pain intensity that is substantially greater compared to the controls.[46] The pain reduction in PEA-treated patients was 1.04 points every two weeks with a 35% response variance explained by the linear model. Conversely, in the control groups, pain reduction intensity was 0.20 points every two weeks with only 1% of the total variance explained by the regression. Pain scores on the Kaplan-Meier estimator was ≤3 in 81% of patients given PEA whereas only 40% of control subjects had a score ≤3 60 days after the beginning of the trial. The researchers concluded, "These results confirm that PEA might represent an exciting, new therapeutic strategy to manage chronic and neuropathic pain associated with neuroinflammation."

CONCLUSION

Chronic pain is a debilitating condition that is widespread among the population. Regulating the endocannabinoid system through the use of phytocannabinoids and PEA is an alternative to other pain control approaches associated with potentially dangerous side effects. The use of these agents is associated with improvements in pain caused by various forms of neuropathy, joint problems, and other pain disorders. The benefits are achieved through modulation of not only the endocannabinoid system but also indirect influence on opioid receptors.

REFERENCES

1. Nahin RL. Estimates of pain prevalence and severity in adults: United States, 2012. *J Pain*. 2015 Aug;16(8):769–80.
2. Casey SL, Vaughan CW. Plant-based cannabinoids for the treatment of chronic neuropathic pain. Medicines (Basel). 2018 Jul 1;5(3):E67.
3. Turk DC, Audette J, Levy RM, et al. Assessment and treatment of psychosocial comorbidities in patients with neuropathic pain. *Mayo Clin Proc*. 2010 Mar;85(3 Suppl):S42–50.
4. Dworkin RH, O'Connor AB, Audette J, et al. Recommendations for the pharmacological management of neuropathic pain: An overview and literature update. *Mayo Clin Proc*. 2010 Mar;85(3 Suppl):S3–14.
5. Zhang Y, Jordan JM. Epidemiology of osteoarthritis. *Clin Geriatr Med*. 2010 Aug;26(3):355–69.
6. Hogg-Johnson S, van der Velde G, Carroll LJ, et al. The burden and determinants of neck pain in the general population: results of the Bone and Joint Decade 2000–2010 Task Force on neck pain and its associated disorders. *J Manipulative Physiol Ther*. 2009 Feb;32(2 Suppl):S46–60.
7. American Chiropractic Association. www.acatoday.org/Patients/Health-Wellness-Information/Back-Pain-Facts-and-Statistics. Accessed August 1, 2018.
8. Centers for Disease Control and Prevention. www.cdc.gov/drugoverdose/data/prescribing.html. Accessed August 1, 2018.

9. U.S. drug overdose deaths continue to rise; increase fueled by synthetic opioids. Press Release. Centers for Disease Control and Prevention. March 29, 2018. www.cdc.gov/media/releases/2018/p0329-drug-overdose-deaths.html. Accessed August 2, 2018.

10. Miller RJ, Miller RE. Is cannabis an effective treatment for joint pain? *Clin Exp Rheumatol*. 2017 Sep–Oct;35(Suppl 107(5)):59–67.

11. Manzanares J, Julian MD, Carrascosa A. Role of the cannabinoid system in pain control and therapeutic implications for the management of acute and chronic pain episodes. *Curr Neuropharmacol*. 2006 Jul;4(3):239–57.

12. Malan TP, Ibrahim MM, Deng H, et al. CB2 cannabinoid receptor-mediated peripheral antinociception. *Pain*. 2001 Sep;93(3):239–45.

13. Clayton N, Marshall FH, Bountra C, et al. CB1 and CB2 cannabinoid receptors are implicated in inflammatory pain. *Pain*. 2002 Apr;96(3):253–60.

14. Nackley AG, Makriyannis A, Hohmann AG. Selective activation of cannabinoid CB(2) receptors suppresses spinal fos protein expression and pain behavior in a rat model of inflammation. *Neuroscience*. 2003;119(3):747–57.

15. Quartilho A, Mata HP, Ibrahim MM, et al. Inhibition of inflammatory hyperalgesia by activation of peripheral CB2 cannabinoid receptors. *Anesthesiology*. 2003 Oct;99(4):955–60.

16. Ibrahim MM, Deng H, Zvonok A, et al. Activation of CB2 cannabinoid receptors by AM1241 inhibits experimental neuropathic pain: pain inhibition by receptors not present in the CNS. *Proc Natl Acad Sci USA*. 2003 Sep 2;100(18):10529–33.

17. O'Hearn S, Diaz P, Wan BA, et al. Modulating the endocannabinoid pathway as treatment for peripheral neuropathic pain: A selected review of preclinical studies. *Ann Palliat Med*. 2017 Dec;6(Suppl 2):S209–14.

18. Klinger-Gratz PP, Ralvenius WT, Neumann E, et al. Acetaminophen relieves inflammatory pain through CB1 cannabinoid receptors in the rostral ventromedial medulla. *J Neurosci*. 2018 Jan 10;38(2):322–34.

19. Păunescu H, Coman OA, Coman L, et al. Cannabinoid system and cyclooxygenases inhibitors. *J Med Life*. 2011 Jan–Mar;4(1): 11–20.

20. Huang WJ, Chen WW, Zhang X. Endocannabinoid system: Role in depression, reward and pain control (review). *Mol Med Rep*. 2016 Oct;14(4):2899–903.

21. Ibrahim MM, Porreca F, Lai J, et al. CB2 cannabinoid receptor activation produces antinociception by stimulating peripheral release of endogenous opioids. *Proc Natl Acad Sci USA*. 2005 Feb 22;102(8):3093–8.

22. Jennings EA, Vaughan CW, Christie MJ. Cannabinoid actions on rat superficial medullary dorsal horn neurons in vitro. *J Physiol*. 2001 Aug 1;534(Pt 3):805–12.

23. Mao J, Price DD, Lu J, et al. Two distinctive antinociceptive systems in rats with pathological pain. *Neurosci Lett*. 2000 Feb 11;280(1):13–6.

24. Breivogel CS, Griffin G, Di Marzo V, et al. Evidence for a new G protein-coupled cannabinoid receptor in mouse brain. *Mol Pharmacol*. 2001 Jul;60(1):155–63.

25. Hájos N, Ledent C, Freund TF. Novel cannabinoid-sensitive receptor mediates inhibition of glutamatergic synaptic transmission in the hippocampus. *Neuroscience*. 2001;106(1):1–4.

26. Bhattacharyya S, Egerton A, Kim E, et al. Acute induction of anxiety in humans by delta-9-tetrahydrocannabinol related to amygdalar cannabinoid-1 (CB1) receptors. *Sci Rep*. 2017 Nov 3;7(1):15025.

27. Toth CC, Jedrzejewski NM, Ellis CL, et al. Cannabinoid-mediated modulation of neuropathic pain and microglial accumulation in a model of murine type I diabetic peripheral neuropathic pain. *Mol Pain*. 2010 Mar 17;6:16.

28. Leweke FM, Piomelli D, Pahlisch F, et al. Cannabidiol enhances anandamide signaling and alleviates psychotic symptoms of schizophrenia. *Transl Psychiatry*. 2012 Mar 20;2:e94.

29. Russo E, Guy GW. A tale of two cannabinoids: the therapeutic rationale for combining tetrahydrocannabinol and cannabidiol. *Med Hypotheses*. 2006;66(2):234–46.

30. Casey SL, Atwal N, Vaughan CW. Cannabis constituent synergy in a mouse neuro-pathic pain model. *Pain*. 2017 Dec;158(12):2452–60.
31. Costa B, Trovato AE, Comelli F, et al. The non-psychoactive cannabis constituent cannabidiol is an orally effective therapeutic agent in rat chronic inflammatory and neuropathic pain. *Eur J Pharmacol*. 2007 Feb 5;556(1–3):75–83.
32. Harris HM, Sufka KJ, Gul W, et al. Effects of delta-9-tetrahydrocannabinol and cannabidiol on cisplatin-induced neuropathy in mice. *Planta Med*. 2016 Aug;82(13):1169–72.
33. King KM, Myers AM, Soroka-Monzo AJ, et al. Single and combined effects of Δ^9-tetrahydrocannabinol and cannabidiol in a mouse model of chemotherapy-induced neuropathic pain. *Br J Pharmacol*. 2017 Sep;174(17):2832–41.
34. Russo M, Naro A, Leo A, et al. Evaluating Sativex® in neuropathic pain management: A clinical and neurophysiological assessment in multiple sclerosis. *Pain Med*. 2016 Jun;17(6):1145–54.
35. Nurmikko TJ, Serpell MG, Hoggart B, et al. Sativex successfully treats neuropathic pain characterised by allodynia: A randomised, double-blind, placebo-controlled clinical trial. *Pain*. 2007 Dec 15;133(1–3):210–20.
36. Hoggart B, Ratcliffe S, Ehler E, et al. A multicentre, open-label, follow-on study to assess the long-term maintenance of effect, tolerance and safety of THC/CBD oromucosal spray in the management of neuropathic pain. *J Neurol*. 2015 Jan;262(1):27–40.
37. Dunn SL, Wilkinson JM, Crawford A, et al. Expression of cannabinoid recep-tors in human osteoarthritic cartilage: Implications for future therapies. *Cannabis Cannabinoid Res*. 2016 Jan 1;1(1):3–15.
38. O'Brien M, McDougall JJ. Cannabis and joints: Scientific evidence for the alleviation of osteoarthritis pain by cannabinoids. *Curr Opin Pharmacol*. 2018 Apr 7;40:104–9.
39. Philpott HT, O'Brien M, McDougall JJ. Attenuation of early phase inflammation by cannabidiol prevents pain and nerve damage in rat osteoarthritis. *Pain*. 2017 Dec;158(12):2442–51.
40. Malfait AM, Gallily R, Sumariwalla PF, et al. The nonpsychoactive cannabis constitu-ent cannabidiol is an oral anti-arthritic therapeutic in murine collagen-induced arthritis. *Proc Natl Acad Sci USA*. 2000 Aug 15;97(17):9561–6.
41. La Porta C, Bura SA, Negrete R, et al. Involvement of the endocannabinoid system in osteoarthritis pain. *Eur J Neurosci*. 2014 Feb;39(3):485–500.
42. Skrabek RQ, Galimova L, Ethans K, et al. Nabilone for the treatment of pain in fibromyalgia. *J Pain*. 2008 Feb;9(2):164–73.
43. Cuñetti L, Manzo L, Peyraube R, et al. Chronic pain treatment with cannabidiol in kidney transplant patients in Uruguay. *Transplant Proc*. 2018 Mar;50(2):461–4.
44. Palmieri B, Laurino C, Vadalà M. Short-term efficacy of CBD-enriched hemp oil in girls with dysautonomic syndrome after human papillomavirus vaccination. *Isr Med Assoc J*. 2017 Feb;19(2):79–84.
45. Shaladi AM, Crestani F, Tartari S, et al. [Cannabinoids in the control of pain]. [Article in Italian, Abstract in English]. *Recenti Prog Med*. 2008 Dec;99(12):616–24.
46. Paladini A, Fusco M, Cenacchi T, et al. Palmitoylethanolamide, a special food for medical purposes, in the treatment of chronic pain: A pooled data meta-analysis. *Pain Physician*. 2016;19:11–24.
47. Facci L, Dal Toso R, Romanello S, et al. Mast cells express a peripheral cannabinoid receptor with differential sensitivity to anandamide and palmitoylethanolamide. *Proc Natl Acad Sci USA*. 1995 Apr 11;92(8):3376–80.
48. Franklin A, Parmentier-Batteur S, Walter L, et al. Palmitoylethanolamide increases after focal cerebral ischemia and potentiates microglial cell motility. *J Neurosci*. 2003 Aug 27;23(21):7767–75.

7 Hemp Oil in the Management of Pain, Inflammation, & Stress*

Chris D. Meletis
Naturopathic Physician

CONTENTS

The endocannabinoid system is a fascinating regulator of many aspects of our health. Endogenous endocannabinoids that are produced within the body including anandamide (arachidonylethanolamide) and 2-arachidonoylglycerol (2-AG) are able to activate receptors in this system. Phytocannabinoids, such as Δ^9-tetrahydrocannabinol (THC), the psychoactive component of cannabis sativa plant, and cannabidiol (CBD), a non-psychoactive component, are also able to activate endocannabinoid receptors. Additionally, synthetic cannabinoids have been synthesized and have an effect on endocannabinoid system pathways.

Two of the main receptors in the endocannabinoid system are CB_1 and CB_2. CB_1 is the primary receptor in the nervous system. It is also found in the adrenal gland, adipose tissue, heart, liver, lungs, prostate, uterus, ovary, testis, bone marrow, thymus, and tonsils.[1] Its expression is weak in the areas of the brain stem that regulate respiration, which is why respiratory depression, a potentially fatal adverse effect of opioid drugs, does not occur when using phytocannabinoids as painkillers.[1]

The CB_2 receptor is typically not expressed in neurons, which is why it was originally called the peripheral cannabinoid receptor. The immune system is the primary

---

* Author Note: Reprinted from *Townsend Letter*, June 2018, http://www.townsendletter.com/). Permission to reuse granted by *Townsend Letter, The Examiner of Alternative Medicine.*

site of its expression. However, its presence has been detected in dorsal root ganglia, a cluster of cells in spinal nerves.[2] CB_2 receptors can also be expressed in bone, the gastrointestinal tract, and in activated microglia in the central nervous system.[2] Microglia are cells found in the brain and spinal column that defend the central nervous system against immune assaults. Because antibodies are too large to penetrate the blood brain barrier, microglia serve as the last defense against pathogens that enter the brain. Activated microglia, sometimes referred to as reactive microglia, create an inflammatory response linked to diseases of the brain.[3] The presence of CB_2 receptors in activated microglia indicates they may be involved in blocking the effect of painful stimuli in inflammatory processes of the nervous system.[4]

Different phytocannabinoids have different effects on endocannabinoid receptors. THC directly acts on CB_1 receptors of the endocannabinoid system,[5] which are primarily expressed in the brain. CBD indirectly acts on the CB_1 receptors by suppressing the enzymatic breakdown of the endogenous cannabinoid anandamide, increasing the duration of time it stays in the system.[6] CBD's effects on the CB_1 receptor counteract the psychoactive effects of THC.[7] CBD thus inhibits adverse effects of THC including intoxication, sedation, and tachycardia.[7] CBD also acts on the CB_2 receptor, which is expressed in the periphery and is involved in immunity.[8]

FROM FETUS TO NEWBORN: THE ENDOCANNABINOID SYSTEM'S IMPORTANT ROLE

The endocannabinoid system plays an important role in our health long before we are born. The endocannabinoid system has been observed in cell types that play a role in male reproduction.[9]

Endocannabinoids and cannabinoid receptors have been detected in testicular tissue, including Sertoli and Leydig cells and spermatozoa.[10] The endocannabinoid system also is involved in the hypothalamus-pituitary-gonadal (HPG) axis.[10] The anandamide-degrading enzyme FAAH regulates key steps in sperm biology pathways, and this action involves the CB_1 receptor.[10]

Furthermore, the endocannabinoid system is important and highly expressed during fetal development. Too much cannabinoid resulting in the over expression of anandamide could lead to negative outcomes such as ectopic pregnancy.[11] Therefore, anandamide concentrations in the uterus must be tightly regulated for conception to occur.[12] During vaginal birth, the newborn's exposure to high endocannabinoid levels assists with the transition from fetus to becoming an infant. During birth, the levels of anandamide and an anti-inflammatory fatty acid amide known as palmitoylethanolamide (PEA) are markedly higher in vaginally delivered babies compared with infants delivered by cesarean section,[13] indicating that vaginally born infants would have a naturally higher degree of protection against pain and inflammation.

Another rodent study serving as a good example of the importance of the endocannabinoid system in prenatal and postnatal health involved female rats who were subjected to dietary restriction involving 20% fewer calories than a normal diet during pre-gestation and gestation. At birth, a significant decline in the levels of anandamide, 2-AG, and PEA were detected in the hypothalamus of the offspring of the calorie-restricted rodents. As adults, these offspring were more likely to gain excessive weight and body weight and be overweight as well as have increased anxiety-related responses.[14]

Furthermore, endocannabinoids have been detected in breast milk, and activation of CB_1 receptors was found to be critically important for milk sucking by newborn mice, helping them to develop oral-motor musculature.[15] This means that if a baby is delivered by C-section and then is bottle fed, he or she may be seriously depleted in endocannabinoids and may be at a disadvantage both as infants and later in life both mentally and physically. CB_1 receptors are temporarily present in white matter regions of the pre- and postnatal nervous system.[15] This implies that CB_1 receptors have a part to play in brain development and endocannabinoid deprivation in newborns can therefore be especially concerning.

The importance of the endocannabinoid system to infants is supported by a study showing that anandamide was neuroprotective against lesions induced in perinatal rodents.[16]

Another study demonstrated that in rats that receive poor rearing during the neonatal timeframe, the neuroendocrine response to early life stress is reduced. Increasing anandamide levels ameliorates these stress-induced changes in glucocorticoid synthesis in these rats.[17]

BEYOND CB_1 AND CB_2 RECEPTORS

Research is beginning to look beyond the classical CB_1 and CB_2 receptors as potential mediators of some of the beneficial effects of phytocannabinoids. Other receptors targeted by phytocannabinoids include G-protein coupled receptors (GP—CRs: GPR_{18}, GPR_{55}, and GPR_{119}). Both GPR_{18} and GPR_{55} may recognize the phytocannabinoid CBD. Evidence indicates this phytocannabinoid serves as a GPR_{55} antagonist, as well as a weak partial agonist.[1] GPR_{18} is expressed primarily in immune cells, while GPR_{55} is expressed in several brain regions as well as in the dorsal root ganglia in neurons with larger diameters, the hippocampus, frontal cortex, cerebellum, striatum, and hypothalamus. GPR_{55} may also be expressed in the immune system as well as in the microglia and bone.[1]

Research suggests that type 1 vanilloid receptors ($TRPV_1$) may regulate some cannabinoid effects. The $TRPV_1$ receptor has been identified in neurons that play a role in pain signaling.[18] Other undiscovered cannabinoid receptors may exist, and these receptors may partly mediate some of the analgesic effects associated with cannabinoids.[19,20]

INTERACTION OF CBD RECEPTORS AND OTHER PHYSIOLOGICAL PATHWAYS

The role of endocannabinoids and phytocannabinoids in mood enhancement and reduction of pain and inflammation cannot be completely explained by their effects on CB_1 and CB_2 receptors alone as well as the other receptors mentioned above. Cannabinoids influence other pathways, and their effects on these pathways may play a role in their myriad health benefits. Peroxisome proliferator-activated receptor gamma (PPAR-gamma) is one of those pathways. PPAR-gamma is a nuclear receptor whose actions include regulation of glucose homeostasis and inflammatory processes and connective tissue health.[21] Mice experiencing a loss of PPAR-gamma function in fibroblasts were more likely to suffer from skin fibrosis.[21] Some endocannabinoids and associated signaling lipids as well as certain natural and synthetic cannabinoids can activate PPAR-gamma including THC and CBD.[22] The anti-inflammatory effects of anandamide and 2-arachidonoylglycerol are mediated by PPAR-gamma.[22]

Moreover, CBD blocks microglial activation in vitro through a mechanism that involves the activation of PPAR-gamma.[23] This effect was mediated by the inhibition of the inflammatory nuclear kappa factor beta (NF-KB) pathway.[23] The ability of cannabinoids to target both CB receptors and PPAR-gamma may explain their regulation of a number of processes including neuroprotection, inflammation, immunomodulation, and vascular responses.[24]

Cannabinoids also interact with 5HT1A serotonin receptors. It has been shown that the anxiety-reducing effects of CBD are dependent upon neurotransmission that is mediated by 5HT1A.[23] It is thought that CBD indirectly influences the 5HT1A receptors through interactions with the receptor binding site and/or modulating intracellular pathways.[23] CBD's effects on stress-reduction and anxiety as well as its mood-enhancing abilities are also mediated through the 5HT1A receptor.[23] Furthermore, CBD's ability to reduce brain tissue damage in mice caused by cerebral artery occlusion is blocked when 5HT1A receptors are inactivated.[25] The fact that CBD interacts with multiple receptors was shown in an animal study where CBD's ability to prevent hypoxic-induced brain damage was dependent upon both 5HT1A and CB2 receptors.[26]

CB_2 receptors themselves are able to indirectly stimulate opioid receptors located in primary afferent pathways, and this may be a means by which CBD inhibits pain.[27]

ENDOCANNABINOID SYSTEM BURDENS

A number of factors can interfere with the proper functioning of the endocannabinoid system, throwing the body out of homeostasis. For example, obesity is associated with an over activated endocannabinoid system in adult subjects.[28] Moreover, offspring of female rodents that consumed a high-fat diet during pregnancy were obese with fat cell hypertrophy and buildup of lipids in brown adipose tissue.[29] These effects correlated with alterations in the endocannabinoid system of the rat pups. In male offspring of mothers fed a high-fat diet, CB_1 and CB_2 receptor levels declined in subcutaneous adipose tissue. In female offspring of mothers fed a high-fat diet, visceral CB_1 levels increased while subcutaneous concentrations decreased. CB_1 concentrations increased in brown adipose tissue from both male and female offspring of mothers that consumed the high-fat diet.

Toxins can serve as another disrupter of the endocannabinoid system. For example, the mechanism by which BPA causes fatty liver is thought to involve up-regulation of the endocannabinoid system.[30]

An imbalance of the gut microbiota known as dysbiosis is another threat to the optimal functioning of the endocannabinoid system. A rodent study found that dysbiosis of the gut microbiota led to changes in the endocannabinoid system.[31] In this study, researchers administered antimicrobials to mice for two weeks in order to cause dysbiosis. Afterward, the animals were given 10^9 CFU/day of *Lactobacillus casei* DG or a placebo for up to a week. Antimicrobial administration resulted in dysbiosis of the microbiota. At the same time, there was a general inflammatory state and changes in some aspects of the endocannabinoid system in the gut. These changes were accompanied by behavioral alterations, including increased immobility in the tail suspension test (an indicator of depression), as well as biochemical and functional changes in the brain such as neuronal firing in the hippocampus and rearrangements of non-neuronal cells in brain regions controlling emotional behavior. Probiotic intake eliminated most of these changes.

SEX HORMONES AND CANNABINOIDS

The association between the endocannabinoid system and estrogen indicates that declining estrogen levels with menopause may disrupt this system. The endocannabinoid system has an under-recognized role in male and female health. Cannabinoids and sex hormones influence common molecular pathways involved in cell proliferation.[32] Furthermore, estrogen plays an important role in the endocannabinoid system expression in the female reproductive tract.[12] Administering the estrogen estradiol to ovariectomized rats caused a marked increase in CB_1, CB_2, the anandamide-degrading enzyme fatty acid amide hydrolase (FAAH), and COX-2 expression.[12] These effects were estrogen-receptor dependent. Anandamide levels also increased in the plasma after estradiol treatment. According to the study authors, "Thus, estradiol may have a direct regulatory role in the modulation of ECS [the endocannabinoid system] in female reproductive tissues."

These findings may explain anecdotal reports of CBD oil reducing hot flashes and other symptoms of surgically induced menopause in women.

AN IMBALANCED ENDOCANNABINOID AND PSYCHOLOGICAL STRESS

One characteristic of an imbalanced endocannabinoid system is the inability to cope with stress.[33–35] That's why this system is often dysfunctional in people with posttraumatic stress disorder. Stimulation of the endocannabinoid system inhibits the activation of the hypothalamus-pituitary-adrenal axis that occurs after stress.[33–35] In this way, this system helps us recover from anxious experiences and brings us back to homeostasis. In male rodents, when the CB_1 receptor is blocked, it takes longer for the HPA axis to recover from stress.[36]

Significant concentrations of nitric oxide (NO) are found in the brain and adrenal glands, and NO may be involved in the stress response. During stress, anandamide suppresses the activity of the nitric oxide synthase enzyme, indicating that endocannabinoids may reduce stress by inhibiting the generation of NO in the hypothalamus and adrenals.[37]

An impaired endocannabinoid system may also be one of the reasons why stress impacts gastrointestinal function.[38] The endocannabinoid system in the gastrointestinal tract regulates motility, secretion, sensation, emesis, satiety, and inflammation. It also influences visceral sensation.

Beyond stress, there are many other consequences of a dysfunctional endocannabinoid system including pain, cognitive dysfunction, depression, epilepsy, and more.

IMPROVING ENDOCANNABINOID SYSTEM FUNCTION WITH CANNABINOID-RICH HEMP OIL

Cannabinoid-rich hemp oil is an ideal choice to optimize the endocannabinoid system. Throughout the remainder of this chapter and the next part of this chapter we will discuss the justification for using hemp oil in a variety of clinical applications. The primary cannabinoid in hemp oil is CBD. However, it also contains other phytocannabinoids as well as terpenes, which work with CBD to support endocannabinoid system function and therefore make hemp oil uniquely suited to enhance areas of health regulated by the endocannabinoid system. The entourage effect—sometimes called the "hemptourage effect"—refers to the ability of other more minor components of hemp oil such as the terpenes to support the activity of its main player, CBD. For example, the terpenes limonene, pinene, and linalool can provide a complimentary action to CBD's cognitive-enhancing abilities by improving mood.[39] Pinene is also known to enhance mental clarity, thus acting synergistically to CBD.[39] The entourage effect is a fascinating aspect of cannabinoid therapy, and Dr. Chris Meletis explores this effect in more detail in the ICCT medical certification program.

Like so many herbals that are popularly used around the world, hemp has been employed for centuries with many health benefits. The moment we start eliminating certain constituents we may lose certain therapeutic benefits often attributed to the entourage or hemptourage effect. Yet, even with that said, we still don't fully know all the effects of the cannabinoids and terpenes either as standalone substances or in concert.

CANNABINOID-RICH HEMP OIL AND PAIN CONTROL

As noted earlier, various receptors in the endocannabinoid system are involved in the regulation of pain including CB_1, CB_2, and $TRPV_1$. Pain is a common complaint among patients as evidenced by the fact sales of opioid drugs almost quadrupled from 1999 to 2014.[40] CB_2 indirectly activates opioid receptors, thus blocking painful stimuli.[41] In part through this mechanism, cannabinoids reduce inflammatory and neuropathic pain, which are notoriously difficult to successfully treat.[42] Animal models, human studies, and experience from clinical practice indicate that cannabinoid-rich hemp oil or CBD are useful in various types of pain. In a rodent model of osteoarthritis, CBD administered locally to the area surrounding the joint reduced the initial inflammatory response and thus subsequent pain and inflammation.[43] Furthermore, cannabinoid-rich hemp oil reduced body pain and improved other symptoms in girls who had an adverse reaction to the human papillomavirus (HPV) vaccine.[44] Other evidence indicates the oil of cannabis seeds reduces pain in patients with chronic musculoskeletal inflammation, an effect attributed to the ideal omega-3/omega-6 ratio content.[45]

Treating pain properly involves addressing more than just physical discomfort. Pain is a multidimensional problem that also encompasses impairments in mood, cognition, and function. This is one way where management of pain with opioids goes wrong as opioids can actually worsen all of these components of pain. Phytocannabinoids found in hemp oil, on the other hand, can improve all of these accompanying mental health factors as we will discuss in the next part of this chapter.

PROPER DOSING IS CRUCIAL

Before concluding this chapter, we want to caution that it is important to keep in mind proper dosing protocols when employing cannabinoid-rich hemp oil. CBD is less potent than THC, and much higher doses may be needed for its beneficial effects on pain and inflammation. At the same time, it's crucial not to over activate the endocannabinoid system as scientists at the ICCT have found that overdosing on CBD can worsen certain conditions such as epilepsy. It's best to begin dosing at modest levels and then increase the dose slowly over two weeks.

Diligent education and a conservative approach to dose for each individual patient and the patient pool in general needs to be in the forefront of the prescriber. As Dr. Meletis has shared in the classroom setting as an associate professor of natural pharmacology, if a natural substance is strong enough to nudge a biochemical pathway towards optimized homeostasis, it also holds the potential to disturb homeostasis when not employed judiciously. Keeping up with the rapidly growing and burgeoning research field on hemp is critical.

CONCLUSION

From long before birth, our bodies are dependent upon the homeostasis provided by the endocannabinoid system, which casts a wide net over various aspects of health including pain management and control of psychological stress, among many others. The endocannabinoid system functions through the activation of a number of receptors. Endocannabinoids as well as phytocannabinoids such as those found in hemp oil interact with these receptors. Consequently, supporting the function of the endocannabinoid system is an under recognized way to enhance virtually every aspect of health.

REFERENCES

1. Miller RJ, Miller RE. Is cannabis an effective treatment for joint pain? *Clin Exp Rheumatol.* 2017 Sep-Oct;35(Suppl 107(5)):59–67.
2. Atwood BK, Mackie K. CB2: a cannabinoid receptor with an identity crisis. *Br J Pharmacol.* 2010 Jun;160(3):467–79.
3. Lowry JR, Klegeris A. Emerging roles of microglial cathepsins in neurodegenerative disease. *Brain Res Bull.* 2018 Feb 15. [Epub ahead of print.]
4. Manzanares J, Julian MD, Carrascosa A. Role of the cannabinoid system in pain control and therapeutic implications for the management of acute and chronic pain episodes. *Curr Neuropharmacol.* 2006 Jul;4(3):239–57.
5. Bhattacharyya S, Egerton A, Kim E, et al. Acute induction of anxiety in humans by delta-9-tetrahydrocannabinol related to amygdalar cannabinoid-1 (CB1) receptors. *Sci Rep.* 2017 Nov 3;7(1):15025.
6. Leweke FM, Piomelli D, Pahlisch F, et al. Cannabidiol enhances anandamide signaling and alleviates psychotic symptoms of schizophrenia. *Transl Psychiatry.* 2012 Mar 20;2:e94.
7. Russo E, Guy GW. A tale of two cannabinoids: the therapeutic rationale for combining tetrahydrocannabinol and cannabidiol. *Med Hypotheses.* 2006;66(2):234–46.
8. Shannon S, Opila-Lehman J. Effectiveness of cannabidiol oil for pediatric anxiety and insomnia as part of posttraumatic stress disorder: A case report. *Perm J.* 2016 Fall;20(4): 108–11.

9. du Plessis SS, Agarwal A, Syriac A. Marijuana, phytocannabinoids, the endocannabinoid system, and male fertility. *J Assist Reprod Genet.* 2015 Nov;32(11):1575–88.
10. Lewis SE, Maccarrone M. Endocannabinoids, sperm biology and human fertility. *Pharmacol Res.* 2009 Aug;60(2):126–31.
11. Gebeh AK, Willets JM, Marczylo EL. Ectopic pregnancy is associated with high anandamide levels and aberrant expression of FAAH and CB1 in fallopian tubes. *J Clin Endocrinol Metab.* 2012 Aug;97(8):2827–35.
12. Maia J, Almada M, Silva A. The endocannabinoid system expression in the female reproductive tract is modulated by estrogen. *J Steroid Biochem Mol Biol.* 2017 Nov;174:40–7.
13. Jokisch V, Kroll R, Lutz B, et al. Endocannabinoid levels in newborns in relation to the mode of delivery. *Am J Perinatol.* 2015 Oct;32(12):1145–50.
14. Ramírez-López MT, Vázquez M, Bindila L, et al. Maternal caloric restriction implemented during the preconceptional and pregnancy period alters hypothalamic and hippocampal endocannabinoid levels at birth and induces overweight and increased adiposity at adulthood in male rat offspring. *Front Behav Neurosci.* 2016 Nov 1;10:208.
15. Fride E. The endocannabinoid-CB(1) receptor system in pre- and postnatal life. *Eur J Pharmacol.* 2004 Oct 1;500(1–3):289–97.
16. Shouman B, Fontaine RH, Baud O, et al. Endocannabinoids potently protect the newborn brain against AMPA-kainate receptor-mediated excitotoxic damage. *Br J Pharmacol.* 2006 Jun;148(4):442–51.
17. McLaughlin RJ, Verlezza S, Gray JM, et al. Inhibition of anandamide hydrolysis dampens the neuroendocrine response to stress in neonatal rats subjected to suboptimal rearing conditions. *Stress.* 2016;19(1):114–24.
18. O'Hearn S, Diaz P, Wan BA, et al. Modulating the endocannabinoid pathway as treatment for peripheral neuropathic pain: a selected review of preclinical studies. *Ann Palliat Med.* 2017 Dec;6(Suppl 2):S209–14.
19. Breivogel CS, Griffin G, Di Marzo V, et al. Evidence for a new G protein-coupled cannabinoid receptor in mouse brain. *Mol Pharmacol.* 2001 Jul;60(1):155–63.
20. Hájos N, Ledent C, Freund TF. Novel cannabinoid-sensitive receptor mediates inhibition of glutamatergic synaptic transmission in the hippocampus. *Neuroscience.* 2001;106(1):1–4.
21. del Río C, Navarrete C, Collado JA, et al. The cannabinoid quinol VCE-004.8 alleviates bleomycin-induced scleroderma and exerts potent antifibrotic effects through peroxisome proliferator-activated receptor-γ and CB2 pathways. *Sci Rep.* 2016 Feb 18;6:21703.
22. O'Sullivan SE. Cannabinoids go nuclear: evidence for activation of peroxisome proliferator-activated receptors. *Br J Pharmacol.* 2007 Nov;152(5):576–82.
23. Campos AC, Fogaça MV, Sonego AB, et al. Cannabidiol, neuroprotection and neuropsychiatric disorders. *Pharmacol Res.* 2016 Oct;112:119–27.
24. del Río C, Navarrete C, Collado JA. The cannabinoid quinol VCE-004.8 alleviates bleomycin-induced scleroderma and exerts potent antifibrotic effects through peroxisome proliferator-activated receptor-γ and CB2 pathways. *Sci Rep.* 2016; 6:21703.
25. Mishima K, Hayakawa K, Abe K, et al. Cannabidiol prevents cerebral infarction via a serotonergic 5-hydroxytryptamine1A receptor-dependent mechanism. *Stroke.* 2005 May;36(5):1077–82.
26. Pazos MR, Mohammed N, Lafuente H, et al. Mechanisms of cannabidiol neuroprotection in hypoxic-ischemic newborn pigs: role of 5HT(1A) and CB2 receptors. *Neuropharmacology.* 2013 Aug;71:282–91.
27. Ibrahim MM, Porreca F, Lai J, et al. CB2 cannabinoid receptor activation produces antinociception by stimulating peripheral release of endogenous opioids. *Proc Natl Acad Sci U S A.* 2005 Feb 22;102(8):3093–8.

28. Engeli S, Heusser K, Janke J, et al. Peripheral endocannabinoid system activity in patients treated with sibutramine. *Obesity (Silver Spring)*. 2008 May;16(5):1135–7.

29. Almeida MM, Dias-Rocha CP, Souza AS, et al. Perinatal maternal high-fat diet induces early obesity and sex-specific alterations of the endocannabinoid system in white and brown adipose tissue of weanling rat offspring. *Br J Nutr*. 2017 Nov;118(10):788–803.

30. Martella A, Silvestri C, Maradonna F, et al. Bisphenol A induces fatty liver by an endocannabinoid-mediated positive feedback loop. *Endocrinology*. 2016 May; 157(5):1751–63.

31. Guida F, Turco F, Iannotta M, et al. Antibiotic-induced microbiota perturbation causes gut endocannabinoidome changes, hippocampal neuroglial reorganization and depression in mice. *Brain Behav Immun*. 2018 Jan;67:230–45.

32. Dobavišek L, Hojnik M, Ferk P. Overlapping molecular pathways between cannabinoid receptors type 1 and 2 and estrogens/androgens on the periphery and their involvement in the pathogenesis of common diseases (Review). *Int J Mol Med*. 2016 Dec;38(6):1642–51.

33. Ganon-Elazar E, Akirav I. Cannabinoid receptor activation in the basolateral amygdala blocks the effects of stress on the conditioning and extinction of inhibitory avoidance. *J Neurosci*. 2009 Sep 9;29(36):11078–88.

34. Hill MN, McLaughlin RJ, Morrish AC, et al. Suppression of amygdalar endocannabinoid signaling by stress contributes to activation of the hypothalamic-pituitary-adrenal axis. *Neuropsychopharmacology*. 2009 Dec;34(13):2733–45.

35. Patel S, Roelke CT, Rademacher DJ, et al. Endocannabinoid signaling negatively modulates stress-induced activation of the hypothalamic-pituitary-adrenal axis. *Endocrinology*. 2004 Dec;145(12):5431–8.

36. Hill MN, McLaughlin RJ, Pan B, et al. Recruitment of prefrontal cortical endocannabinoid signaling by glucocorticoids contributes to termination of the stress response. *J Neurosci*. 2011 Jul 20;31(29):10506–15.

37. Surkin PN, Gallino SL, Luce V, et al. Pharmacological augmentation of endocannabinoid signaling reduces the neuroendocrine response to stress. *Psychoneuroendocrinology*. 2018 Jan;87:131–40.

38. Storr MA, Sharkey KA. The endocannabinoid system and gut-brain signalling. *Curr Opin Pharmacol*. 2007 Dec;7(6):575–82.

39. Russo EB. Taming THC: potential cannabis synergy and phytocannabinoid-terpenoid entourage effects. *Br J Pharmacol*. 2011 Aug;163(7):1344–64.

40. Centers for Disease Control and Prevention. www.cdc.gov/drugoverdose/data/prescribing.html. Accessed March 2, 2018.

41. Ibrahim MM, Porreca F, Lai J, et al. CB2 cannabinoid receptor activation produces antinociception by stimulating peripheral release of endogenous opioids. *Proc Natl Acad Sci U S A*. 2005 Feb 22;102(8):3093–8.

42. Manzanares J, Julian MD, Carrascosa A. Role of the cannabinoid system in pain control and therapeutic implications for the management of acute and chronic pain episodes. *Curr Neuropharmacol*. 2006 Jul;4(3):239–57.

43. Philpott HT, O'Brien M, McDougall JJ. Attenuation of early phase inflammation by cannabidiol prevents pain and nerve damage in rat osteoarthritis. *Pain*. 2017 Dec;158(12):2442–51.

44. Palmieri B, Laurino C, Vadalà M. Short-term efficacy of CBD-enriched hemp oil in girls with dysautonomic syndrome after human papillomavirus vaccination. *Isr Med Assoc J*. 2017 Feb;19(2):79–84.

45. Shaladi AM, Crestani F, Tartari S, et al. [Cannabinoids in the control of pain]. [Article in Italian, Abstract in English]. *Recenti Prog Med*. 2008 Dec;99(12):616–24.

8 Many Applications of Hemp in Neurological & Gut-Brain Axis*

Chris D. Meletis
Naturopathic Physician

CONTENTS

THE ENDOCANNABINOID SYSTEM AND NEUROLOGICAL DISEASES

An impaired endocannabinoid system may play a role in neurodegenerative disorders including Alzheimer's, Parkinson's, and Huntington's disease. Endogenous cannabinoid signaling performs many functions in the central nervous system (CNS), such as modulating neuroinflammation and neurogenesis, as well as regulating synaptic plasticity, and the response to stress.[1,2] Furthermore, upregulation of type-2 cannabinoid (CB$_2$) receptors is associated with many neurodegenerative disorders. Consequently, influencing CB$_2$ receptor signaling may be neuroprotective.[2]

Endocannabinoids possess a broad-spectrum of activity,[2] which is advantageous in neurodegenerative diseases where neural dysfunction is caused by a combination of different factors including protein misfolding, neuroinflammation, excitotoxicity, oxidative stress, and mitochondrial dysfunction.[2] The endocannabinoid signaling system is thought to regulate each of these factors.[2] The endocannabinoid system also modulates brain tissue homeostasis during aging and/or neuroinflammation.[2]

CB$_2$ receptors exert neuroprotective properties through their ability to suppress inflammation.[3] Activation of CB$_2$ receptors regulates the production of cytokines, proteins that play a significant role in immune function and inflammatory

---

* Author Note: Reprinted from *Townsend Letter*, October 2018, http://www.townsendletter.com/). Permission to reuse granted by *Townsend Letter, The Examiner of Alternative Medicine*.

responses.[4] Conversely, rather than inhibiting neurodegenerative diseases via an immunological pathway, the CB_1 receptor suppresses cell death through protecting against excitotoxicity, overstimulation of excitatory receptors, and simultaneous calcium release.[2]

In the neurons of healthy brains, there is a lower expression of CB_2 receptors. However, a significant increase in expression of these receptors is noted in reactive microglia and activated astrocytes during neuroinflammation.[5,6] Microglia are cells in the brain and spinal cord. When they become reactive, it is associated with neurodegenerative diseases. Activated microglia modulate inflammatory responses to pathogens and injury by signaling the synthesis of pro-inflammatory cytokines. Similarly, diseases that impact the central nervous system activate astrocytes. The fact that CB_2 receptors are highly expressed when both these types of cells are activated may indicate they are needed to combat inflammation. This led researchers to conclude, "Therefore, the CB_2 receptors have the potential to restrain the inflammatory processes that contribute to the declines in neural function occurring in a number of neurodegenerative disorders."[2]

The involvement of CB_2 receptors in Alzheimer's disease was demonstrated in a number of human studies. Inspections of post-mortem brains from individuals with Alzheimer's disease showed that CB_2 receptors are upregulated in cells that are linked to amyloid beta (Aβ)-enriched neuritic plaques.[7–10] The deposition of amyloid beta plaques in the brain is involved in Alzheimer's disease pathology. Other researchers found markedly higher CB_2 receptor levels in individuals with severe Alzheimer's disease compared with age-matched controls or people with moderate Alzheimer's.[11] Activation of the CB_2 receptor has resulted in beneficial effects in Alzheimer's disease, including the inhibition of microglial activation in mice.[12]

Further support for the role of the endocannabinoid system in Alzheimer's is provided by preclinical studies showing that cannabidiol, the non-psychoactive component of cannabis sativa, may be beneficial in Alzheimer's. In one of these studies, mice inoculated with Aβ then injected with CBD (2.5 or 10 mg/kg) for 7 days had anti-inflammatory and neuroprotective effects as evidenced by its ability to suppress a marker of activated astrocytes.[13] A rat model of Alzheimer's-related neuroinflammation further elucidated the role CBD may play in Alzheimer's. In this study, adult, male rats were inoculated with human $Aβ_{42}$ in the hippocampus.[14] Then, for 15 days, they were given 10 mg/kg CBD either with or without a PPAR-γ or PPAR-α receptor antagonist. CBD counteracted many of the pathogenic mechanisms of Aβ and its effects involved the regulation of PPAR-γ. This makes sense since PPAR-γ receptors are increased in people with Alzheimer's disease.

PARKINSON'S DISEASE

The progressive loss of dopaminergic neurons primarily in the substantia nigra (SN) is the distinguishing characteristic of Parkinson's disease. This dopaminergic neuron loss impairs the basal ganglia leading to bradykinesia (slowness of movement), rigidity, and tremors. Inflammation is a prominent player in Parkinson's disease pathogenesis. Post-mortem evaluations of Parkinson's disease patients observed microglia activation in the SN.[15] Structural brain imaging studies have also shown that activated microglia and an increase of pro-inflammatory cytokines occur in the nigrostriatal system of Parkinson's disease patients.[16,17] A post-mortem study indicated that individuals with Parkinson's disease have increased expression of CB_2 receptors in microglial cells of the SN.[18] This and other evidence suggests that targeting the CB_2 receptor may serve as an anti-inflammatory approach in Parkinson's.[2]

In support of the idea that modulating the endocannabinoid system is beneficial in Parkinson's disease are a number of small studies investigating the use of cannabidiol in this group of patients. In a double-blind, placebo-controlled study of 21 Parkinson's patients without dementia or comorbid psychiatric conditions, 300 mg/day cannabidiol enhanced well-being and quality of life.[19] In an open-label pilot study, six Parkinson's disease outpatients (four men and two women) who suffered from psychosis for at least three months received CBD starting with an oral dose of 150 mg/day for 4 weeks combined with their usual therapy.[20] CBD intervention resulted in a marked decline in psychotic symptoms as measured by the Brief Psychiatric Rating Scale and the Parkinson Psychosis Questionnaire. CBD also lowered the total scores of the Unified Parkinson's Disease Rating Scale. Furthermore, cannabidiol significantly reduced the frequency of sleep behavior disorder (RBD) in four patients with Parkinson's disease.[21]

ANXIETY AND POST-TRAUMATIC STRESS DISORDER

The endocannabinoid system regulates stress and anxiety, and modulation of the endocannabinoid system has been found to reduce anxiety. Repeated injections of cannabidiol to mice exposed to chronic unpredictable stress reduced anxiety in the animals.[22] This effect was mediated by CB_1, CB_2, and serotonin ($5HT_{1A}$) receptors. In a double-blind randomized trial investigating subjects with generalized social anxiety disorder not receiving medication, 600 mg of cannabidiol reduced anxiety and cognitive impairment caused by simulated public speaking and improved the participants' comfort level in their speech performance.[23] Another study of 10 individuals with generalized social anxiety disorder observed that 400 mg of cannabidiol was associated with markedly reduced subjective anxiety.[24] Furthermore, advanced imaging studies indicate that the endocannabinoid system is underactive in post-traumatic stress disorder.[25] Preliminary studies in humans have observed that cannabinoids may improve PTSD symptoms such as sleep quality and hyperarousal.[26] Nabilone, a synthetic cannabinoid, reduced PTSD-related nightmares in a small group of Canadian military personnel.[27] In an animal model, cannabinoids given shortly after experiencing a traumatic event blocked the development of a PTSD-like phenotype.[26]

DEPRESSION

Dysregulation of the endocannabinoid system may be involved in the development of depression. Suppressing the CB_1 receptor results in a phenotypic state that is comparable to melancholic depression, with identical symptoms such as decreased appetite, increased anxiety, arousal, and wakefulness, an inability to release aversive memories, and increased sensitivity to stress.[28] Furthermore, some antidepressant medications enhance endocannabinoid activity.[28]

One mechanism by which CBD reduces depression may be via its ability to protect against the effects of stress. Stress can lead to anxiety and depression. In animal models, CBD lowers autonomic indices of stress and behavioral effects of depression and anxiety and improves the delayed emotional consequences of stress via mechanisms that involve serotonin receptors.[29,30] CBD is also thought to reduce depressive symptoms by enhancing hippocampal neurogenesis. Ongoing administration of CBD in mice undergoing chronic unpredictable stress improved depressive- and anxiety-like behaviors and triggered hippocampal progenitor proliferation and neurogenesis.[31]

CBD is thought to stimulate neurogenesis by elevating hippocampal levels of the endocannabinoid anandamide (AEA). A clinical study found that higher serum concentrations of AEA were associated with reduced anxiety in patients with major depression, although in this group of patients AEA levels were not associated with major depressive symptoms.[32] Conversely, in people with minor depression, AEA concentrations were elevated compared to controls, suggesting that these levels might be raised as the body's way to compensate for the depression and that they may have a neuroprotective role in patients with less severe depressive symptoms.

The role of cannabinoids in depression is a vast topic and we recommend that you enroll in the ICCT medical certification program to understand how phytocannabinoids can be safely used in depression.

GUT-BRAIN AXIS AND ENDOCANNABINOIDS

The gut-brain axis refers to the bidirectional interplay between the gut microbiota and the nervous system whereby the gut microbiota can impact behavior and cognition and the central nervous system can influence enteric microbiota composition. The gut-brain axis is thought to explain the association between chronic inflammatory bowel disease and depression.[33]

Accumulating evidence points to the endocannabinoid system's important role in both normal gastrointestinal function and gastrointestinal pathology.[34] The endocannabinoid system is involved in the regulation of motility, gut-brain mediated fat intake and hunger signaling, and inflammation and gut permeability.[34] The endocannabinoid system also works together with the gut microbiota to maintain gut health.[34] Additionally, cannabinoids help recruit immune cells to the site of intestinal inflammation.[35] In models of colitis, cannabidiol also has been shown to suppress the synthesis of pro-inflammatory cytokines, such as TNF-α and IFN-γ.[35–38] This anti-inflammatory role in gut health was also reflected in a study where intestinal tissues of individuals with ulcerative colitis had concentrations of the endocannabinoid PEA that were 1.8 fold higher compared with healthy patients, likely in an attempt to help heal the inflammation.[39] The anti-inflammatory effect of cannabinoids in the gastrointestinal system may be mediated by the gut microbiota. In mice, dysbiosis of the microbiota caused by antibiotics resulted in a general inflammatory state and altered endocannabinoids in the gut.[33] (The concept of an Endocannabinoidome will be addressed in much further detail in the ICCT certification program). Mitochondrial transport in enteric nerves may also be controlled by CB_1 receptors, further lending support to the role of cannabinoids in gut health.[40]

The interplay between the gut, the brain, and the endocannabinoid system is involved in the development and progression of inflammatory bowel disease and irritable bowel syndrome. CB_1 receptors in sensory ganglia modulate visceral sensation. During ongoing psychological stress, epigenetic pathways change the transcription of CB_1 receptors, a mechanism which may explain the link between stress and abdominal pain.[41] Furthermore, in rodent models, the endocannabinoid system is altered by early-life stress, leading to the development of irritable bowel syndrome (IBS).[42,43]

In tissue from humans with inflammatory bowel disease, there is elevated epithelial CB_2 receptor expression.[44] This indicates that CB_2 receptors modulate immunity in this disorder.[45] The CB_2 receptors impact mucosal immunity and act together with CB_1 receptors in the colonic epithelium to encourage epithelial wound healing.[44]

Research suggests that type 1 vanilloid receptors ($TRPV_1$) may regulate some cannabinoid effects. One study observed a 3.5-fold increase in TRPV1-immunoreactive nerve fibers in biopsies from IBS sufferers compared with controls.[45] This elevation may promote visceral hypersensitivity and pain in IBS.[45] One scientist concluded, "Thus, a rationale exists for therapeutic interventions that would boost AEA levels or desensitize TRPV1, such as cannabidiol (CBD), to treat the condition [IBS]."[25]

CANNABINOIDS, AUTOIMMUNITY, STROKES, EPILEPSY, AND OTHER DISORDERS

Cannabidiol may have a role to play in autoimmune health. Animal models indicate it exerts beneficial actions in a number of autoimmune disorders including multiple sclerosis (MS), type 1 diabetes, and autoimmune myocarditis.[46,47] Autoimmune disease develops due to transformed subsets of T cells into autoreactive memory T cells. These cells are falsely directed to target the body's own cells resulting in tissue degeneration and autoimmune disease development such as type 1 diabetes, rheumatoid arthritis, and MS.[46] CBD is able to modulate autoreactive T cell function.[46] In one study it weakened the function of encephalitogenic Th17 cells.[46] CBD also increased anti-inflammatory actions in activated memory T cells including enhanced synthesis of the anti-inflammatory IL-10 cytokine.[48] Furthermore, CBD produced anti-inflammatory effects in animal models of T cell-mediated collagen-induced arthritis,[49] autoimmune diabetes,[50] and autoimmune hepatitis.[51] It also has reversed the development of type 1 diabetes mellitus in mice.[52] Most of the human studies showing cannabinoids are beneficial in multiple sclerosis have used a pharmaceutical combination of THC and CBD.[53,54]

Cannabinoids are important to other aspects of immunity. Specifically, they possess strong antibacterial activity. All five major cannabinoids (cannabidiol, cannabichromene, cannabigerol, Delta (9)-tetrahydrocannabinol, and cannabinol) significantly inhibited a number of methicillin-resistant *Staphylococcus aureus* (MRSA) strains.[55] THC use by itself, however, was associated with increased susceptibility of mice to infection with the pathogen *Legionella pneumophila*.[56]

Another application of CBD may include protection against stroke.[57] In vivo and in vitro stroke models indicate cannabidiol reduces infarct size.[57] A study of human brain microvascular endothelial cells and human astrocyte co-cultures suggests that CBD can prevent permeability changes in the blood brain barrier.[57]

Another promising role for cannabidiol is in the improvement of schizophrenia. Modulating the endocannabinoid system using THC, the main psychoactive component in cannabis, can cause acute psychotic effects and cognitive impairment in schizophrenia patients.[58] Conversely, CBD may possess antipsychotic actions and may have a role to play in supporting schizophrenia patients. Evidence to this effect is emerging thanks to small-scale clinical studies with CBD for the treatment of patients with psychotic symptoms.[59] The results demonstrated that CBD is effective, safe, and well-tolerated in patients with schizophrenia, although large randomized clinical trials are needed.[59]

Cannabidiol has also been used successfully in clinical practice and in human studies in patients with epilepsy. It has been found to improve brain tumor-related seizures.[60] Additionally, patients with Sturge-Weber syndrome, a disorder characterized by medically refractory epilepsy, stroke, and cognitive impairments, experienced up to a 50% reduction in seizures after supplementation with cannabidiol.[61] It's important to note that CBD supplementation can alter the serum levels of certain anti-epilepsy medications. This is not always a bad thing as CBD may reduce the side effects of some epilepsy medications by lowering their dosage.[62] However, the blood levels of these pharmaceuticals should be monitored when taking CBD.

Dr. Meletis will discuss these and other clinical applications of CBD in the ICCT medical certification course and will also talk about the proper dosing to ensure that doctors who suggest CBD aren't doing more harm than good. This is especially important in regard to seizures as too much CBD may actually cause seizures.

DOSING, SIDE EFFECTS, AND DRUG INTERACTIONS

Cannabidiol is a safe substance, with a half-life of 18–32 hours,[63] but it can have minor adverse effects in some people. Potential side effects are dry mouth, low blood pressure, light headedness, drowsiness, tiredness, diarrhea, and changes of appetite or weight.[62,64] There is also cross-reactivity between medical marijuana and certain foods including molds, dust mites, plants, and cat dander.[65] It's unclear whether these same reactions occur with cannabidiol. In fact, one mouse study indicated CBD in a dose-dependent manner markedly reduced inflammatory reactions associated with delayed type hypersensitivity reactions.[66] These are allergic reactions that develop days after exposure to the offending substance.

It is also important to keep in mind that cannabidiol can affect levels of medications. This is indicated by the fact it is an inhibitor of multiple cytochrome P450 enzymes, which are involved in the metabolism of drugs.[67]

REFERENCES

1. Lu HC, Mackie K. An introduction to the endogenous cannabinoid system. *Biol Psychiatry*. 2016 Apr 1;79(7):516–25.
2. Cassano T, Calcagnini S, Pace L, et al. Cannabinoid receptor 2 signaling in neuro-degenerative disorders: from pathogenesis to a promising therapeutic target. *Front Neurosci*. 2017 Feb 2;11:30.
3. Benito C, Tolón RM, Pazos MR, et al. Cannabinoid CB2 receptors in human brain inflammation. *Br J Pharmacol*. 2008 Jan;153(2):277–85.

4. Turcotte C, Blanchet MR, Laviolette M, et al. The CB2 receptor and its role as a regulator of inflammation. *Cell Mol Life Sci*. 2016 Dec;73(23):4449–70.
5. Stella N. Cannabinoid and cannabinoid-like receptors in microglia, astrocytes, and astrocytomas. *Glia*. 2010 Jul;58(9):1017–30.
6. Onaivi ES, Ishiguro H, Gu S, et al. CNS effects of CB2 cannabinoid receptors: beyond neuro-immuno-cannabinoid activity. *J Psychopharmacol*. 2012 Jan;26(1):92–103.
7. Benito C, Núñez E, Tolón RM, et al. Cannabinoid CB2 receptors and fatty acid amide hydrolase are selectively overexpressed in neuritic plaque-associated glia in Alzheimer's disease brains. *J Neurosci*. 2003 Dec 3;23(35):11136–41.
8. Ramírez BG, Blázquez C, Gómez del Pulgar T, et al. Prevention of Alzheimer's disease pathology by cannabinoids: neuroprotection mediated by blockade of microglial activation. *J Neurosci*. 2005 Feb 23;25(8):1904–13.
9. Grünblatt E, Bartl J, Zehetmayer S, et al. Gene expression as peripheral biomarkers for sporadic Alzheimer's disease. *J Alzheimers Dis*. 2009;16(3):627–34.
10. Solas M, Francis PT, Franco R, et al. CB2 receptor and amyloid pathology in frontal cortex of Alzheimer's disease patients. *Neurobiol Aging*. 2013 Mar;34(3):805–8.
11. Halleskog C, Mulder J, Dahlström J, et al. WNT signaling in activated microglia is proinflammatory. *Glia*. 2011 Jan;59(1):119–31.
12. Ehrhart J, Obregon D, Mori T, et al. Stimulation of cannabinoid receptor 2 (CB2) suppresses microglial activation. *Neuroinflammation*. 2005 Dec 12;2:29.
13. Esposito G, Scuderi C, Savani C, et al. Cannabidiol in vivo blunts beta-amyloid induced neuroinflammation by suppressing IL-1beta and iNOS expression. *Br J Pharmacol*. 2007 Aug;151(8):1272–9.
14. Esposito G, Scuderi C, Valenza M, et al. Cannabidiol reduces Aβ-induced neuroinflammation and promotes hippocampal neurogenesis through PPARγ involvement. *PLoS One*. 2011;6(12):e28668.
15. McGeer PL, Itagaki S, Boyes BE, et al. Reactive microglia are positive for HLA-DR in the substantia nigra of Parkinson's and Alzheimer's disease brains. *Neurology*. 1988 Aug;38(8):1285–91.
16. Ouchi Y, Yoshikawa E, Sekine Y, et al. Microglial activation and dopamine terminal loss in early Parkinson's disease. *Ann Neurol*. 2005 Feb;57(2):168–75.
17. Gerhard A, Pavese N, Hotton G, et al. In vivo imaging of microglial activation with [11C](R)-PK11195 PET in idiopathic Parkinson's disease. *Neurobiol Dis*. 2006 Feb;21(2):404–12.
18. Gómez-Gálvez Y, Palomo-Garo C, Fernández-Ruiz J, et al. Potential of the cannabinoid CB(2) receptor as a pharmacological target against inflammation in Parkinson's disease. *Prog Neuropsychopharmacol Biol Psychiatry*. 2016 Jan 4;64:200–8.
19. Chagas MH, Zuardi AW, Tumas V, et al. Effects of cannabidiol in the treatment of patients with Parkinson's disease: an exploratory double-blind trial. *J Psychopharmacol*. 2014 Nov;28(11):1088–98.
20. Zuardi AW, Crippa JA, Hallak JE, et al. Cannabidiol for the treatment of psychosis in Parkinson's disease. *J Psychopharmacol*. 2009 Nov;23(8):979–83.
21. Chagas MH, Eckeli AL, Zuardi AW, et al. Cannabidiol can improve complex sleep-related behaviours associated with rapid eye movement sleep behaviour disorder in Parkinson's disease patients: a case series. *J Clin Pharm Ther*. 2014 Oct;39(5):564–6.
22. Fogaça MV, Campos AC, Coelho LD, et al. The anxiolytic effects of cannabidiol in chronically stressed mice are mediated by the endocannabinoid system: role of neurogenesis and dendritic remodeling. *Neuropharmacology*. 2018 Mar 3;135:22–33.
23. Bergamaschi MM, Queiroz RH, Chagas MH. Cannabidiol reduces the anxiety induced by simulated public speaking in treatment-naïve social phobia patients. *Neuropsychopharmacology*. 2011 May;36(6):1219–26.

24. Crippa JA, Derenusson GN, Ferrari TB, et al. Neural basis of anxiolytic effects of cannabidiol (CBD) in generalized social anxiety disorder: a preliminary report. *J Psychopharmacol*. 2011 Jan;25(1):121–30.

25. Russo EB. Clinical endocannabinoid deficiency reconsidered: current research supports the theory in migraine, fibromyalgia, irritable bowel, and other treatment-resistant syndromes. *Cannabis Cannabinoid Res*. 2016 Jul 1;1(1):154–65.

26. Mizrachi Zer-Aviv T, Segev A, Akirav I. Cannabinoids and post-traumatic stress disorder: clinical and preclinical evidence for treatment and prevention. *Behav Pharmacol*. 2016 Oct;27(7):561–9.

27. Jetly R, Heber A, Fraser G, et al. The efficacy of nabilone, a synthetic cannabinoid, in the treatment of PTSD-associated nightmares: a preliminary randomized, double-blind, placebo-controlled cross-over design study. *Psychoneuroendocrinology*. 2015 Jan;51:585–8.

28. Hill MN, Gorzalka BB. Is there a role for the endocannabinoid system in the etiology and treatment of melancholic depression? *Behav Pharmacol*. 2005 Sep;16(5–6):333–52.

29. Resstel LB, Tavares RF, Lisboa SF, et al. 5-HT1A receptors are involved in the cannabidiol-induced attenuation of behavioural and cardiovascular responses to acute restraint stress in rats. *Br J Pharmacol*. 2009 Jan;156(1):181–8.

30. Granjeiro EM, Gomes FV, Guimarães FS, et al. Effects of intracisternal administration of cannabidiol on the cardiovascular and behavioral responses to acute restraint stress. *Pharmacol Biochem Behav*. 2011 Oct;99(4):743–8.

31. Campos AC, Ortega Z, Palazuelos J, et al. The anxiolytic effect of cannabidiol on chronically stressed mice depends on hippocampal neurogenesis: involvement of the endocannabinoid system. *Int J Neuropsychopharmacol*. 2013 Jul;16(6):1407–19.

32. Hill MN, Miller GE, Ho WS, et al. Serum endocannabinoid content is altered in females with depressive disorders: a preliminary report. *Pharmacopsychiatry*. 2008 Mar;41(2):48–53.

33. Guida F, Turco F, Iannotta M, et al. Antibiotic-induced microbiota perturbation causes gut endocannabinoidome changes, hippocampal neuroglial reorganization and depression in mice. *Brain Behav Immun*. 2017 Sep 7. pii: S0889-1591(17)30417-8. [Epub ahead of print.]

34. DiPatrizio NV. Endocannabinoids in the Gut. *Cannabis Cannabinoid Res*. 2016 Feb;1(1):67–77.

35. Alhouayek M, Lambert DM, Delzenne NM, et al. Increasing endogenous 2-arachidonoylglycerol levels counteracts colitis and related systemic inflammation. *FASEB J*. 2011 Aug;25(8):2711–21.

36. Schicho R, Bashashati M, Bawa M, et al. The atypical cannabinoid O-1602 protects against experimental colitis and inhibits neutrophil recruitment. *Inflamm Bowel Dis*. 2011 Aug;17(8):1651–64.

37. Borrelli F, Aviello G, Romano B, et al. Cannabidiol, a safe and non-psychotropic ingredient of the marijuana plant Cannabis sativa, is protective in a murine model of colitis. *J Mol Med (Berl)*. 2009 Nov;87(11):1111–21.

38. De Filippis D, Esposito G, Cirillo C, et al. Cannabidiol reduces intestinal inflammation through the control of neuroimmune axis. *PLoS One*. 2011;6(12):e28159.

39. Darmani NA, Izzo AA, Degenhardt B, et al. Involvement of the cannabimimetic compound, N-palmitoyl-ethanolamine, in inflammatory and neuropathic conditions: review of the available pre-clinical data, and first human studies. *Neuropharmacology*. 2005 Jun;48(8):1154–63.

40. Boesmans W, Ameloot K, van den Abbeel V, et al. Cannabinoid receptor 1 signalling dampens activity and mitochondrial transport in networks of enteric neurones. *Neurogastroenterol Motil*. 2009 Sep;21(9):958–e77.

41. Sharkey KA, Wiley JW. The role of the endocannabinoid system in the brain-gut axis. *Gastroenterology*. 2016 Aug;151(2):252–66.

42. Marco EM, Echeverry-Alzate V, López-Moreno JA, et al. Consequences of early life stress on the expression of endocannabinoid-related genes in the rat brain. *Behav Pharmacol.* 2014 Sep;25(5–6):547–56.

43. Moloney RD, Stilling RM, Dinan TG, et al. Early-life stress-induced visceral hypersensitivity and anxiety behavior is reversed by histone deacetylase inhibition. *Neurogastroenterol Motil.* 2015 Dec;27(12):1831–6.

44. Wright K, Rooney N, Feeney M, et al. Differential expression of cannabinoid receptors in the human colon: cannabinoids promote epithelial wound healing. *Gastroenterology.* 2005 Aug;129(2):437–53.

45. Akbar A, Yiangou Y, Facer P, et al. Increased capsaicin receptor TRPV1-expressing sensory fibres in irritable bowel syndrome and their correlation with abdominal pain. *Gut.* 2008 Jul;57(7):923–9.

46. Kozela E, Juknat A, Gao F, et al. Pathways and gene networks mediating the regulatory effects of cannabidiol, a nonpsychoactive cannabinoid, in autoimmune T cells. *J Neuroinflammation.* 2016 Jun 3;13(1):136.

47. Lee WS, Erdelyi K, Matyas C, et al. Cannabidiol limits Tcell-mediated chronic autoimmune myocarditis: implications to autoimmune disorders and organ transplantation. *Mol Med.* 2016 Jan 8. [Epub ahead of print.]

48. Kozela E, Juknat A, Kaushansky N, et al. Cannabidiol, a non-psychoactive cannabinoid, leads to EGR2-dependent anergy in activated encephalitogenic T cells. *J Neuroinflammation.* 2015 Mar 15;12:52.

49. Malfait AM, Gallily R, Sumariwalla PF, et al. The nonpsychoactive cannabis constituent cannabidiol is an oral anti-arthritic therapeutic in murine collagen-induced arthritis. *Proc Natl Acad Sci U S A.* 2000 Aug 15;97(17):9561–6.

50. Weiss L, Zeira M, Reich S, et al. Cannabidiol lowers incidence of diabetes in non-obese diabetic mice. *Autoimmunity.* 2006 Mar;39(2):143–51.

51. Hegde VL, Nagarkatti PS, Nagarkatti M. Role of myeloid-derived suppressor cells in amelioration of experimental autoimmune hepatitis following activation of TRPV1 receptors by cannabidiol. *PLoS One.* 2011 Apr 1;6(4):e18281.

52. Weiss L, Zeira M, Reich S, et al. Cannabidiol arrests onset of autoimmune diabetes in NOD mice. *Neuropharmacology.* 2008 Jan;54(1):244–9.

53. Vaney C, Heinzel-Gutenbrunner M, Jobin P, et al. Efficacy, safety and tolerability of an orally administered cannabis extract in the treatment of spasticity in patients with multiple sclerosis: a randomized, double-blind, placebo-controlled, crossover study. *Mult Scler.* 2004 Aug;10(4):417–24.

54. Leocani L, Nuara A, Houdayer E, et al. Sativex(®) and clinical-neurophysiological measures of spasticity in progressive multiple sclerosis. *J Neurol.* 2015 Nov;262(11):2520–7.

55. Appendino G, Gibbons S, Giana A, et al. Antibacterial cannabinoids from Cannabis sativa: a structure-activity study. *J Nat Prod.* 2008 Aug;71(8):1427–30.

56. Smith MS, Yamamoto Y, Newton C, et al. Psychoactive cannabinoids increase mortality and alter acute phase cytokine responses in mice sublethally infected with Legionella pneumophila. *Proc Soc Exp Biol Med.* 1997 Jan;214(1):69–75.

57. Hind WH, England TJ, O'Sullivan SE. Cannabidiol protects an in vitro model of the blood-brain barrier from oxygen-glucose deprivation via PPARγ and 5-HT1A receptors. *Br J Pharmacol.* 2016 Mar;173(5):815–25.

58. Ceskova E, Silhan P. Novel treatment options in depression and psychosis. *Neuropsychiatr Dis Treat.* 2018;14:741–7.

59. Leweke FM, Mueller JK, Lange B. Therapeutic potential of cannabinoids in psychosis. *Biol Psychiatry.* 2016 Apr 1;79(7):604–12.

60. Warren PP, Bebin EM, Nabors LB, et al. The use of cannabidiol for seizure management in patients with brain tumor-related epilepsy. *Neurocase.* 2017 Oct–Dec;23(5–6):287–91.

61. Kaplan EH, Offermann EA, Sievers JW, et al. Cannabidiol treatment for refractory seizures in Sturge-Weber syndrome. *Pediatr Neurol.* 2017 Jun;71:18–23.

62. Iffland K, Grotenhermen F. An update on safety and side effects of cannabidiol: a review of clinical data and relevant animal studies. *Cannabis Cannabinoid Res.* 2017;2(1):139–54.

63. Devinsky O, Cilio MR, Cross H, et al. Cannabidiol: pharmacology and potential therapeutic role in epilepsy and other neuropsychiatric disorders. *Epilepsia.* 2014 Jun;55(6):791–802.

64. WebMD. www.webmd.com/vitamins-supplements/ingredientmono-1439-cannabidiol.aspx?activeingredientid=1439&activeingredientname=cannabidiol. Accessed April 3, 2018.

65. Min JY, Min KB. Marijuana use is associated with hypersensitivity to multiple allergens in US adults. *Drug Alcohol Depend.* 2018 Jan 1;182:74–7.

66. Liu DZ, Hu CM, Huang CH, et al. Cannabidiol attenuates delayed-type hypersensitivity reactions via suppressing T-cell and macrophage reactivity. *Acta Pharmacol Sin.* 2010 Dec;31(12):1611–7.

67. Zhornitsky S, Potvin S. Cannabidiol in humans—the quest for therapeutic targets. *Pharmaceuticals* (Basel). 2012 May;5(5):529–52.

9 Endocannabinoid Role in Gut Health*

Chris D. Meletis
Naturopathic Physician

CONTENTS

Cannabis has been used medicinally for centuries in people suffering from disorders associated with the gastrointestinal tract (GI), including abdominal pain, cramps, diarrhea, nausea, and vomiting.[1,2] An extensive amount of recent research offers justification for the traditional use of not only cannabis but also other phytocannabinoids such as cannabidiol (CBD) for GI health. This research points to a strong connection between the endocannabinoid system and various aspects of gut health. The gut-brain axis, which refers to the ability of intestinal function to alter various aspects of mental and cognitive health, has drawn considerable attention in the medical literature. New research indicates that actions of the gut-brain axis may be in part mediated by the endocannabinoid system.[3]

The endocannabinoid system refers to cannabinoids produced within the body (endocannabinoids), neurotransmitters that bind to cannabinoid receptors 1 and 2 (CB_1 and CB_2), thus regulating many aspects of health. Enzymes that play an important role in the synthesis and breakdown of endocannabinoids and molecules required for endocannabinoid uptake and transport are also involved in the endocannabinoid system. Phytocannabinoids like CBD may exert their health benefits in part through their actions on this system. It has long been known that the endocannabinoid system regulates many functions in the body including mental health and pain control. Its role in other areas of health has only recently begun to be appreciated. One of those areas is the role it plays in the intestines.

---

* Author Note: Reprinted from *Townsend Letter*, July 2018, http://www.townsendletter.com/). Permission to reuse granted by *Townsend Letter, The Examiner of Alternative Medicine.*

THE ENDOCANNABINOID SYSTEM'S ROLE IN GUT HEALTH

An extensive amount of evidence indicates the endocannabinoid system plays a significant role in intestinal health. High concentrations of the endocannabinoids 2-arachidonoylglycerol (2-AG) and anandamide are observed in the colon along with significant fatty acid amide hydrolase (FAAH) activity,[4] which is involved in the breakdown of anandamide.

The enteric nervous system (ENS) of the GI tract contains approximately 500 million nerve endings.[5] The highest levels of immune cells in the body are also found in the gastrointestinal tract.[5] Roughly 20% of the nerves in the GI tract are intrinsic primary afferent neurons, which alert the brain when subtle changes within the GI tract occur.[5] This communication occurs through the vagus nerve. Endocannabinoids may regulate neurotransmission in the gut, as indicated by the presence of the CB_2 receptor on enteric neurons and its expression by immune and epithelial cells in the GI tract.[6,7] Furthermore, altering the activity of CB_1 receptors can regulate sensory processing from the gut, brain integration of the brain-gut axis, extrinsic control of the gut, and intrinsic control by the enteric nervous system.[4]

The effect of both endocannabinoids and phytocannabinoids on colon carcinogenesis in rodents further supports the role of the endocannabinoid system in gut health. Studies using CBD or a cannabis sativa extract with high cannabidiol content inhibited the initiation of aberrant crypt foci, polyps, and tumors in the colon of mice.[8,9] Cannabidiol also suppressed cell proliferation in colorectal carcinoma cell lines.[8]

THE ENDOCANNABINOID SYSTEM AND GUT MOTILITY

Endocannabinoids are known to regulate gut motility, the time it takes for food to move through the intestines. Slow gut motility is more commonly called constipation, and fast gut motility is known as diarrhea. Evidence indicates that the endocannabinoid system plays an important role in gut motility. In obese mice fed high-fat diets, the endocannabinoid system in the gut underwent alterations, leading to an increase in gut motility.[10] Many studies also indicate that CB_1 receptor activation suppresses peristalsis and gastrointestinal contraction. The CB_1 receptor is activated by THC, the psychoactive component in marijuana.[11,12] Because CBD does not activate the CB_1 receptor, it may be less likely to produce constipation. This was indicated in a mouse model of sepsis, which demonstrated that CBD slowed gastrointestinal motility in the animals with sepsis but did not affect motility in normal mice.[13] Furthermore, CBD regulates the activity of FAAH, an enzyme involved in gastrointestinal motility through its actions on anandamide.[13] Additional evidence that the endocannabinoid system is involved in gut motility was provided by a mouse model of constipation in which inhibiting diacylglycerol lipase (DGL), the enzyme responsible for the synthesis of the endocannabinoid 2-AG, improves gut motility.[14]

ENDOCANNABINOIDS, THE GUT, AND OBESITY

Through pathways associated with the gut-brain axis, alterations in the endocannabinoid system can result in obesity and accompanying inflammation.[15]

Endocannabinoid signaling in the gut may modulate food intake and energy balance by indirectly interacting with the vagus nerve,[16] which permits neurotransmission between the gut and brain.[17]

A rodent model found fasting leads to the synthesis of 2-AG and activates the CB_1 receptor through efferent vagal activation of receptors in the small intestine, which may signal hunger.[18]

The endocannabinoid system's role in food intake was shown in a study demonstrating increased endocannabinoid signaling occurs after hedonic eating (consuming food for pleasure).[18] In both normal-weight and obese humans, thinking about eating or eating a highly palatable food, such as chocolate or pudding, leads to circulating levels of endocannabinoids that are higher compared with a nonpalatable control diet.[19–21]

THE ENDOCANNABINOID SYSTEM AND INFLAMMATORY BOWEL DISEASE

Endocannabinoids and phytocannabinoids are involved in inflammatory regulation in the gut. Endocannabinoids help signal immune cell movement to intestinal inflammation sites.[22,23] Cannabidiol has been shown to suppress the synthesis of proinflammatory cytokines, such as TNF-α and IFN-γ, and reduce intestinal inflammation.[24,25] Due to its role in regulating gut inflammation, it's not surprising that the endocannabinoid system has also been shown to modulate inflammatory bowel disease (IBD) and irritable bowel syndrome (IBS). Tissue from humans with IBD is characterized by increased epithelial CB_2 receptor expression, suggesting CB_2 receptors act in an immunomodulatory capacity in this disorder.[26] This in turn affects mucosal immunity in the inflamed colon and interacts with the actions of CB_1 receptors in the colonic lining to promote wound healing.[26] In fact, CB_1 receptors play an important role in gut health as evidenced by the increased incidence of diarrhea in people administered CB_1 receptor antagonists.[27]

Other evidence supporting the endocannabinoid system's role in modulating colonic inflammation was provided by rodent models showing that suppressing FAAH, leading to a rise in anandamide levels, stops the development of colitis.[28,29] Likewise, inhibiting FAAH and the inflammatory enzyme cyclooxygenase (COX) in mice with colitis reduces the severity of the disease by elevating anandamide levels and acting on the CB_1 receptor.[30] Blocking FAAH and COX correlated with higher concentrations of the endocannabinoids palmitoylethanolamide (PEA) and oleoylethanolamide. In intestinal tissue from ulcerative colitis patients, PEA levels are 1.8-fold higher compared with healthy patients, likely a result of the PEA attempting to help heal the inflammation.[31] PEA has pronounced anti-inflammatory properties that inhibit features of colitis in mice as well as the synthesis of inflammatory cytokines.[32]

The phytocannabinoids CBD, THC, and cannabigerol have significantly reduced intestinal inflammation in animal models. In one of those models, both CBD and THC proved beneficial.[33] However, THC was the most effective in rats with experimental colitis, although CBD enhanced the effects of an ineffective THC dose to the point where the combination of CBD and lower-dose THC was the equivalent of a higher THC-only dose.[33] The phytocannabinoid cannabigerol (CBG) has also proved beneficial in rodent models of colitis. In one study, CBG inhibited colitis in mice and lowered the synthesis of reactive oxygen species in intestinal epithelial cells.[34]

Polymorphisms in the gene encoding CB_1 receptors are associated with irritable bowel syndrome, further establishing the link between the endocannabinoid system and this disease.[35] Variants of the CB_1 receptor gene (CNR1) and FAAH genes have been noted in individuals with diarrhea-predominant and alternating forms of IBS.[36,37] In intestinal tissues of patients with constipation-predominant IBS, lower levels of FAAH mRNA were observed.[38] In a study of patients with constipation-predominant IBS (C-IBS), diarrhea-predominant IBS (D-IBS), and mixed IBS (M-IBS) who suffered from chronic abdominal pain and functional dyspepsia, there was a relationship between the non-wild type FAAH genotype and functional bowel disease phenotypes and with increased colonic transit in IBS-D patients.[39] Likewise, in another study, there was a pronounced association between a polymorphism in the cannabinoid receptor 1 (CNR1) gene and IBS symptoms, colonic transit in IBS-D, and intestinal gas.[40] However, pain was not associated with this polymorphism. Furthermore, researchers found that the CNR1 mutations correlated with the emergence of IBS symptoms, as observed in two studies of a Korean and Chinese population with IBS.[41,37]

Human research using a CBD supplement further corroborates the potential benefits of modulating the endocannabinoid system in IBD/IBS. In a 10-week study of patients with ulcerative colitis given a CBD-rich botanical extract, the primary endpoint of percentage of patients in remission after treatment was similar between the placebo and CBD group.[42] However, subjective physician's global assessment of illness severity, subject global impression of change, and patient-reported quality-of-life outcomes were improved in the CBD group. Additionally, the placebo group experienced more gastrointestinal-associated adverse effects. Furthermore, in human colonic cultures derived from ulcerative colitis patients, CBD suppressed enteric reactive gliosis and reduced inflammation, thus inhibiting intestinal damage.[25] The researchers concluded, "Our results therefore indicate that CBD indeed unravels a new therapeutic strategy to treat inflammatory bowel diseases." Clearly, as another group of researchers stated, the endocannabinoid system "in the gut is a potential therapeutic target for IBS and other functional bowel disorders."

PSYCHOLOGICAL STRESS AND THE ENDOCANNABINOID SYSTEM

The endocannabinoid system regulates abdominal pain (visceral hyperalgesia) caused by chronic stress and may explain, at least in part, the relationship between chronic stress and IBD/IBS.[27,43] Rodent models indicate that early-life stress alters the endocannabinoid system, which increases the susceptibility to IBS.[44] The endocannabinoid system is a key player in the regulation of visceral pain and the means by which psychological stress impairs GI function may involve this system.[44] Chronic stress reduces levels of the endocannabinoid anandamide while elevating 2-AG in the brain and downregulating CB_1 receptors in sensory ganglia, which regulate visceral pain.[45] During chronic psychological stress, CB_1 receptor activity is altered through epigenetic pathways, which may explain the association between stress and abdominal pain.[46] Epigenetics refers to the alteration of gene expression through pathways other than the genetic code. It refers to the changes that occur in our genes due to lifestyle or environmental factors. Through these epigenetic actions, chronic stress affects the CB_1 gene promoter, leading to lower levels of CB_1 in sensory neurons that innervate the colon and other pelvic organs.[47]

THE MICROBIOTA AND THE ENDOCANNABINOID SYSTEM

Perhaps one of the most interesting aspects of the endocannabinoid system's role in gut health is its interaction with the gut microbiota. The gut microbiota can modulate intestinal endocannabinoid tone.[48] A microbiota profile associated with obesity also correlates with an increased intestinal concentration of anandamide, which leads to increased gut permeability (leaky gut).[48] In fact, the link between the gut microbiota and obesity may be mediated by the endocannabinoid system.[48] The results of a study where the bacterium, *Akkermansia muciniphila*, was administered to obese and type 2 diabetic mice daily support this concept.[49] In that study, the bacterium reversed diet-caused obesity. It accomplished this by increasing intestinal levels of endocannabinoids that control inflammation, the gut barrier, and gut peptide secretion.

On the other end of the spectrum, endocannabinoids from adipose tissue can also modulate the composition of the gut microbiota.[35] This indicates there is bidirectional communication between the microbiota and the endocannabinoid system.[35] Evidence of this cross-talk between the endocannabinoid system and the microbiota is reinforced by studies showing that the beneficial effects of probiotic supplementation on gut health may in part involve this system. The probiotic *Lactobacillus* given orally to rodents reduced visceral pain while simultaneously upregulating CB_2 receptors in the intestinal epithelium.[50] Inhibiting CB_2 eliminated the beneficial effects of the probiotic. In a model of chronic colonic hypersensitivity, *Lactobacillus acidophilus* NCFM resulted in analgesia.[50] This study also indicated that CB_2 receptors may be involved in the association between gut microbiota and visceral hypersensitivity. Furthermore, dysbiosis of the gut microbiota caused by antibiotics correlates with a general inflammatory state and alteration of certain endocannabinoids in the gut of mice as well as accompanying depression.[51] However, in a human study of individuals consuming *Lactobacillus acidophilus* NCFM over a period of 21 days, CB_2 receptors were not upregulated in colonic mucosal biopsies.[52]

CONCLUSION

An abundance of evidence is pointing to the conclusion that the endocannabinoid system is involved in gut health and that it may even be an important mediator of the actions of the gut-brain axis. The damaging effects of chronic psychological stress on the intestinal tract may also be driven by the endocannabinoid system. Targeting this system by the use of CBD oil or other phytocannabinoids may be one way to reduce colonic inflammation and reduce the effects of stress on the gut.

REFERENCES

1. DiPatrizio NV. Endocannabinoids in the Gut. *Cannabis Cannabinoid Res.* 2016 Feb;1(1):67–77.
2. Sharkey KA, Wiley JW. The role of the endocannabinoid system in the brain-gut axis. *Gastroenterology.* 2016 Aug;151(2):252–66.
3. Hasenoehrl C, Taschler U, Storr M, et al. The gastrointestinal tract - a central organ of cannabinoid signaling in health and disease. *Neurogastroenterol Motil.* 2016 Dec;28(12):1765–80.
4. Hornby PJ, Prouty SM. Involvement of cannabinoid receptors in gut motility and visceral perception. *Br J Pharmacol.* 2004 Apr;141(8):1335–45.
5. Furness JB, Kunze WAA, Clerc N. Nutrient tasting and signaling mechanisms in the gut II. The intestine as a sensory organ: neural, endocrine, and immune responses. *Am J Physiol Gastrointest Liver Physiol.* 1999 Nov;277(5 Pt 1):G922–8.
6. Trautmann SM, Sharkey KA. The endocannabinoid system and its role in regulating the intrinsic neural circuitry of the gastrointestinal tract. *Int Rev Neurobiol.* 2015;125:85–126.
7. Wright K, Rooney N, Feeney M, et al. Differential expression of cannabinoid receptors in the human colon: cannabinoids promote epithelial wound healing. *Gastroenterology.* 2005 Aug;129(2):437–53.
8. Aviello G, Romano B, Borrelli F, et al. Chemopreventive effect of the non-psychotropic phytocannabinoid cannabidiol on experimental colon cancer. *J Mol Med (Berl).* 2012 Aug;90(8):925–34.
9. Romano B, Borrelli F, Pagano E, et al. Inhibition of colon carcinogenesis by a standardized Cannabis sativa extract with high content of cannabidiol. *Phytomedicine.* 2014 Apr 15;21(5):631–9.
10. Izzo AA, Piscitelli F, Capasso R, et al. Peripheral endocannabinoid dysregulation in obesity: relation to intestinal motility and energy processing induced by food deprivation and re-feeding. *Br J Pharmacol.* 2009 Sep;158(2):451–61.
11. Márquez L, Abanades S, Andreu M. [Endocannabinoid system and bowel inflammation]. [Article in Spanish]. *Med Clin (Barc).* 2008 Oct 18;131(13):513–7.
12. Krowicki ZK, Moerschbaecher JM, Winsauer PJ, et al. Delta9-tetrahydrocannabinol inhibits gastric motility in the rat through cannabinoid CB1 receptors. *Eur J Pharmacol.* 1999 Apr 29;371(2–3):187–96.
13. de Filippis D, Iuvone T, d'amico A, et al. Effect of cannabidiol on sepsis-induced motility disturbances in mice: involvement of CB receptors and fatty acid amide hydrolase. *Neurogastroenterol Motil.* 2008 Aug;20(8):919–27.
14. Bashashati M, Nasser Y, Keenan CM, et al. Inhibiting endocannabinoid biosynthesis: a novel approach to the treatment of constipation. *Br J Pharmacol.* 2015 Jun;172(12):3099–111.
15. Cluny NL, Reimer RA, Sharkey KA. Cannabinoid signalling regulates inflammation and energy balance: the importance of the brain-gut axis. *Brain Behav Immun.* 2012 Jul;26(5):691–8.
16. DiPatrizio NV, Piomelli D. The thrifty lipids: endocannabinoids and the neural control of energy conservation. *Trends Neurosci.* 2012 Jul;35(7):403–11.
17. Berthoud HR. The vagus nerve, food intake and obesity. *Regul Pept.* 2008 Aug 7;149(1–3):15–25.
18. DiPatrizio NV, Igarashi M, Narayanaswami V, et al. Fasting stimulates 2-AG biosynthesis in the small intestine: role of cholinergic pathways. *Am J Physiol Regul Integr Comp Physiol.* 2015 Oct 15;309(8):R805–13.

19. Monteleone P, Piscitelli F, Scognamiglio P, et al. Hedonic eating is associated with increased peripheral levels of ghrelin and the endocannabinoid 2-arachidonoyl-glycerol in healthy humans: a pilot study. *J Clin Endocrinol Metab.* 2012 Jun;97(6):E917–24.

20. Rigamonti AE, Piscitelli F, Aveta T, et al. Anticipatory and consummatory effects of (hedonic) chocolate intake are associated with increased circulating levels of the orexigenic peptide ghrelin and endocannabinoids in obese adults. *Food Nutr Res.* 2015 Nov 4;59:29678.

21. Mennella I, Ferracane R, Zucco F, et al. Food liking enhances the plasma response of 2-arachidonoylglycerol and of pancreatic polypeptide upon modified sham feeding in humans. *J Nutr.* 2015 Sep;145(9):2169–75.

22. Alhouayek M, Lambert DM, Delzenne NM, et al. Increasing endogenous 2-arachidonoylglycerol levels counteracts colitis and related systemic inflammation. *FASEB J.* 2011 Aug;25(8):2711–21.

23. Schicho R, Bashashati M, Bawa M, et al. The atypical cannabinoid O-1602 protects against experimental colitis and inhibits neutrophil recruitment. *Inflamm Bowel Dis.* 2011 Aug;17(8):1651–64.

24. Borrelli F, Aviello G, Romano B, et al. Cannabidiol, a safe and non-psychotropic ingredient of the marijuana plant Cannabis sativa, is protective in a murine model of colitis. *J Mol Med (Berl).* 2009 Nov;87(11):1111–21.

25. De Filippis D, Esposito G, Cirillo C, et al. Cannabidiol reduces intestinal inflammation through the control of neuroimmune axis. *PLoS One.* 2011;6(12):e28159.

26. Wright K, Rooney N, Feeney M, et al. Differential expression of cannabinoid receptors in the human colon: cannabinoids promote epithelial wound healing. *Gastroenterology.* 2005 Aug;129(2):437–53.

27. Izzo AA, Sharkey KA. Cannabinoids and the gut: new developments and emerging concepts. *Pharmacol Ther.* 2010 Apr;126(1):21–38.

28. Massa F, Marsicano G, Hermann H, et al. The endogenous cannabinoid system protects against colonic inflammation. *J Clin Invest.* 2004 Apr;113(8):1202–9.

29. Storr MA, Keenan CM, Emmerdinger D, et al. Targeting endocannabinoid degradation protects against experimental colitis in mice: involvement of CB1 and CB2 receptors. *J Mol Med (Berl).* 2008 Aug;86(8):925–36.

30. Sasso O, Migliore M, Habrant D, et al. Multitarget fatty acid amide hydrolase/cyclo-oxygenase blockade suppresses intestinal inflammation and protects against nonsteroidal anti-inflammatory drug-dependent gastrointestinal damage. *FASEB J.* 2015 Jun;29(6):2616–27.

31. Darmani NA, Izzo AA, Degenhardt B, et al. Involvement of the cannabimimetic compound, N-palmitoyl-ethanolamine, in inflammatory and neuropathic conditions: review of the available pre-clinical data, and first human studies. *Neuropharmacology.* 2005 Jun;48(8):1154–63.

32. Borrelli F, Romano B, Petrosino S, et al. Palmitoylethanolamide, a naturally occurring lipid, is an orally effective intestinal anti-inflammatory agent. *Br J Pharmacol.* 2015 Jan;172(1):142–58.

33. Jamontt JM, Molleman A, Pertwee RG, et al. The effects of delta-tetrahydrocannabinol and cannabidiol alone and in combination on damage, inflammation and in vitro motility disturbances in rat colitis. *Br J Pharmacol.* 2010 Jun;160(3):712–23.

34. Borrelli F, Fasolino I, Romano B, et al. Beneficial effect of the non-psychotropic plant cannabinoid cannabigerol on experimental inflammatory bowel disease. *Biochem Pharmacol.* 2013 May 1;85(9):1306–16.

35. Sharkey KA, Wiley JW. The role of the endocannabinoid system in the brain-gut axis. *Gastroenterology.* 2016 Aug;151(2):252–66.

36. Camilleri M, Kolar GJ, Vazquez-Roque MI, et al. Cannabinoid receptor 1 gene and irritable bowel syndrome: phenotype and quantitative traits. *Am J Physiol Gastrointest Liver Physiol.* 2013 Mar 1;304(5):G553–60.
37. Park JM, Choi MG, Cho YK, et al. Cannabinoid receptor 1 gene polymorphism and irritable bowel syndrome in the Korean population: a hypothesis-generating study. *J Clin Gastroenterol.* 2011 Jan;45(1):45–9.
38. Fichna J, Wood JT, Papanastasiou M, et al. Endocannabinoid and cannabinoid-like fatty acid amide levels correlate with pain-related symptoms in patients with IBS-D and IBS-C: a pilot study. *PLoS One.* 2013 Dec 27;8(12):e85073.
39. Camilleri M, Carlson P, McKinzie S, et al. Genetic variation in endocannabinoid metabolism, gastrointestinal motility, and sensation. *Am J Physiol Gastrointest Liver Physiol.* 2008 Jan;294(1):G13–9.
40. Camilleri M, Kolar GJ, Vazquez-Roque MI, et al. Cannabinoid receptor 1 gene and irritable bowel syndrome: phenotype and quantitative traits. *Am J Physiol Gastrointest Liver Physiol.* 2013 Mar 1;304(5):G553–60.
41. Jiang Y, Nie Y, Li Y, et al. Association of cannabinoid type 1 receptor and fatty acid amide hydrolase genetic polymorphisms in Chinese patients with irritable bowel syndrome. *J Gastroenterol Hepatol.* 2014 Jun;29(6):1186–91.
42. Irving PM, Iqbal T, Nwokolo C, et al. A randomized, double-blind, placebo-controlled, parallel-group, pilot study of cannabidiol-rich botanical extract in the symptomatic treatment of ulcerative colitis. *Inflamm Bowel Dis.* 2018 Mar 10. [Epub ahead of print.]
43. Storr MA, Sharkey KA. The endocannabinoid system and gut-brain signalling. *Curr Opin Pharmacol.* 2007 Dec;7(6):575–82.
44. Marco EM, Echeverry-Alzate V, López-Moreno JA, et al. Consequences of early life stress on the expression of endocannabinoid-related genes in the rat brain. *Behav Pharmacol.* 2014 Sep;25(5–6):547–56.
45. Morena M, Patel S, Bains JS, et al. Neurobiological interactions between stress and the endocannabinoid system. *Neuropsychopharmacology.* 2016 Jan;41(1):80–102.
46. Hong S, Zheng G, Wiley JW. Epigenetic regulation of genes that modulate chronic stress-induced visceral pain in the peripheral nervous system. *Gastroenterology.* 2015 Jan;148(1):148–57.
47. Muccioli GG, Naslain D, Bäckhed F, et al. The endocannabinoid system links gut microbiota to adipogenesis. *Mol Syst Biol.* 2010 Jul;6:392.
48. Everard A, Belzer C, Geurts L, et al. Cross-talk between Akkermansia muciniphila and intestinal epithelium controls diet-induced obesity. *Proc Natl Acad Sci U S A.* 2013 May 28;110(22):9066–71.
49. Rastelli M, Knauf C, Cani PD. Gut microbes and health: a focus on the mechanisms linking microbes, obesity, and related disorders. *Obesity* (Silver Spring). 2018 May;26(5):792–800.
50. Rousseaux C, Thuru X, Gelot A, et al. Lactobacillus acidophilus modulates intestinal pain and induces opioid and cannabinoid receptors. *Nat Med.* 2007 Jan;13(1):35–7.
51. Guida F, Turco F, Iannotta M, et al. Antibiotic-induced microbiota perturbation causes gut endocannabinoidome changes, hippocampal neuroglial reorganization and depression in mice. *Brain Behav Immun.* 2017 Sep 7. Epub ahead of print.
52. Ringel-Kulka T, Goldsmith JR, Carroll IM, et al. Lactobacillus acidophilus NCFM affects colonic mucosal opioid receptor expression in patients with functional abdominal pain - a randomised clinical study. *Aliment Pharmacol Ther.* 2014 Jul;40(2):200–7.

10 Cannabidiol in Mental Health Disorders

Alline C. de Campos, Felipe V. Gomes, Samia R. Joca, and Francisco S. Guimarães
University of Sao Paulo

CONTENTS

BRIEF HISTORY OF CANNABIDIOL

Cannabidiol (CBD) was initially isolated from the cannabis sativa plant in the 1940s by Adams and Todd (for a detailed revision, see Adams, 1941; Todd, 1946). Later, Raphael Mechoulam's laboratory characterized its chemical structure (Mechoulam and Shvo, 1963). In the following year, his group identified delta-9-tetrahydrocannabinol (THC) as the primary psychoactive compound present in the plant, starting a new era of cannabinoid research (Gaoni and Mechoulam 1964). Because CBD did not mimic most of the THC effects, it was initially thought to be an inactive cannabinoid. However, pioneer studies by Elisardo Carlini's group in Brazil and others described that CBD could modify THC effects by pharmacokinetic and pharmacodynamic interactions (for review, see Zuardi, 2008, Figure 10.1). Regarding the latter, CBD decreased some, but not all, THC effects, indicating that it was not an antagonist of (at that time) a putative THC receptor (Zuardi, 2008). As will be discussed below, the antagonism of the anxiogenic and psychotomimetic effects of high doses of THC gave the first clue that CBD could be useful for the treatment of mental health disorders (Zuardi, 2008). Since then, the interest in the possible

1940	Adams, Tood. CBD isolated from Cannabis preparations
1963	Mechoulan and Shvo, CBD structure identified
1974	Karniol et al., CBD interfered with THC effects in humans
1975	Hine et al., CBD (together with THC) decreased morphine withdrawal symptoms in rats with
1982	Zuardi et al., CBD decreased the anxiogenic and psychotomimetic effects of THC in humans
1990	Guimaraes al., CBD produced anxiolytic-like effects in rats tested in the elevated-plus maze rats
1991	Zuardi et al., CBD produced antipsychotic-like effects similar to clozapine in rats
1993	Zuardi et al., CBD decreased anxiety in volunteers in a simulated public speaking test
1995	Zuardi et al., CBD decreased psychotic symptoms in a schizophrenia patient
2004	Crippa et al., CBD reduced anxiety affected cerebral blood flow in healthy volunteers
2010	Zanelati et al., CBD produced antidepressant-like effects in mice
2011	Bergamaschi et al. CBD reduced anxiety induced by simulated public speaking in social phobia patients
2012	Leweke et al. CBD reduced symptoms in schizophrenia in a double-blind trial

FIGURE 10.1 Cannabidiol in mental disorders: key discoveries.

therapeutic properties of CBD in these disorders has been growing exponentially. Figure 10.2 shows the number of studies in the literature (PUBMED) regarding the psychotherapeutic effects of CBD.

MULTIPLE MECHANISMS INVOLVED WITH CBD EFFECTS: POSSIBLE TARGETS DESCRIBED BY *IN VITRO* STUDIES

CBD has evolved from an inactive cannabinoid to a promising multi-spectrum medicine for several pathological conditions such as cancer, neuropsychiatric disorders, skin disorders, and periodontal disease (Crippa et al., 2018). The mechanisms of

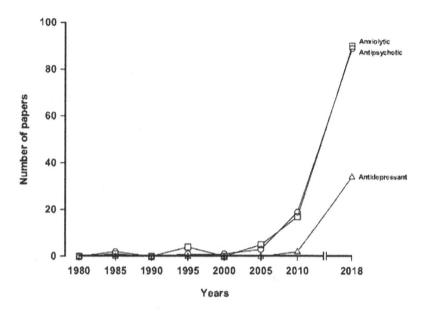

FIGURE 10.2 Papers on the potential therapeutic effects of CBD in mental disorders.

action responsible for CBD effects, however, remain poorly understood, challenging pharmacologists, biochemists, cell biologists, and other fields of biomedical research.

In the past 20 years, several results based on *in vitro* approaches have been trying to shade light into the possible targets of CBD (Campos et al., 2012; Ibeas Bih et al., 2015).

In the 1980s, a series of well-conducted studies by Dr. Howlett's group demonstrated that THC interacts with a specific G-coupled receptor in the brain, later cloned and named cannabinoid type 1 receptor, CB_1 (Howlett, 1985; Devane et al., 1988; Matsuda et al., 1990). Given that CBD could antagonize some of the THC effects *in vivo* (Zuardi et al., 1982; Crippa et al., 2018), it was reasonable to infer that CBD was an antagonist of CB_1 receptors. Initial observations of Dr. Pertwee's group indicated that CBD could indeed produce an opposite effect when compared with a synthetic agonist of CB_1 receptors in the mouse vas deferens (Pertwee et al., 2002). Moreover, in preparations of mouse brains and Chinese Hamster Ovarian cells (CHO) expressing human CB_1 and the cannabinoid type 2 receptor (CB_2), CBD acted as a potent antagonist of CB_1 receptor and an inverse agonist of CB_2 receptors (Thomas et al., 2007).

However, the picture proved to be more complicated. In 1996, Watanabe and colleagues suggested that CBD was more potent than THC to inhibit the enzyme responsible for anandamide hydrolysis (the fatty acid amide hydrolase—FAAH). Anandamide (AEA), described for the first time in 1992 (Devane et al., 1992), and 2-arachidonoylglycerol (2AG) are the most important lipid-derived endocannabinoid present in mammals. In 2001, another talented group in the field of cannabinoid research added an essential piece in the multiple and puzzled mechanism of action of CBD. Bisogno and colleagues demonstrated that in human embryonic kidney 293 cells (HEK293) overexpressing the transient vanilloid receptor type 1 ($TRPV_1$) and in rat basophilic leukemia (RBL—2H3) cells, CBD acted as a $TRPV_1$ antagonist and increased levels of endogenous anandamide (AEA) (Bisogno et al., 2001). CBD effects on increasing AEA levels were attributed to its actions as a FAAH inhibitor (Bisogno et al., 2001). Additionally, CBD-induced neural stem cells (NSC) proliferation *in vitro* seems also to involve its inhibitory action on the FAAH enzyme. Using embryonic neural stem cells derived from the mouse hippocampus, Campos and colleagues (2013b) demonstrated that, at the concentration of 100nM, CBD increases NSC proliferation. The effects of CBD on cell proliferation were blocked entirely in NSC overexpressing FAAH, suggesting that its effects depended on increased AEA levels (Campos et al., 2013b). Lately, Elmes and colleagues (2015) showed that CBD inhibits the Fatty acid-binding protein (FABP) molecule, a carrier that mediates the transport of AEA to the FAAH enzyme in the cytoplasm of *HeLa (Henrietta Lacks)* cells overexpressing the transporter FABP5.

Recently, new evidence indicated that the actions of CBD at cannabinoid receptors could be even more complex (Laprairie et al., 2015; Navarro et al., 2018). In HEK293 cells overexpressing human CB_1 receptors, CBD can act as a non-competitive negative allosteric modulator, which could explain its positive effects on CB_1 receptors without causing psychotomimetic effects (Laprairie et al., 2015). On the other hand, Navarro and colleagues (2018), using similar *in vitro* approach, suggested that CBD behaves as an allosteric modulator, modifying the efficacy and facilitating biased agonism of different cannabinoid receptor agonists. In this work, it was demonstrated that AEA appears to be more biased to β-arrestin than the full CB_1 and CB_2 receptors agonist ACEA. In the presence of CBD, AEA and ACEA increase their bias agonism toward signaling at cannabinoid receptors (Navarro et al., 2018).

Besides its effects on the endocannabinoid system, CBD also influences the actions of other neurotransmitters. Using CHO cultured cells overexpressing serotonin-1A ($5-HT_{1A}$) receptors, Russo and colleagues (2005) observed that CBD, at μM range, displaces OH-DPAT, a selective $5-HT_{1A}$-receptor agonist (Russo et al., 2005). In the brain, $5-HT_{1A}$-receptors are present in presynaptic membranes, as autosomic receptors in the raphe nuclei, and also expressed postsynaptically in other brain regions (Piñeyro and Blier, 1999; Kia et al., 1996). It was also demonstrated in rat brain membrane preparations that CBD enhances the ability of 8-OH-DPAT to stimulate the second messenger cascade induced by the activation of $5-HT_{1A}$-receptors at relatively low concentrations (100nM) (Rock et al., 2012). In a co-culture of human brain microvascular endothelial cell (HBMEC) and human astrocyte, used as an *in vitro* model of blood-brain barrier permeability induced by oxygen–glucose deprivation (OGD), CBD prevented OGD-induced permeability partially due its activation of $5-HT_{1A}$-receptors (Hind et al., 2016). Interestingly, the neuroprotective effects of CBD in this *in vitro* model were entirely blocked by an antagonist of another receptor, the peroxisome proliferator-activated receptors gamma (PPAR-γ) (Hind et al., 2016). PPAR-γ is a nuclear receptor that, once activated, controls the expression of several genes in the target cell, being essential for processes such as cell growth and proliferation (Michalik et al., 2016). More recently, Sonego et al. (2018) showed that in cultured microglia activated by LPS, CBD attenuated the pro-inflammatory profile of these cells by activating PPAR-γ. CBD also seems to mitigate *in vitro* microglial phagocytosis via TRPV1 receptors (Hassan et al., 2014). On the other hand, in rat primary culture of glial cells and microglial cell lines activated by ATP/Ca^{2+}, CBD reduced microglia activation via CB_1 and adenosine A2A receptors (Martín-Moreno et al., 2011). In addition, Carrier and colleagues (2006) showed that, in cultured murine microglia and macrophages, CBD decreases the uptake of [3H] adenosine, unveiling the capacity of this phytocannabinoid to inhibit adenosine transporter.

Antioxidant properties could also be involved in the neuroprotective effects of CBD. For example, it protected oligodendrocytes progenitors from oxidative and pro-inflammatory insults by blocking endoplasmic reticulum and oxidative stress (Mecha et al., 2012). In brain slices containing the hippocampus, CBD positively modulates intracellular Ca^{2+} stores and L-type mediated Ca^{2+} entry into the neurons (Drysdale et al., 2006). The same group demonstrated that in the SH-SY5Y neuroblastoma human cells, CBD prevented toxin-induced mitochondrial damage by restoring the intracellular Ca^{2+} homeostasis (Ryan et al., 2009). These effects are part of the well-described antioxidant properties of CBD. They seem to involve its chemical structure rather than a receptor-mediated action (Campos et al., 2017).

Several other putative molecular targets for CBD (such as antagonism of G protein-coupled receptor 55 or interaction with ion channels such as voltage-dependent anion channel 1, CaV3.x, etc.) have been described, and their number (already more than 60, Ibeas Bih et al., 2015) does not seem to stop growing. The extent of their association with the *in vivo* effects of CBD, however, remains poorly known. The next sessions will present studies that tried to investigate this problem, using animal models employed for the study of neuropsychiatric disorders.

CBD AS AN ANXIOLYTIC AND ANTI-STRESS DRUG

The initial clinical observation that CBD, in healthy volunteers, prevented the anxiogenic effects of high doses of THC (Zuardi et al., 1982), prompted Brazilian researchers to investigate if it could induce anxiolytic effects by itself in rodents. The initial results, however, were contradictory (see Table 10.1). While Silveira Filho and Tufik (1981) failed to show any behavioral effects of CBD (at the dose of 100mg/kg) in the Geller-Seifter model, Zuardi and Karniol (1983) demonstrated that a lower dose of CBD (10 mg/kg) attenuated conditioned emotional responses in rats. Later, using the elevated plus maze (EPM), Guimarães and colleagues (Guimarães et al., 1991) showed that acutely administered CBD did produce anti-anxiety effects, but with an inverted U-shaped dose-response curve. In rats, only low doses of CBD caused anxiolytic effects. These results were later extended to mice and other animal models of general anxiety (Onaivi et al., 1990; Moreira et al., 2006; Resstel et al., 2006; Campos et al., 2012) (Table 10.1). Recently, Zuardi's group showed that the acute anxiolytic effects of CBD were also associated with an inverted U-shaped dose-response curve in humans (Linares et al., 2018; Zuardi et al., 2017, Table 10.2).

In addition to acute effects in these models, CBD was similarly effective in rodents tested in animal models associated with specific anxiety and stressful disorders (Bitencourt et al., 2008; Campos et al., 2013a; Hsiao et al., 2012; Stern et al., 2012). CBD prevented acute restraint-induced autonomic changes and the delayed increase in anxiety observed one week after stress in the EPM (Resstel et al., 2009; Vila-Verde et al., 2016).

TABLE 10.1

Pre-clinical Studies Investigating the Anxiolytic Properties of Cannabidiol

Study	Species	Tested Doses	Model	Effects	Proposed Mechanisms
Silveira Filho and Tufik (1981)	Male Wistar rats	100 mg/kg, i.p.	Geller-Seifter conflict test	None	n.i.
Zuardi and Karniol (1983)	Male Wistar rats	10 mg/kg, i.p.	Conditioned emotional response	Anxiolytic	n.i.
Guimaraes et al. (1990)	Male Wistar rats	2.5, 5.0, 10.0, and 20.0 mg/kg, i.p.	EPM	Anxiolytic	n.i.
Onaivi et al. (1990)	Male ITC mice	0.01, 0.1, 0.5, 1.0, 2.5, 5.0, 10.0, 50.0, and 100.0 mg/kg, i.p.	EPM	Anxiolytic	n.i.
Moreira and Guimarães (2006)	Male Wistar rats	2.5, 5.0, and 10.0 mg/kg, i.p.	Vogel's conflict test	Anxiolytic	n.i.
Resstel et al. (2006)	Male Wistar rats	10 mg/kg, i.p.	Contextual fear conditioning	Anxiolytic	n.i.
Campos and Guimarães (2008)	Male Wistar rats	15–60 nmol, intra-dPAG	EPM and Vogel's conflict test	Anxiolytic	Activation of 5-HT_{1A}-receptors
Bitencourt et al. (2008)	Male Wistar rats	20 µg, i.c.v.	Contextual fear conditioning	Enhanced fear extinction	Activation of CB_1 receptors
Campos and Guimarães (2009)	Male Wistar rats	30–60 nmol, intra-dPAG	EPM	Anxiolytic	Lack of the higher dose effect depended on TRPV1 activation
Long et al. (2010)	Male C57BL/6JArc mice	1–50 mg/kg acute or repeated daily for 8 weeks, i.p.	OFT, LDT, EPM	No acute and anxiolytic after chronic treatment	effect n.i.
Resstel et al. (2009)	Male Wistar rats	1, 10, and 20 mg/kg, i.p.	Contextual fear conditioning	Anxiolytic	Activation of 5-HT_{1A}-receptors
Soares et al. (2010)	Male Wistar rats	15–60 nmol, intra-dPAG	Elevated T maze and aversive brain stimulation	Anxiolytic and panicolytic	Activation of 5-HT_{1A}-receptors

(Continued)

TABLE 10.1 (*Continued*)
Pre-clinical Studies Investigating the Anxiolytic Properties of Cannabidiol

Study	Species	Tested Doses	Model	Effects	Proposed Mechanisms
Lemos et al. (2010)	Male Wistar rats	10 mg/kg (i.p.) and 15–60 nmol intra-PL and IL	Contextual fear conditioning	Anxiolytic	n.i.
Casarotto et al. (2010)	Male C57BL/6J mice	15, 30, and 60 mg/kg, i.p.	Marble-burying test	Anti-compulsive	Activation of CB_1 receptors
Gomes et al. (2011)	Male Wistar rats	15, 30, and 60 nmol intra-BNST	EPM/Vogel's conflict test	Anxiolytic	Activation of $5\text{-}HT_{1A}$-receptors
Gomes et al. (2012)	Male Wistar rats	15, 30, and 60 nmol intra-BNST	Contextual fear conditioning	Anxiolytic	Activation of $5\text{-}HT_{1A}$-receptors
Deiana et al. (2012)	Male Swiss mice	120 mg/kg, i.p. and P.O.	Marble-burying test	Anti-compulsive	n.i.
Uribe-Mariño et al. (2012)	Male Wistar rats	0.3, 3.0, and 30 mg/kg, i.p.	Prey-predator paradigm	Anxiolytic	n.i.
Hsiao et al. (2012)	Male Wistar rats	0.5–1 µg, intra-central amygdala	OFT, EPM	Anxiolytic	n.i.
Stern et al. (2012)	Male Wistar rats	3–30 mg/kg	Contextual fear conditioning	Impaired fear reconsolidation	Activation of CB_1 receptors
Campos et al. (2012)	Male Wistar rats	5 mg/kg/ daily, for 7 days, i.p.	Prey-predator paradigm	Anxiolytic	Activation of $5\text{-}HT_{1A}$-receptors
ElBatsh et al. (2012)	Male Lister-hooded rats	10 mg/kg/ daily for 14 days, i.p.	Contextual fear conditioning	Anxiogenic	n.i.
Do Monte et al. (2013)	Male Long–Evans hooded rats	0.1–0.4 µg, intra-PL	Contextual fear conditioning	Enhanced fear extinction	Activation of CB_1 receptors
Campos et al. (2013a)	Male Wistar rats	5–20 mg/kg, acute or repeated, 5 mg/kg/daily for 14 days, i.p.	Elevated T maze	Panicolytic after repeated treatment	Activation of $5\text{-}HT_{1A}$-receptors
Almeida et al. (2013)	Male SHR and Wistar rats	1–60 mg/kg, i.p.	Social interaction	Low (1 mg/kg) dose was anxiolytic in SHR	n.i.
Campos et al. (2013b)	Male C57BL/6J and GFAP-TK transgenic mice	30 mg/kg/ daily for 14 days, i.p.	CUS/NSF/EPM	Anxiolytic	Activation of CB_1 receptors

(*Continued*)

TABLE 10.1 (*Continued*)

Pre-clinical Studies Investigating the Anxiolytic Properties of Cannabidiol

Study	Species	Tested Doses	Model	Effects	Proposed Mechanisms
Twardowschy et al. (2013)	Male Swiss mice	3 mg/kg i.p.	Prey-predator paradigm	Anxiolytic	Activation of $5\text{-}HT_{1A}$-receptors
Nardo et al. (2014)	Male Swiss mice	15 mg/kg, i.p.	Marble-burying test	Anti-compulsive	n.i.
Fogaça et al. (2014)	Male Wistar rats	Intra-PL	EPM/contextual fear conditioning/ restraint stress + EPM	Anxiolytic in previously stressed animals	Activation of $5\text{-}HT_{1A}$-receptors
Marinho et al. (2015)	Male Wistar rats	15–60 nmol intra-PL and IL	EPM/contextual fear conditioning/ restraint stress + EPM	Anxiolytic or anxiogenic depending on the region and previous stress exposure	Activation of $5\text{-}HT_{1A}$-receptors
Song et al. (2016)	Male Lister-hooded rats	10 mg/kg, i.p.	Contextual fear conditioning	Anxiolytic under strong fear conditioning and anxiogenic under low fear conditioning	n.i.
Rock et al. (2017)	Male Sprague-Dawley rats	5 mg/kg, i.p.	LDT 24 hours after foot shock stress	Anxiolytic	n.i.
Stern et al. (2017)	Male Wistar rats	3–30 mg/kg, i.p.	Contextual fear conditioning	Impaired fear reconsolidation	Activation of CB_1 and CB_2 receptors in the dorsal hippocampus
Fogaça et al. (2018)	Male C57/BL7 mice	30 mg/kg, i.p.	CUS/NSF/EPM	Anxiolytic	Activation of CB_1 and CB_2 receptors
De Gregorio et al. (2019)	Male Wistar rats	5 mg/kg/ daily for 7 days, s.c.	OFT, EPM, and NSF after nerve injury	Anxiolytic	Activation of $5\text{-}HT_{1A}$-receptors

Abbreviations: BNST: bed nucleus of the stria terminalis, CUS: chronic unpredictable stress, dPAG: dorsal periaqueductal gray, EPM: elevated plus-maze, LDT: IL: infralimbic cortex, i.c.v.: intracerebro-ventricular, i.p.: intraperitoneal, LDT: light-dark test, NSF: novelty suppressed feeding, OFT: open field test, n.i.: not investigated, PL: prelimbic cortex, s.c.: subcutaneous.

TABLE 10.2
Clinical Studies Investigating the Anxiolytic Properties of CBD

Study	Subjects	Tested Doses	Effects
Zuardi et al. (1982)	Healthy volunteers	1 mg/kg, P.O.	Decreased STAI scores elevation induced by THC
Zuardi et al. (1993)	Healthy volunteers	300 mg, P.O.	Decreased VAS factor anxiety scores after simulated public speaking
Crippa et al. (2004)	Healthy volunteers	400 mg, P.O.	Decreased VAS factor anxiety scores before SPECT procedure
Fusar-Poli et al. (2009)	Healthy volunteers	600 mg, P.O.	Decreased skin conductance fluctuation in task with fearful faces during an fMRI procedure
Crippa et al. (2011)	Social phobia patients	400 mg, P.O.	Decreased VAS factor anxiety scores before SPECT procedure
Bergamaschi et al. (2011)	Social phobia patients	600 mg, P.O.	Decreased VAS factor anxiety scores after simulated public speaking
Zuardi et al. (2017)	Healthy volunteers	150–600 mg P.O	Decreased VAS factor anxiety scores after real public speaking with a U-shaped dose-response curve (300 mg anxiolytic)
Elms et al. (2019)	Retrospective study with PTSD patients	Variable	10/11 (91%) patients showed a decrease in PTSD symptoms after 8 weeks
Hundal et al. (2018)	Healthy volunteers with high trait paranoia	600 mg, P.O.	No effect in anxiety induced by virtual-reality
Shannon et al. (2019)	Retrospective study in patients with primary concerns of anxiety or poor sleep	Variable	79.2% of patients improved in the first month
Linares et al. (2018)	Healthy volunteers	150–600 mg P.O.	Decreased VAS factor anxiety scores after simulated public speaking with a U-shaped dose-response curve (300 mg anxiolytic)

Abbreviations: fMRI: functional magnetic resonance imaging, SPCT: single-photon spectroscopy, STAI: state-train anxiety inventory, VAS: visual analogue scale.

Repeated CBD treatment (7 daily injections) also attenuated the long-lasting anxiogenic consequence of a single predator exposure in a posttraumatic stress disorder (PTSD) animal model (Campos et al., 2013a). Likewise, this drug impaired fear reconsolidation and accelerates extinction, two processes associated with PTSD symptoms in humans (Bitencourt et al., 2008; Stern et al., 2012; Hsiao et al., 2012).

Regarding panic disorder, acute and chronic CBD treatment attenuated defensive behaviors in two different models of this disorder, the elevated T-maze (ETM) and the electrical stimulation of the dorsal portions of the periaqueductal gray matter (Campos et al., 2013a, Soares et al., 2010). In these models, the effect was similar to the antidepressant fluoxetine (Campos et al., 2013a). Also, CBD reduced marble-burying behavior, suggesting that it could be effective against disorders associated with compulsive behaviors such as obsessive-compulsive disorder (OCD—Casarotto et al., 2010; Nardo et al., 2014).

The effects of repeated administration of CBD in chronic stress have also been investigated. CBD (30 mg/kg/daily for 14 days) prevented the anxiogenic effect of chronic unpredictable stress in mice tested in the EPM and novelty suppressed feeding tests (Campos et al., 2013b; Fogaça et al., 2018).

In a double-blind placebo-controlled clinical study performed in healthy volunteers submitted to a public speaking simulation test (SPS), CBD (300 mg, P.O.) prevented the test-induced anxiogenic effect. This effect was similar to that induced by the 5-HT_{1A} partial agonist ipsapirone (5 mg, P.O.) and diazepam (10 mg) (Zuardi et al., 1993). As pointed out above, this original result was recently replicated by two distinct clinical studies (Linares et al., 2018; Zuardi et al., 2017) that showed, in addition, that the drug dose-response curve is bell-shaped. Corroborating these data, CBD (400 mg, P.O.) attenuated the anxiety induced in healthy volunteers by a brain imaging procedure (insertion of the venous cannula, tracer injection, and scanning inside the machine) (Crippa et al., 2004). Acute anxiolytic effects of CBD have also been demonstrated in patients with social anxiety disorder (SAD). The drug (600 mg, P.O.) significantly reduced the anxiety induced by a simulated public speaking (Bergamaschi et al., 2011). Although data investigating the safety of long-term CBD administration in humans are still sparse (Crippa et al., 2018), in the studies reported above no significant side effect of CBD was found.

Possible Mechanisms of the Anxiolytic Effects of CBD

Similar to its other effects, CBD anxiolytic action seems to involve several targets depending on drug concentrations, species, and animal models being tested (Campos et al., 2013; Campos et al., 2016, 2017). The typical bell-shaped dose-response curves produced by this phytocannabinoid further complicated this issue (Campos et al., 2008; Guimaraes et al., 1990; Linares et al., 2018).

In 2008, we found that the anxiolytic effects of CBD observed after direct injection into the dorsal portions of the periaqueductal gray matter (dPAG) were not mediated by CB_1 receptors. Considering that CBD can inhibit the FAAH enzyme (Bisogno et al., 2001), this result came as a surprise for us. We had previously found that AEA, injected into the same site, caused a CB_1-mediated anxiolytic response (Moreira et al., 2007). We went on to test if, as had been suggested by Russo et al. (2005), CBD could be acting through 5-HT_{1A} receptors. We found that WAY100635, a 5-HT_{1A}-receptor antagonist, prevented the anxiolytic effects of CBD when injected into this region (Campos and Guimarães, 2008). This antagonist also abolished the panicolytic-like effects of intra-dPAG CBD injections (Soares et al., 2010; Campos et al., 2013a). Since then, 5-HT_{1A}-receptors have been found to mediate CBD acute anti-aversive effects in several other studies using systemic or intra-cerebral (into the prelimbic prefrontal cortex and bed nucleus of the stria terminalis) administration (Fogaça et al., 2014; Gomes et al., 2011, 2012; Zanelati et al., 2010).

The mechanisms of CBD interaction with 5-HT_{1A}-receptors remain obscure (for review, see Fogaça et al. 2016). We failed to find an increase in serotonin release in the dPAG in rats treated acutely or sub-chronically with CBD (Campos et al., 2013a).

More recently, however, Linge and colleagues (2015) did demonstrate that CBD increases serotonin release in the prefrontal cortex of bulbectomized rodents. On the other hand, as discussed above, Rock and colleagues showed in rat brain stem membranes that CBD potentiates the ability of a 5-HT$_{1A}$-agonist to stimulate [35S] GTPγS (Rock et al., 2012). In this study, however, CBD failed to displace the binding of this 5-HT$_{1A}$ agonist even at high concentrations. Although these results have not been fully explained, they suggest that CBD modulation of 5-HT$_{1A}$-receptors is complicated and could involve allosteric interactions.

Another important mechanism that might contribute to CBD anxiolytic effects involves a complex action of this cannabinoid on the endocannabinoid system. CB$_1$ receptors seem to mediate the positive effects of CBD on processes related to aversive memories, such as extinction and reconsolidation (Bitencourt et al., 2008; Do Monte et al., 2013; Stern et al., 2012). Also, the inverse agonist of CB$_1$ receptors, AM251, but not a 5-HT$_{1A}$ receptor antagonist, prevented CBD effects in the marble-burying model (Casarotto et al., 2010). CB$_1$-mediated effects of CBD seems to be indirect, involving FAAH inhibition. Chronic systemic treatment with CBD increased hippocampal levels of AEA, but 2-AG, in mice. This increase was associated with the pro-neurogenic and anti-stress-induced synaptic remodeling in this region (Campos et al., 2013b; Fogaça et al., 2018). These two processes have been associated with the pathogenesis of anxiety disorders and depression (Samuels and Hen, 2011), and at least some of the behavioral effects of antidepressant drugs depend on their facilitation (Santarelli et al., 2003). Accordingly, the anxiolytic effects of repeated CBD (30 mg/kg/daily for 14 days) in mice submitted to a chronic unpredictable stress model were abolished in mice lacking adult proliferation and differentiation of adult stem cells (Campos et al., 2013b) or treated concomitantly with CB$_1$ or CB$_2$ antagonists (Fogaça et al., 2018). Further implicating the endocannabinoid system in these effects, Wolf et al. (2010) showed that the pro-neurogenic effect of CBD was absent in CB$_1$-knockout mice. In addition to the endocannabinoids and cannabinoid receptors, the activation of peroxisome proliferator-activated receptors could also be of particular importance for the pro-neurogenic actions of CBD during neuroimmune modulation induced by neurodegenerative processes (Esposito et al., 2011).

CBD can also act as an agonist of transient receptor potential (TRP) channels. Activation of TRPV1 receptors in the central nervous system can increase glutamate release, which usually enhances anxiety in animal models (Guimarães et al., 1991). Campos and Guimarães (2009) suggested that TRPV1 activation could explain, at least partially, the inverted U-shaped dose-response observed after local CBD infusion into the dPAG. They demonstrated that intra-dPAG injections of an ineffective dose of the TRPV1 antagonist, capsazepine, turned a higher, ineffective dose (60 nmol) of CBD, into an anxiolytic one (Campos and Guimarães, 2009). TRPV1 blocked is also involved in the bell-shaped dose-response curves produced by other cannabinoids such as the AEA analog Win55, 212-2 (Rubino et al., 2008; Campos and Guimarães, 2009).

CBD AS AN ANTIDEPRESSANT

Antidepressant-like effects of drugs that facilitate 5-HT$_{1A}$-mediated neurotransmission have been described for quite a long time (Graeff et al., 1996; Blier and

El-Mansari, 2013; Delgado et al., 1990; Carr and Lucki, 2011). Based on the finding that CBD acts as a 5-HT$_{1A}$ agonist (Russo et al., 2005) and that the anxiolytic-like effect of CBD could be mediated by the activation of post-synaptic 5-HT$_{1A}$-receptors (Campos and Guimarães, 2008), Zanelati and colleagues (2010) tested CBD in mice submitted to the forced swimming test, an animal model predictive of antidepressant effects (Cryan et al., 2002; Nestler and Hyman, 2010). CBD (30 mg/kg) decreased immobility time in this model, an effect similar to the prototype antidepressant imipramine. Moreover, as previously described for the anxiolytic effects (see above), CBD produced a bell-shaped dose-response curve (Table 10.3), and its effect was blocked by a 5-HT$_{1A}$-antagonist. Since then, several studies have also described the antidepressant-like effects of CBD in different species and animal models, as described in Table 10.3. For instance, El-Alfy and colleagues (2010) showed that

TABLE 10.3
Pre-clinical Studies Investigating the Anxiolytic Properties of Cannabidiol

Study	Species	Tested Doses	Model	Effects	Proposed Mechanisms
Zanelati et al. (2010)	Male Swiss mice	3, 10, 30, and 100 mg/kg, i.p.	FST	Antidepressant effect at the dose of 30 mg/kg	Activation of 5-HT$_{1A}$ receptor
El-Alfy et al. (2010)	Male Swiss Webster mice	20, 100, and 200 mg/kg, i.p.	FST	Antidepressant effect at the dose of 200 mg/kg	n.i.
	Male DBA/2	20, 100, and 200 mg/kg i.p.	TST	No effect	n.i.
Réus et al. (2011)	Male Wistar rats	15, 30, and 60 mg/kg (Acute and 14d treatment), i.p.	FST	Antidepressant effect at the dose of 30 mg/kg	BDNF levels were unchanged in PFC, HPC, and amygdala
Campos et al. (2013)	Male C57BL/6J mice	30 mg/kg (14 days), i.p.	CUS + EPM and NSF	Anti-stress effect	Increased AEA levels and neurogenesis in the hippocampus Effects independent of 5-HT$_{1A}$ and dependent on CB$_1$ activation

(Continued)

TABLE 10.3 (*Continued*)

Pre-clinical Studies Investigating the Anxiolytic Properties of Cannabidiol

Study	Species	Tested Doses	Model	Effects	Proposed Mechanisms
Schiavon et al. (2016)	Male Swiss albino mice	3, 10, and 30 mg/kg (Acute), i.p.	TST	Antidepressant effect at the doses of 10 and 30 mg/kg	n.i.
		3 and 30 mg/kg (15 days), i.p.	TST	Antidepressant effect	Dual effects on neurogenesis (increase with 3 and decreased with 30 mg/kg)
Linge et al. (2016)	Male C57BL6 mice	50 mg/kg (Acute), i.p.	Olfactory bulbectomy + OFT	Antidepressant effect	Increase 5-HT and glutamate in vmPFC dependent of $5\text{-}HT_{1A}$ receptor activation Independent of CB_1 receptor antagonism (AM251)
		50 mg/kg (7 days), i.p.	Olfactory bulbectomy + OFT	Antidepressant effect	Increase 5-HT and glutamate in vmPFC
			Olfactory bulbectomy + SPT	Prohedonic effect	Restored functionality of $5\text{-}HT_{1A}$ receptor (CA_1 and CA_2 hippocampus, DRN, amygdala)
Shoval et al. (2016)	Wistar-Kyoto rats	15, 30, and 45 mg/kg, oral	SPT	Prohedonic effect at the dose of 30 mg/kg	n.i.
Sartim et al. (2016)	Male Wistar rats	10, 30, and 60 nmol/0.2 µl/ side of the vmPFC	FST	Antidepressant effect at 30 and 60 nmol/0.2 ul	Activation of $5\text{-}HT_{1A}$ and CB_1 receptors

(Continued)

TABLE 10.3 (*Continued*)

Pre-clinical Studies Investigating the Anxiolytic Properties of Cannabidiol

Study	Species	Tested Doses	Model	Effects	Proposed Mechanisms
Fogaça et al. (2018)	Male C57BL6 mice	30 mg/kg (14 days), i.p.	CUS + EPM and NSF	Anti-stress effect	Decrease FAAH expression and activation of CB_1 and CB_2 receptors Increase neurogenesis in SGZ of DG and increased synaptogenesis in the HPC
Sartim et al. (2018)	Male Swiss mice	10, 30, and 60 nmol/0.2 μl/ side of the dHPC	FST	Antidepressant effect	Dependent on TrkB and mTOR activation in the HPC
		10 mg/kg, i.p.	FST	Antidepressant effect	Increased BDNF levels in the HPC
Sales et al. (2018)	Male Swiss mice	7, 10, and 30 mg/kg, i.p.	FST	Acute and sustained antidepressant effect with 10 mg/kg	Rapid increase in BDNF-TrkB and mTOR signaling in PFC Increased PSD95 and synaptophysin in the PFC Increase number of dendritic spines in PL and IL mPFC
		50, 150, 300 nmol/μl/i.c.v.	FST	Antidepressant effect	n.i.
	Male Wistar rats	10, 30 mg/kg, i.p.	LH	Rapid antidepressant effect with 30 mg/kg	n.i.
	Male FSL and FRL rats	10 and 30 mg/ kg, i.p.	FST	Rapid antidepressant effect	n.i.

(*Continued*)

TABLE 10.3 (*Continued*)
Pre-clinical Studies Investigating the Anxiolytic Properties of Cannabidiol

Study	Species	Tested Doses	Model	Effects	Proposed Mechanisms
Sales et al. (2018)	Male Swiss mice	3, 7, and 10 mg/kg, i.p.	FST	Antidepressant effect with 10 mg/kg	Effect is dependent on brain serotonin levels
De Morais et al. (2018)	Male Wistar rats	0.3, 3, 10, 30, and 60 mg/kg (Acute), i.p.	FST	Antidepressant effect with 30 mg/kg	n.i.
		0.3, 3, 10, and 60 mg/kg (subchronic, 24, 5 and 1 hour before the test), i.p.	FST	Antidepressant effect with 30 mg/kg	n.i.
Shbiro et al. (2019)	Wistar-Kyoto and FSL rats (males and females)	30 mg/kg, oral	SPT	Prohedonic effect at the dose of 30 mg/kg in males (WKY and FSL) and females (WKY)	n.i.

Abbreviations: 2AG: arachidonoylglycerol, 5-HT: serotonin, 5-HT$_{1A}$: serotonin receptor type 1A, AEA: anandamide, BDNF: brain-derived neurotrophic factor, BrdU: 5-bromo-2'-deoxyuridine, CB$_1$: cannabinoid receptor type 1, CB$_2$: cannabinoid receptor type 2, CUS: chronic unpredictable stress, DCX: doublecortin, EPM: elevated plus maze, FAAH: fatty acid amide hydrolase, FRL rats: flinders resistant line, FSL rats: flinders sensitive line, FST: forced swimming test, GSK-3β: glycogen synthase kinase 3β, HPC: hippocampus, i.c.v.: intracerebroventrcular, i.p.: intraperitoneal, intra-dHPC: intra-dorsal hippocampus, intra-IL mPFC: intra-infralimbic medial prefrontal cortex, intra-PL mPFC: intra-prelimbic medial prefrontal cortex, LH: learned helplessness, MAGL: monoacylglycerol lipase, mTOR: mammalian target of rapamycin, n.i.: not investigated, NSF: novelty suppressed feeding, OFT: open field test, p-Akt: phospho protein kinase B, PEA: palmitoylethanolamide, PFC: prefrontal cortex, PSD-95: post-synaptic density 95, SPT: sucrose preference test, SGZ: subgranular zone, TST: tail suspension test, TrkB: tropomyosin receptor kinase B, WKY: Wistar-Kyoto rats.

a single systemic administration of CBD (200 mg/kg) induced antidepressant-like effect in Swiss mice submitted to the FST and the tail suspension test (TST). Repeated treatment with CBD (30 mg/kg/daily for 15 days) has also been effective in Swiss albino mice tested in the TST (Schiavon et al., 2016) and male Wistar rats tested in the FST (Réus et al., 2011).

More recently, studies have confirmed the antidepressant properties of CBD in other animal models, including the learned helplessness in rats (LH, Sales et al., 2019) and the olfactory bulbectomy in C57BL6J mice (OBM; 50 mg/kg, Linge et al., 2016).

Altogether, the above findings suggest that CBD has antidepressant properties in different rodent models, using distinct species and strains of mice and rats. Moreover, both acute and chronic treatments with CBD are effective. This evidence highlights the importance of further investigating CBD effects, both in animals and in humans, and study its mechanism of action as an attempt to pave the way for better and more effective antidepressant treatments.

Despite the antidepressant-like effects of CBD observed in pre-clinical works, few studies have investigated the effects of this drug in depressed patients, and no clinical trial in depression has been published so far. Sub-euphoric doses of THC have shown antidepressant effects in humans (Ashton et al., 2005) and in animal studies (El-Alfy et al., 2010; Häring et al., 2013). It has been argued, however, that some of the mood-improving effects attributed to the use of the cannabis plant are due to its CBD content (Ashton et al., 2005). More recently, Corroon and Phillips (2018) reported that approximately 30% of the individuals who have used CBD for treating other medical conditions declared mood-improving effects of the compound with 17% of the patients reporting that the drug worked "very well by itself." Since the study did not discriminate the different sources of CBD (natural vs. synthetic), it is possible that THC content on CBD formulations might have contributed to the observed effects. Therefore, controlled clinical trials assessing CBD effects in depressed patients are needed. Despite that, only two randomized placebo-controlled trials of adjunctive CBD in bipolar depression are currently being carried out (EUCTR 2015-000465-31-DE, 2018; NCT03310593, 2017). No trials on CBD effects in unipolar depression have been registered so far.

Possible Mechanisms of the Antidepressant Effects of CBD

The molecular and neurochemical mechanisms involved in CBD antidepressant effects are still poorly understood. The initial evidence showed that the antidepressant-like effect of CBD in the forced swimming could be blocked by pretreatment with a selective 5-HT_{1A}-antagonist, thus indicating that it was dependent on activation of these receptors (Zanelati et al., 2010). A subsequent study reported that direct administration of CBD into the ventromedial prefrontal cortex (vmPFC) induced antidepressant-like effect, which was also blocked by local administration of 5-HT_{1A}-antagonist (Sartim et al., 2016). This finding is consistent with previous studies showing that 5-HT_{1A}-activation in the PFC promotes stress-coping behavior and sustained antidepressant effects (Fukumoto et al., 2018). Activation of post-synaptic 5-HT_{1A}-receptors in limbic brain regions, including the PFC, has been widely accepted as an important mechanism involved in the behavioral effect of antidepressant drugs (for a complete review, see Blier and El-Mansari, 2013; Carr and Lucki, 2011). Moreover, impaired 5-HT_{1A}-signaling has been described in limbic brain regions of stressed animals and in depressed individuals, further corroborating 5-HT_{1A}-involvement in the neurobiology of depression and the therapeutic effects of antidepressant drugs (reviewed by Kaufman et al., 2016). Pretreatment with a CB_1 receptor antagonist in the vmPFC, however, also blocked local CBD effects in rats submitted to the FST (Sartim et al., 2016). Since, as discussed above, CBD has low affinity for CB_1 receptors but may increase AEA levels by inhibiting its reuptake (Bisogno et al., 2001), it was hypothesized that CBD effects would result from increased AEA signaling in the vmPFC. Corroborating this hypothesis, administration of AEA into the vmPFC induced antidepressant-like effect in the FST, which was blocked by local administration of the 5-HT_{1A}-antagonist WAY100635 (Sartim et al., 2016). This result suggests that CBD effect on 5-HT_{1A}-signaling in the vmPFC would be secondary to increased AEA signaling. This hypothesis is further supported by previous evidence that increasing AEA levels in the vmPFC by locally administering the FAAH inhibitor URB597 induced antidepressant-like effects in the FST, which was associated with the increased firing rate of serotonergic neurons within the DRN and subsequent increased serotonin levels in the vmPFC (McLaughlin et al., 2012). Since the effects above were blocked by both CB_1 antagonist administration and by serotonin depletion, the authors suggested that increased AEA signaling in the vmPFC would facilitate stress-coping behaviors through CB_1-mediated disinhibition of the DRN, with a subsequent increase in serotonin levels in limbic brain regions (McLaughlin et al., 2012). In line with this evidence, a recent study demonstrated that CBD effects in the FST are dependent on brain serotonin levels, since depletion of this neurotransmitter abolished the behavioral effects induced by CBD (Sales et al., 2018).

In another study, Linge and colleagues (2016) reported that the rapid behavioral effects of CBD in bulbectomized mice were associated with increased extracellular serotonin and glutamate levels in the vmPFC. Moreover, the impaired 5-HT_{1A} signaling observed in the DRN, hippocampus, amygdala, and vmPFC of bulbectomized mice was reversed by chronic CBD treatment (Linge et al., 2016). The neurochemical and the behavioral effects induced by CBD were counteracted by the co-administration of a 5-HT_{1A}, but not CB_1, receptor antagonist. Based on these data, the authors suggested that CBD activates 5-HT_{1A} on GABAergic interneurons, disinhibition local glutamate release, which in turn could result in stimulation of the DRN and increased serotonergic drive into the vmPFC (Linge et al., 2016).

More recently, evidence has indicated that neuroplastic mechanisms are involved in CBD-induced behavioral effects in animal models predictive of antidepressant effects. For instance, CBD administration rapidly increased brain-derived neurotrophic (BDNF) levels within mice PFC and hippocampus (Sales et al., 2019). BDNF is a neurotrophin fundamental for synaptogenesis, cell proliferation, and repair in developing and adult central nervous system (Castrén and Rantamäki, 2010a, b). The behavioral effects of CBD in the FST were blocked by intracerebroventricular administration of an antagonist of the TrkB receptor, BDNF main receptor in the adult brain (Sales et al., 2018). This result provided a causal link between increased BDNF signaling and the behavioral effects induced by CBD in the FST. In agreement with that, CBD increased the expression of synaptophysin and PSD95, as well as increased dendritic spine density in the mPFC of mice (Sales et al., 2018). These effects depended on BDNF signaling and are also observed in response to fast-acting antidepressant drugs (Gerhard and Duman, 2018). Similar to other antidepressant drugs (Li et al., 2010), inhibition of TrkB and mTOR signaling in the hippocampus also blocked the behavioral effects of CBD in the FST (Sartim et al., 2018). Together, these results suggest that CBD induces rapid BDNF-TrkB-mTOR signaling with subsequent synaptic changes in the PFC and hippocampus, favoring fast behavioral adaptation to stress and antidepressant effects. As both 5-HT_{1A} (Zhou et al., 2014) and endocannabinoid

(Bambico et al., 2016) signaling can modulate BDNF levels in limbic brain regions, it can be hypothesized that both systems are involved in the acute neuroplastic effects induced by CBD.

As it has been discussed above, in the CUS model, chronic administration of CBD promoted stress-coping behavior in the novelty suppressed feeding test associated with increased AEA levels in the hippocampus, increased hippocampal neurogenesis, and reduced stress-induced dendritic remodeling (Campos et al., 2013, 2017, Fogaça et al., 2018). CBD effects were sensitive to CB_1 and CB_2 antagonists, but not a 5-HT_{1A}-antagonist. Moreover, CBD increased proliferation of embryonic hippocampal HiB5 cells was abolished by CB_1 and CB_2, but not by 5-HT_{1A}-antagonists (Campos et al., 2013, Fogaça et al., 2018). The stress-coping behavior observed after repeated CBD administration was associated with decreased FAAH expression in the hippocampus (Fogaça et al., 2018), which may contribute to the increased AEA levels in this region previously after CBD chronic treatment (Campos et al., 2013). Therefore, similar to antidepressant drugs, (Bambico and Belzung, 2013; Dwyer and Duman, 2013, Tanti and Belzung, 2013), the stress-coping effects induced by CBD may also involve increased hippocampal neurogenesis. These results fit well with reports showing that sustained increase in endocannabinoid signaling promotes hippocampal neurogenesis and induces antidepressant-like effects in pre-clinical models through CB_1 and CB_2 receptors (Bambico and Gobbi, 2008; Fogaça et al., 2018; Zhang et al., 2015).

Additional evidence, however, suggests that the involvement of neurogenesis on CBD effects seems to be rather complicated and might depend on treatment duration and the behavioral paradigm used. For instance, Schiavon and colleagues (2016) reported that chronic (15 days; 3 and 30 mg/kg) treatment with CBD caused an antidepressant-like effect in the TST. However, the higher CBD dose tested decreased neurogenesis, thus revealing that it can induce antidepressant-like effects even under conditions of decreased hippocampal neurogenesis.

In conclusion, CBD induces antidepressant-like effects in a variety of animal models. The mechanisms responsible for these effects seem to depend on several factors such as treatment duration (acute vs. chronic stress) and the experimental paradigm used.

CBD AS AN ANTIPSYCHOTIC

Zuardi et al. (1982) observed that CBD inhibits THC-induced anxiety and psychotic-like symptoms such as disconnected thoughts, perceptual disturbance, and depersonalization. Because experimental evidence available by that time indicated that the antagonistic effect of CBD did not result from a pharmacokinetic interaction between the two cannabinoids (Hunt et al., 1981), these initial observations led to the hypothesis that CBD could possess antipsychotic properties. This proposal was later confirmed by studies with animal models and schizophrenia patients.

In pre-clinical studies, it has been observed that CBD attenuates several schizophrenia-related behavioral abnormalities (i.e., psychostimulant-induced hyperlocomotion and stereotypies, decreased sensorimotor gating, cognitive deficits, social withdrawal) in pharmacological, genetic, and neurodevelopmental animal models (Zuardi et al., 1991; Moreira and Guimaraes, 2005; Long et al., 2012; Levin et al., 2014; Pedrazzi et al., 2015; Gomes et al., 2015, Table 10.4).

TABLE 10.4
Pre-clinical Studies Investigating the Antipsychotic Properties of Cannabidiol

Study	Species	Tested Doses	Model	Effects	Proposed Mechanisms
Zuardi et al. (1991)	Male Wistar rats	15, 30, and 60 mg/kg, i.p.	Apomorphine-induced stereotyped behavior	Antipsychotic-like effect at 60 mg/kg	n.i.
Moreira and Guimarães, 2006	Male Swiss mice	15, 30, and 60 mg/kg, i.p.	D-amphetamine- and ketamine-induced hyperlocomotion	Decreased amphetamine-induced hyperlocomotion at 30 and 60 mg/kg and ketamine-induced hyperlocomotion at 30 mg/kg	n.i.
Long et al. (2006)	Male Swiss mice	1, 5, and 15 mg/kg, i.p.	MK-801-induced disruption of PPI	Antipsychotic-like effect at 5 mg/kg	Activation of TRPV1 receptors
Long et al. (2010)	C57BL/6JArc mice	1, 5, 10, and 50 mg/kg, i.p. (21 days)	D-amphetamine-induced hyperlocomotion	Antipsychotic-like effect at 50 mg/kg	n.i.
Gururajan et al. (2011)	Male Sprague-Dawley rats	3, 10, and 30 mg/kg, i.p.	MK-801-induced social withdrawal, hyperlocomotion, and PPI disruption	CBD inhibited MK-801-induced social withdrawal at 3 and 10 mg/kg	n.i.
Long et al. (2012)	Nrg 1 mutant mouse	1, 50, and 100 mg/kg, i.p.	Locomotor hyperactivity and PPI	No effect	n.i.
Gomes et al. (2014, 2015)	Male C57BL/6J mice	15, 30, and 60 mg/kg, i.p. (21 days)	Deficits in PPI, NOR, and social interaction induced by repeated treatment with MK-801 (28 days)	Antipsychotic-like effect at 30 and 60 mg/kg	Attenuated the changes in the expression of glial markers, deltaFosB and number of parvalbumin-positive cells in the mPFC induced by MK-801

(*Continued*)

TABLE 10.4 (*Continued*)
Pre-clinical Studies Investigating the Antipsychotic Properties of Cannabidiol

Study	Species	Tested Doses	Model	Effects	Proposed Mechanisms
Pedrazzi et al. (2015)	Male Swiss mice	15, 30, and 60 mg/kg, i.p. and intra-NAc (60 nmol)	D-amphetamine-induced disruption of PPI	Antipsychotic-like effect at 30 and 60 mg/kg and intra-NAc	n.i.
Deiana et al. (2015)	Male Wistar rats	5, 12, and 30 mg/kg, i.p.	MK-801-induced deficits in social recognition	No effect	n.i.
Renard et al., 2016	Male Sprague-Dawley rats	100 ng/0.5 µl/side, Intra-NAc shell	Amphetamine-induced Sensitization	CBD attenuated amphetamine-induced hyperlocomotion	Dependent upon the mTOR/p70S6K signaling pathway
Osborne et al. (2017)	Male Sprague-Dawley rats	10 mg/kg, i.p. (3 weeks)	Maternal immune activation model (with Poly:IC)	Attenuated the social interaction and cognitive deficits induced by prenatal poly I:C	n.i.
Peres et al. (2018)	Male spontaneously hypertensive rat (SHR)	0.5, 1, or 5 mg/kg, i.p., from PD30 to P60	SHR rats	Prevented the emergence of SHRs' hyperlocomotor activity and deficits in PPI at PD90	Increased the PFC 5-HIAA/serotonin ratio and the levels of 5-HIAA
Stark et al. (2019)	Male Sprague-Dawley rats	30 mg/kg/day, i.p., from PD19 to P39 (peripuberty)	MAM model	Prevented the emergence of schizophrenia-like deficits in adult MAM rats	Decreased 2-AG levels and CB$_1$ receptor expression in the mPFC of adult MAM rats

Abbreviations: 2-AG: 2-arachidonoylglycerol, i.p.: intraperitoneal, MAM: methylazoxymethanol, mPFC: medial prefrontal cortex, mTOR: mammalian target of rapamycin, NAc: Nucleus accumbens, n.i.: not investigated, NOR: novel object recognition test, Nrg 1: neuroregulin 1, PD: post-natal day, PPI: prepulse inhibition, TRPV$_1$: transient receptor potential vanilloid 1.

While typical antipsychotics, such as haloperidol, induce abnormal motor behaviors (i.e., catalepsy, tardive dyskinesia) and increases in prolactin levels, atypical antipsychotics, such as clozapine, do not (Miller, 2009). CBD shows a profile similar to atypical antipsychotics (Zuardi et al., 1991; Guimaraes et al., 2004; Moreira and Guimaraes, 2005). Interestingly, we recently observed that CBD was able to attenuate motor impairments induced by haloperidol in mice. Whereas acute CBD treatment prevented and partially reversed catalepsy caused by a single haloperidol administration (Gomes et al., 2013; Sonego et al., 2016), repeated CBD blocked the haloperidol-induced orofacial dyskinesia and inflammatory changes via a mechanism dependent on the activation of PPAR-γ receptors (Sonego et al., 2018).

TABLE 10.5
Clinical Studies Investigating the Antipsychotic Properties of CBD

Study	Subjects	Tested Doses	Effects
Zuardi et al. (1982)	Healthy volunteers (8)	1 mg/kg, P.O.	Decreased psychotic symptoms induced by THC
Zuardi et al. (1995)	Schizophrenia female patient (1)	Increasing oral doses of CBD, reaching 1,500 mg/day, P.O. (4 weeks)	Decreased psychotic symptoms evaluated by the BPRS
Zuardi et al. (2006)	Male patients with treatment-resistant schizophrenia (3)	Increased from 40 up to 1,280 mg/day, P.O. (30 days)	One patient showed mild improvement (BPRS)
Zuardi et al. (2009)	L-dopa-induced psychosis in Parkinson's disease patients (6)	Increased from 150 up to 600 mg/day depending on the clinical response, P.O. (4 weeks)	Decreased psychotic symptoms evaluated by the BPRS and the PPQ
Hallak et al. (2010)	Schizophrenia patients (28)	300 and 600 mg, P.O. (acute)	No effect in the Stroop Color Word Test
Hallak et al. (2011)	Healthy volunteers (10)	600 mg, P.O.	Trend to reduce ketamine-induced psychotic symptoms
Leweke et al. (2012)	Acute paranoid schizophrenia patients (42)	600 mg/day, P.O. (4 weeks)	Decreased BPRS and PANSS scores
Boggs et al. (2018)	Stable antipsychotic-treated patients with chronic schizophrenia (36)	600 mg/day, P.O. (6 weeks)	Add-on CBD was not associated with an improvement in MCCB or PANSS

(Continued)

TABLE 10.5 (*Continued*)
Clinical Studies Investigating the Antipsychotic Properties of CBD

Study	Subjects	Tested Doses	Effects
McGuire et al. (2018)	Schizophrenia patients (43)	1,000 mg/day, P.O. (6 weeks)	Add-on CBD group had lower levels of psychotic symptoms (PANSS) and also improvements in cognitive performance (BACS)
Bhattacharyya et al. (2018)	Antipsychotic medication-naive at clinical high risk (CHR) of psychosis (33)	600 mg, P.O. (acute)	CBD normalized alterations in parahippocampal, striatal, and midbrain function associated with the CHR state

Abbreviations: BACS: brief assessment of cognition in schizophrenia, BPRS: brief psychiatric rating scale, MCCB: MATRICS consensus cognitive battery, PANSS: positive and negative syndrome scale, PPQ: Parkinson psychosis questionnaire, THC: Δ^9-tetrahydrocannabinol.

In humans, the use of CBD in schizophrenia patients was tested for the first time in 1995 (Table 10.5). In an open, case report study, a 19-year-old schizophrenia female patient, who presented marked side effects after treatment with conventional antipsychotics, received increasing oral doses of CBD (up to 1,500 mg/day) for 4 weeks (Zuardi et al., 1995). An important symptom improvement, with no significant side effects, was observed during CBD treatment. In another case study, CBD monotherapy was administered for 30 days to three 22- or 23-year-old male schizophrenia patients who had not responded to typical antipsychotics (Zuardi et al., 2006). One patient showed mild improvement, but only slight or no change was observed in the other two, suggesting that CBD monotherapy may not be effective in patients with treatment-resistant schizophrenia. However, a recent case study reported a patient with treatment-resistant schizophrenia remitting following adjunctive CBD (Makiol and Kluge, 2018).

In support to the idea that CBD has antipsychotic properties, a 4-week double-blind controlled clinical trial in 42 unmedicated individuals with acute schizophrenia or schizophreniform psychosis showed that CBD, similar to the atypical antipsychotic amisulpride, was effective in reducing acute psychotic symptoms after 2 and 4 weeks of treatment. Importantly, compared to amisulpride, CBD caused a lower incidence of extrapyramidal symptoms and increases in prolactin and weight gain (Leweke et al., 2012). More recently, it was reported the effects of CBD on schizophrenia in an exploratory 6-week, multicenter, randomized, double-blind, placebo-controlled clinical trial in 88 schizophrenia patients stably medicated with conventional antipsychotics (mainly atypical antipsychotics). Patients remained on their antipsychotic medication and were randomized to receive CBD or placebo in addition to their antipsychotic medication. The results demonstrate that patients receiving CBD had significantly lower levels of psychotic symptoms, higher clinical improvement scores, and a near-significant trend toward a better cognitive performance (McGuire et al., 2018).

Another potential application of CBD is in people at high-risk for psychosis. An early phase trial in high-risk subjects suggests that a single dose of CBD partially normalize dysfunction in the medial temporal lobe, striatum, and midbrain in individuals at high-risk for psychosis and may reduce presenting symptoms (Bhattacharyya et al., 2018). In this context, pre-clinical studies indicate that CBD administered during adolescence in animal models of schizophrenia based on neurodevelopmental disruption could also prevent the transition to the full-blown psychosis (Peres et al., 2018; Stark et al. 2019).

Possible Mechanisms of the Antipsychotic Effects of CBD

The exact mechanisms by which CBD exert its antipsychotic effects are still unknown. CBD has been reported to up-regulate levels of the endocannabinoid AEA by inhibiting its reuptake and degradation (Bisogno et al., 2001; Elmes et al. 2015). AEA levels are negatively correlated with severity of psychotic symptoms (Giuffrida et al., 2004), and the improvement of psychotic symptoms in patients treated with CBD was associated with increased serum levels of AEA (Leweke et al., 2012). As discussed above, CBD can inhibit FAAH activity and increase AEA levels (Leweke et al., 2012). Thus, by indirectly activating CB_1 receptors via increased AEA levels, CBD could potentially modulate other neurotransmitters systems (Campos et al., 2012). However, other mechanisms could also be involved in the antipsychotic properties of CBD.

Recently, we observed that CBD, as well as the atypical antipsychotic clozapine, attenuated the decreased number of parvalbumin-positive cells in the mPFC of mice submitted to repeated treatment with the NMDA receptor antagonist MK-801, which is used as a mouse model of schizophrenia based on the hypofunction of NMDA receptors (Gomes et al., 2014). Parvalbumin is a calcium binding protein expressed in a subset of GABAergic interneurons. GABAergic interneurons containing parvalbumin are fast-spiking interneurons, which synapse on the cell body or the initial axon segment of glutamate pyramidal neurons, promoting synchronization and temporal control of the information flow through pyramidal neurons (Lewis et al., 2005). Parvalbumin interneurons are selectively altered in schizophrenia patients and can account for abnormal circuit synchrony and several symptoms in this disorder (Lewis et al., 2005; Grace and Gomes, 2019). Similar to patients, different rodent models of schizophrenia show deficits in the function or loss of parvalbumin interneurons. This parvalbumin loss has been associated with increased oxidative stress (Steullet et al., 2017). Thus, the effects of CBD in attenuating the decrease in the number of parvalbumin-positive cells induced by MK-801 could involve mechanisms associated with protection against the damage caused by increased levels of oxidative stress. CBD has pronounced antioxidant properties (Pellati et al., 2018).

Besides the changes in parvalbumin, the MK-801 treatment also increased the expression of astrocyte and microglial cell markers in the mPFC (Gomes et al., 2015), similar to what has been observed in *post-mortem* brain of schizophrenia patients (Radewicz et al., 2000; Catts et al., 2014). These changes were also attenuated by CBD (Gomes et al., 2015) suggesting that anti-inflammatory properties may contribute to the antipsychotic-like effects induced by CBD. Other potential mechanisms can also be involved in these effects, such as the activation of PPAR-γ receptors, 5-HT$_{1A}$-receptors, and CB$_1$ and/or CB$_2$ receptors by the indirect increase in AEA levels (Campos et al., 2012; Campos et al., 2017).

CBD IN DRUG DEPENDENCE

Contrary to THC, CBD has low rewarding properties with minimal abuse potential and does not induce cognitive and psychomotor impairments across a broad dose range in humans (even up to a supratherapeutic dose of 4,500 mg), including in a highly sensitive population of recreational polydrug user (Schoedel et al., 2018). In addition to the potential beneficial effects of CBD in anxiety, depression, and schizophrenia, CBD has recently attracted greater interest as a strategy for treating substance abuse disorders.

Substance abuse disorders are chronic illness characterized not just by the intoxication associated with acute drug use, but also by disruptions of cognition and negative emotional states that trigger craving and relapse, perpetuating the cycle of drug abuse (Leshner, 1997; Koob, 2006). Several factors contribute to the risk of relapse, including susceptibility to stress, craving induced by drug contexts, increased anxiety, and impaired impulse control (Koob, 2006). Evidence indicates that CBD may be effective for targeting these risk states. For example, its anxiolytic (Guimaraes et al., 1990, Bergamaschi et al., 2011), stress-relieving (Resstel et al., 2009; Granjeiro et al., 2011), antidepressant (Zanelati et al., 2010), and anti-compulsive activity (Casarotto et al., 2010; Nardo et al., 2014) may imply therapeutic benefit for affective changes and the compulsive nature of drug seeking in affected individuals. Also, CBD decreases the rewarding proprieties of some drugs of abuse.

Research on CBD and the behavioral effects induced by psychostimulants (i.e., amphetamine and cocaine) has revealed contradictory results. While CBD does not inhibit the reward-facilitating effects of cocaine on intracranial self-stimulation (Katsidoni et al., 2013), it mitigates cocaine-induced conditioned place preference (Lujan et al., 2018). This latter effect is consistent with findings showing that CBD disrupts reconsolidation of cocaine-associated conditioned place preference memories (de Carvalho and Takahashi, 2017) and facilitates extinction of conditioned place preference induced by cocaine and amphetamine (Parker et al., 2004). CBD also blocks amphetamine (Renard et al., 2016), but not cocaine-induced behavioral sensitization (Lujan et al., 2018) in rodents. In addition, repeated CBD attenuates cocaine intake and breaking point values under a progressive ratio reinforcement schedule in a self-administration paradigm, but not alter the reinstatement of cocaine-seeking behavior following extinction training (Lujan et al., 2018). However, a 7-day treatment based on transdermal delivery of CBD attenuated cue-induced reinstatement of cocaine self-administration in rats. Following the termination of CBD treatment, reinstatement remained attenuated up to 5 months (Gonzalez-Cuevas et al., 2018). Together, these findings indicate that CBD could reduce the compulsive and escalating intake of cocaine and cue-induced reinstatement in cocaine-abstinent subjects. Interestingly, these long-lasting effects have been suggested to involve the pro-neurogenic properties of CBD (Gonzalez-Cuevas et al., 2018; Lujan et al., 2018).

In addition to psychostimulants, animal studies have also suggested beneficial effects of CBD to clinical symptoms associated with opioid exposure. Pioneer studies conducted in the 1970s indicated that CBD could attenuate morphine withdrawal symptoms in rats (Hine et al., 1975a, 1975b; Bhargava, 1976). Recently, it was found that CBD inhibits the reward-facilitating effects of morphine on conditioned place preference (Markos et al., 2018) and disrupts reconsolidation of morphine-associated conditioned place preference memories (de Carvalho and Takahashi, 2017). CBD also inhibits the reward-facilitating effects of morphine on intracranial self-stimulation (Katsidoni et al., 2013), an effect blocked by the administration of a 5-HT$_{1A}$-receptor antagonist into the dorsal raphe nucleus. Also, although a single administration of CBD did not alter heroin self-administration in rats, it inhibited cue-induced heroin-seeking behavior. Interestingly, this effect lasted for at least two weeks (Ren et al., 2009). Even when CBD was administered in three consecutive daily injections overlapping with a period of active heroin intake, the inhibition of relapse behavior was still observed weeks after the last CBD administration (Ren et al., 2009). This result suggests that CBD might have anti-relapse properties and could impact the course of opioid abuse even following a potential lapse after a period of abstinence. These effects of CBD may involve normalization of disturbances of AMPA GluR$_1$ and CB$_1$ receptor expression observed in the nucleus accumbens associated with stimulus cue-induced heroin seeking. This finding is important given that several studies have indicated the critical role of mesolimbic AMPA GluR$_1$ in drug-seeking behavior (Anderson et al., 2008; Conrad et al., 2008).

The anti-relapse properties of CBD were also explored in a pilot study with heroin-addicted individuals who are abstinent from heroin use, in which participants were given daily doses of CBD (400 or 800 mg) or placebo for three consecutive days (Hurd et al., 2015). Similar to the animal study, CBD decreased cue-induced and general craving, as well as anxiety induced by heroin cues, with persistent effects of up to 7 days (Hurd et al., 2015). This long-lasting effect is significant since drug craving increases throughout the drug abstinence phase (Hurd, 2017). Additionally, these findings agree with the anxiolytic effects of CBD reported by pre-clinical and clinical studies (see above), suggesting it can attenuate negative states in opioid-dependent individuals. This effect would also reduce craving and, consequently, the likelihood of relapse.

Beneficial effects of CBD may not be limited to opioid abuse disorder since a conceptually analogous, albeit more discrete, effect has also been observed in tobacco smokers (Morgan et al., 2013). In a small, week-long, randomized, double-blind study, smokers who wished to stop smoking were instructed to inhale CBD (metered dose of 400 μg) or placebo when they felt the urge to smoke. CBD reduced the number of cigarettes smoked by approximately 40% during treatment, but this effect was not maintained after the cessation of the treatment. In contrast to the heroin study, CBD did not alter craving, either acutely or chronically (Morgan et al., 2013). Therefore, it is not clear whether CBD has generalized effects on the expression of cue-drug memory to elicit craving and precipitate relapse, or whether its effects are specific to certain classes of substances of abuse. The same group has also evaluated CBD on cannabis abuse. In naturalistic studies with cannabis users, the presence of CBD in smoked cannabis did not attenuate psychotomimetic symptoms in participants when they were acutely intoxicated (Morgan et al., 2010a, b). However, CBD reduced "wanting" and "liking" of the cannabis-related stimuli (Morgan et al., 2010a). In addition, a case report of a 19-year-old female with cannabis dependence, who experienced withdrawal syndrome when she tried to cease cannabis use, indicated that CBD administered for 11 days (300 mg on day 1, 600 mg on days 2–10, and 300 mg on day 11) prevented withdrawal, anxiety, and dissociative symptoms during the treatment, indicating that CBD can be useful for the treatment of cannabis withdrawal syndrome (Crippa et al., 2013). A 6-month follow-up showed a relapse in cannabis use, but at a lower frequency (once or twice a week vs. 7 days a week) (Crippa et al., 2013), suggesting that CBD has also the potential of reducing cannabis use.

Despite some positive findings, pre-clinical and clinical studies investigating the effects of CBD in substance abuse disorders are still scarce. Thus, further studies evaluating the efficacy of this drug at different phases of the drug abuse cycle (i.e., substance abuse, intoxication, withdrawal, and abstinence which include recurrent episode of craving, relapse, compulsive substance use) for different classes of substances of abuse are clearly needed to support the promise of CBD as a treatment for substance abuse disorders.

PROSPECTS AND CONCLUSIONS

In addition to anxiety, psychosis, depression, and drug abuse, CBD could also be useful in other psychiatric disorders, including autism spectrum disorders (ASD). As recently reviewed out by Poleg and colleagues (2018), based on initial pre-clinical studies and clinical reports, CBD could be useful as a possible monotherapy or add-on treatment for these disorders.

Nevertheless, a critical point that needs to be evaluated before the recommendation of any medicine refers to its potential risks. There is now cumulative evidence that CBD has a favorable safety profile in humans. In clinical studies the drug is usually well-tolerated, with somnolence, decreased appetite, diarrhea, and increased serum aminotransferases being the significant side effects (Lattanzi et al., 2018; Taylor et al., 2018). Also, CBD did not potentiate the cognitive impairment induced ethanol (for review, see Turna et al., 2019). However, it inhibits several hepatic cytochrome P450s, important enzymes involved with drug metabolism (Zendulka et al., 2016). Therefore, potential drug interactions should be considered in the clinical use of CBD. Another limitation is the low oral bioavailability of CBD in humans (around 6%, Consroe et al., 1991). At the moment, several studies are trying to develop new drug release approaches or enhance CBD potency to address this problem (Atsmon et al., 2018a, b; Breuer et al., 2016; Cherniakov et al., 2017; Hammell et al., 2016).

In conclusion, pre-clinical and clinical studies indicate that CBD can potentially benefice several mental health disorders. Its use as a medicine, however, still face challenges. As for any drug, clinical recommendations must be based on randomized clinical trials, something that, except for the few examples highlighted in this review, are still lacking. Even so, considering the limitations of the currently available pharmacological treatments for mental health disorders (unacceptable side effect and lack of effectiveness for a considerable number of patients), further efforts should be made to run these much-needed studies.

ACKNOWLEDGMENTS

This work was supported by grants from the National Institute of Science and Translational Medicine, CNPq (465458/2014-9), Coordenação de Aperfeiçoamento de Pessoal de Nível Superior—Brazil (CAPES)—Finance Code 001, FAPESP (2017/24304-0) and AIAS-COFUND fellowship from European Union's Horizon 2020 Research and Innovation Programme under the Marie Skłodowska-Curie agreement (grant #754513). FSG, ACC, and SRJ receive research fellowships from CNPq.

CONFLICT OF INTEREST

FSG is a co-inventor (Mechoulam R, JC, Guimaraes FS, AZ, JH, Breuer A) of the patent "Fluorinated CBD compounds, compositions and uses thereof. Pub. No.: WO/2014/108899. International Application No.: PCT/IL2014/050023" Def. US no. Reg. 62193296; 29/07/2015; INPI on 19/08/2015 (BR1120150164927). The University of São Paulo has licensed the patent to *Phytecs Pharm* (USP Resolution No. 15.1.130002.1.1). The University of São Paulo has an agreement with *Prati-Donaduzzi* (Toledo, Brazil) to "develop a pharmaceutical product containing synthetic cannabidiol and prove its safety and therapeutic efficacy in the treatment of epilepsy, schizophrenia, Parkinson's disease, and anxiety disorders."

REFERENCES

Adams, R. 1941. Marihuana. *Harvey Lect* 37:168–97.
Almeida, V., Levin, R., Peres, F.F., Niigaki, S.T., Calzavara, M.B., Zuardi, A.W., Hallak, J.E., Crippa, J.A., Abílio, V.C. 2013. Cannabidiol exhibits anxiolytic but not antipsychotic property evaluated in the social interaction test. *Prog Neuropsychopharmacol Biol Psychiatry* 41:30–5.
Anderson, S.M., Famous, K.R., Sadri-Vakili, G., Kumaresan, V., Schmidt, H.D., Bass, C.E., Terwilliger, E.F., Cha, J.H., Pierce, R.C. 2008. CaMKII: a biochemical bridge linking accumbens dopamine and glutamate systems in cocaine seeking. *Nat Neurosci* 11 (3):344–53.
Ashton, C.H., Moore, P.B., Gallagher, P., Young, A.H. 2005. Cannabinoids in bipolar affective disorder: a review and discussion of their therapeutic potential. *J Psychopharmacol* 19(3):293–300.
Atsmon, J., Cherniakov, I., Izgelov, D., Hoffman, A., Domb, A.J., Deutsch, L., Deutsch, F., Heffetz, D., Sacks, H. 2018a. PTL401, a new formulation based on pro-nano dispersion technology, improves oral cannabinoids bioavailability in healthy volunteers. *J Pharm Sci* 107(5):1423–29.
Atsmon, J., Heffetz, D., Deutsch, L., Deutsch, F., Sacks, H. 2018b. Single-dose pharmacokinetics of oral cannabidiol following administration of PTL101: a new formulation based on gelatin matrix pellets technology. *Clin Pharmacol Drug Dev* 7(7):751–8.
Bambico, F., Belzung, C. 2013. Novel insights into depression and antidepressants: a synergy between synaptogenesis and neurogenesis? *Curr Top Behav Neurosci* 15:243–91.
Bambico, F.R., Duranti, A., Nobrega, J.N., Gobbi, G. 2016. The fatty acid amide hydrolase inhibitor URB597 modulates serotonin-dependent emotional behaviour, and serotonin1A and serotonin2A/Cactivity in the hippocampus. *Eur Neuropsychopharmacol* 26:578–90.
Bambico, F.R., Gobbi, G. 2008. The cannabinoid CB$_1$ receptor and the endocannabinoid anandamide: possible antidepressant targets. *Expert Opin Ther Targets* 12:1347–66.
Bergamaschi, M.M., Queiroz, R.H., Chagas, M.H., de Oliveira, D.C., De Martinis, B.S., Kapczinski, F., Quevedo, J., Roesler, R., Schroder, N., Nardi, A.E., Martin-Santos, R., Hallak, J.E., Zuardi, A.W., Crippa, J.A. 2011. Cannabidiol reduces the anxiety induced by simulated public speaking in treatment-naive social phobia patients. *Neuropsychopharmacology* 36(6):1219–26.

Bhargava, H.N. 1976. Effect of some cannabinoids on naloxone-precipitated abstinence in morphine-dependent mice. *Psychopharmacology* 49:267–70.

Bhattacharyya, S., Wilson, R., Appiah-Kusi, E., O'Neill, A., Brammer, M., Perez, J., Murray, R., Allen, P., Bossong, M.G., McGuire, P. 2018. Effect of cannabidiol on medial temporal, midbrain, and striatal dysfunction in people at clinical high risk of psychosis: a randomized clinical trial. *JAMA Psychiatry* 75(11):1107–17.

Bisogno, T., Hanus, L., De Petrocellis, L., Tchilibon, S., Ponde, D.E., Brandi, I., Moriello, A.S., Davis, J.B., Mechoulam, R., Di Marzo, V. 2001. Molecular targets for cannabidiol and its synthetic analogues: effect on vanilloid VR1 receptors and on the cellular uptake and enzymatic hydrolysis of anandamide. *Br J Pharmacol.*

Bitencourt, R.M., Pamplona, F.A., Takahashi, R.N. 2008. Facilitation of contextual fear memory extinction and anti-anxiogenic effects of AM404 and cannabidiol in conditioned rats. *Eur Neuropsychopharmacol* 18(12):849–59.

Blier, P., El-Mansari, M., 2013. Serotonin and beyond: therapeutics for major depression. *Philos Trans R Soc B Biol Sci* 3681–7.

Boggs, D.L., Surti, T., Gupta, A., Gupta, S., Niciu, M., Pittman, B., Schnakenberg Martin, A.M., Thurnauer, H., Davies, A., D'Souza, D.C., Ranganathan, M. 2018. The effects of cannabidiol (CBD) on cognition and symptoms in outpatients with chronic schizophrenia a randomized placebo controlled trial. *Psychopharmacology (Berl)* 235(7): 1923–32.

Breuer, A., Haj, C.G., Fogaça, M.V., Gomes, F.V., Silva, N.R., Pedrazzi, J.F., Del Bel, E.A., Hallak, J.C., Crippa, J.A., Zuardi, A.W., Mechoulam, R., Guimarães, F.S. 2016. Fluorinated cannabidiol derivatives: enhancement of activity in mice models predictive of anxiolytic, antidepressant and antipsychotic effects. *PLoS One* 11:1–19.

Campos, A.C., de Paula Soares, V., Carvalho, M.C., Ferreira, F.R., Vicente, M.A., Brandao, M.L., Zuardi, A.W., Zangrossi, H., Jr., Guimaraes, F.S. 2013a. Involvement of serotonin-mediated neurotransmission in the dorsal periaqueductal gray matter on cannabidiol chronic effects in panic-like responses in rats. *Psychopharmacology (Berl)* 226:13–24.

Campos, A.C., Ferreira, F.R., Guimarães, F.S. 2012a. Cannabidiol blocks long-lasting behavioral consequences of predator threat stress: possible involvement of 5-HT$_{1A}$ receptors. *J Psychiatr Res* 46:1501–10.

Campos, A.C., Fogaça, M.V., Scarante, F.F., Joca, S.R.L., Sales, A.J., Gomes, F.V., Sonego, A.B., Rodrigues, N.S., Galve-Roperh, I., Guimarães, F.S. 2017. Plastic and neuroprotective mechanisms involved in the therapeutic effects of cannabidiol in psychiatric disorders. *Front Pharmacol* 8.

Campos, A.C., Fogaça, M.V., Sonego, A.B., Guimarães, F.S. 2016. Cannabidiol, neuroprotection and neuropsychiatric disorders. *Pharmacol Res* 112:119–27.

Campos, A.C., Guimarães, F.S. 2008. Involvement of 5-HT$_{1A}$ receptors in the anxiolytic-like effects of cannabidiol injected into the dorsolateral periaqueductal gray of rats. *Psychopharmacology (Berl)* 199:223–30.

Campos, A.C., Guimarães, F.S. 2009. Evidence for a potential role for TRPV1 receptors in the dorsolateral periaqueductal gray in the attenuation of the anxiolytic effects of cannabinoids. *Prog Neuropsychopharmacol Biol Psychiatry* 33(8):1517–21.

Campos, A.C., Moreira, F.A., Gomes, F.V., Del Bel, E.A., Guimaraes, F.S. 2012b. Multiple mechanisms involved in the large-spectrum therapeutic potential of cannabidiol in psychiatric disorders. *Philos Trans R Soc Lond B Biol Sci* 367(1607):3364–78.

Campos, A.C., Ortega, Z., Palazuelos, J., Fogaca, M.V., Aguiar, D.C., Diaz-Alonso, J., Ortega-Gutierrez, S., Vazquez-Villa, H., Moreira, F.A., Guzman, M., Galve-Roperh, I., Guimaraes, F.S. 2013b. The anxiolytic effect of cannabidiol on chronically stressed mice depends on hippocampal neurogenesis: involvement of the endocannabinoid system. *Int J Neuropsychopharmacol* 16:1407–19.

Carr, G., Lucki, I. 2011. The role of serotonin receptor sutypes in treating depression: a review of animal studies. *Psychopharmacology (Berl)* 213:265–287.

Carrier, E.J., Auchampach, J.A., Hillard, C.J. 2006. Inhibition of an equilibrative nucleoside transporter by cannabidiol: a mechanism of cannabinoid immunosuppression. *Proc Natl Acad Sci U S A* 103(20):7895–900.

Casarotto, P.C., Gomes, F.V., Resstel, L.B., Guimaraes, F.S. 2010. Cannabidiol inhibitory effect on marble-burying behaviour: involvement of CB_1 receptors. *Behav Pharmacol* 21(4):353–8.

Castrén, E., Rantamäki, T. 2010a. Role of brain-derived neurotrophic factor in the aetiology of depression: implications for pharmacological treatment. *CNS Drugs* 24:1–7.

Castrén, E., Rantamäki, T. 2010b. The role of BDNF and its receptors in depression and antidepressant drug action: reactivation of developmental plasticity. *Dev Neurobiol* 70:289–97.

Catts, V.S., Wong, J., Fillman, S.G., Fung, S.J., Shannon Weickert, C. 2014. Increased expression of astrocyte markers in schizophrenia: association with neuroinflammation. *Aust N Z J Psychiatry* 48(8):722–34.

Cherniakov, I., Izgelov, D., Barasch, D., Davidson, E., Domb, A.J., Hoffman, A. 2017. Piperine-pro-nanolipospheres as a novel oral delivery system of cannabinoids: pharmacokinetic evaluation in healthy volunteers in comparison to buccal spray administration. *J Control Release* 266:1–7.

Conrad, K.L., Tseng, K.Y., Uejima, J.L., Reimers, J.M., Heng, L.J., Shaham, Y., Marinelli, M., Wolf, M.E. 2008. Formation of accumbens GluR2-lacking AMPA receptors mediates incubation of cocaine craving. *Nature* 454(7200):118–21.

Consroe, P., Laguna, J., Allender, J., Snider, S., Stern, L., Sandyk, R., Kennedy, K., Schram, K. 1991 Controlled clinical trial of cannabidiol in Huntington's disease. *Pharmacol Biochem Behav* 40(3):701–8.

Corroon, J., Phillips, J.A. 2018. A cross-sectional study of cannabidiol users. *Cannabis Cannabinoid Res* 3:152–161.

Crippa, J.A., Guimarães, F.S., Campos, A.C., Zuardi, A.W. 2018. Translational investigation of the therapeutic potential of cannabidiol (CBD): toward a new age. *Front Immunol* 9:2009.

Crippa, J.A., Hallak, J.E., Machado-de-Sousa, J.P., Queiroz, R.H., Bergamaschi, M., Chagas, M.H., Zuardi, A.W. 2013. Cannabidiol for the treatment of cannabis withdrawal syndrome: a case report. *J Clin Pharm Ther* 38(2):162–4.

Crippa, J.A., Zuardi, A.W., Garrido, G.E., Wichert-Ana, L., Guarnieri, R., Ferrari, L., Azevedo-Marques, P.M., Hallak, J.E., McGuire, P.K., Filho Busatto, G. 2004. Effects of cannabidiol (CBD) on regional cerebral blood flow. *Neuropsychopharmacology* 29(2):417–26.

Cryan, J.F., Markou, A., Lucki, I. 2002. Assessing antidepressant activity in rodents: recent developments and future needs. *TIPS* 23:238–245.

de Carvalho, C.R., Takahashi, R.N. 2017. Cannabidiol disrupts the reconsolidation of contextual drug-associated memories in Wistar rats. *Addict Biol* 22(3):742–751.

De Gregorio, D., McLaughlin, R.J., Posa, L., Ochoa-Sanchez, R., Enns, J., Lopez-Canul, M., Aboud, M., Maione, S., Comai, S., Gobbi, G. 2019. Cannabidiol modulates serotonergic transmission and prevents allodynia and anxiety-like behavior in a model of neuropathic pain. *Pain* 160(1):136–150.

de Morais, H., Chaves, Y.C., Waltrick, A.P.F., Jesus, C.H.A., Genaro, K., Crippa, J.A., da Cunha, J.M., Zanoveli, J.M. 2018. Sub-chronic treatment with cannabidiol but not with URB597 induced a mild antidepressant-like effect in diabetic rats. *Neurosci Lett* 682:62–68.

Deiana, S., Watanabe, A., Yamasaki, Y., Amada, N., Arthur, M., Fleming, S., Woodcock, H., Dorward, P., Pigliacampo, B., Close, S., Platt, B., Riedel, G. 2012. Plasma and brain pharmacokinetic profile of cannabidiol (CBD), cannabidivarine (CBDV), Δ^9-tetrahydrocannabivarin (THCV) and cannabigerol (CBG) in rats and mice following oral and intraperitoneal administration and CBD action on obsessive-compulsive behaviour. *Psychopharmacology (Berl)* 219(3):859–73.

Deiana, S., Watanabe, A., Yamasaki, Y., Amada, N., Kikuchi, T., Stott, C., Riedel, G. 2015. MK-801-induced deficits in social recognition in rats: reversal by aripiprazole, but not olanzapine, risperidone, or cannabidiol. *Behav Pharmacol* 26(8 Spec No):748–65.

Delgado, P.L., Charney, D.S., Price, L.H., Aghajanian, G.K., Landis, H., Heninger, G.R. 1990. Serotonin function and the mechanism of antidepressant action. *Arch Gen Psychiatry* 47: 411–418.

Devane, W.A., Dysarz, F.A. 3rd, Johnson, M.R., Melvin, L.S., Howlett, A.C. 1988. Determination and characterization of a cannabinoid receptor in rat brain. *Mol Pharmacol* 34(5):605–13.

Devane, W.A., Hanus, L., Breuer, A., Pertwee, R.G., Stevenson, L.A., Griffin, G., Gibson, D., Mandelbaum, A., Etinger, A., Mechoulam, R. 1992. Isolation and structure of a brain constituent that binds to the cannabinoid receptor. *Science* 258(5090):1946–9.

Do Monte, F.H., Souza, R.R., Bitencourt, R.M., Kroon, J.A., Takahashi, R.N. 2013. Infusion of cannabidiol into infralimbic cortex facilitates fear extinction via CB_1 receptors. *Behav Brain Res* 250:23–27.

Drysdale, A.J., Ryan, D., Pertwee, R.G., Platt, B. 2006. Cannabidiol-induced intracellular Ca^{2+} elevations in hippocampal cells. *Neuropharmacology* 50(5):621–31.

Dwyer, J.M., Duman, R.S. 2013. Activation of mTOR and synaptogenesis: role in the actions of rapid-acting antidepressants. *Biol Psychiatry* 73:1189–1198.

El-Alfy, A.T., Ivey, K., Robinson, K., Ahmed, S., Radwan, M., Slade, D., Khan, I., ElSohly, M., Ross, S. 2010. Antidepressant-like effect of delta9-tetrahydrocannabinol and other cannabinoids isolated from Cannabis sativa L. *Pharmacol Biochem Behav* 95:434–42.

ElBatsh, M.M., Assareh, N., Marsden, C.A., Kendall, D.A. 2012. Anxiogenic-like effects of chronic cannabidiol administration in rats. *Psychopharmacology (Berl)* 221(2):239–47.

Elmes, M.W., Kaczocha, M., Berger, W.T., Leung, K., Ralph, B.P., Wang, L., Sweeney, J.M., Miyauchi, J.T., Tsirka, S.E., Ojima, I., Deutsch, D.G. 2015. Fatty acid-binding proteins (FABPs) are intracellular carriers for Delta9-tetrahydrocannabinol (THC) and cannabidiol (CBD). *J Biol Chem* 290(14):8711–21.

Elms, L., Shannon, S., Hughes, S., Lewis, N. 2019. Cannabidiol in the treatment of post-traumatic stress disorder: a case series. *J Altern Complement Med* 25(4):392–397.

Esposito, G., Scuderi, C., Valenza, M., Togna, G.I., Latina, V., De Filippis, D., Cipriano, M., Carratù, M.R., Iuvone, T., Steardo, L. 2011. Cannabidiol reduces Aβ-induced neuroinflammation and promotes hippocampal neurogenesis through PPARγ involvement. *PLoS One* 6(12):e28668.

EUCTR 2015-000465-31-DE, 2018. Clinical trials for Cannabidiol [WWW Document]. www.clinicaltrialsregister.eu/ctr-search/search?query=cannabidiol&page=2.

Fogaça, M.V., Campos, A.C., Coelho, L.D., Duman, R.S., Guimarães, F.S. 2018. The anxiolytic effects of cannabidiol in chronically stressed mice are mediated by the endocannabinoid system: role of neurogenesis and dendritic remodeling. *Neuropharmacology* 135:22–33.

Fogaça, M.V., Campos, A.C., Guimaraes, F.S. 2014a. Chapter 70. Cannabidiol and 5-HT$_{1A}$ receptors. In: Preedy, V.R. (ed.) *Neuropathology of Drug Addictions and Substance Misuse. Volume 1: Foundations of Understanding, Tobacco, Alcohol, Cannabinoids and Opioids*. Elsevier, London, pp. 749–759.

Fogaça, M.V., Reis, F.M., Campos, A.C., Guimaraes, F.S. 2014b. Effects of intra-prelimbic prefrontal cortex injection of cannabidiol on anxiety-like behavior: involvement of 5-HT$_{1A}$ receptors and previous stressful experience. *Eur Neuropsychopharmacol* 24(3):410–419.

Fukumoto, K., Iijima, M., Funakoshi, T., Chaki, S. 2018. Role of 5-HT$_{1A}$ receptor stimulation in the medial prefrontal cortex in the sustained antidepressant effects of ketamine. *Int J Neuropsychopharmacol* 21(4):371–381.

Gaoni, Y., Mechoulam, R. 1964. Isolation, structure and partial synthesis of an active constituent of hashish. *J Am Chem Soc* 86:1646.

Gerhard, D.M., Duman, R.S. 2018. Rapid-acting antidepressants: mechanistic insights and future directions. *Curr Behav Neurosci Rep* 5:36–47.

Giuffrida, A., Leweke, F.M., Gerth, C.W., Schreiber, D., Koethe, D., Faulhaber, J., Klosterkotter, J., Piomelli, D. 2004. Cerebrospinal anandamide levels are elevated in acute schizophrenia and are inversely correlated with psychotic symptoms. *Neuropsychopharmacology* 29(11):2108–14.

Gomes, F.V., Del Bel, E.A., Guimaraes, F.S. 2013. Cannabidiol attenuates catalepsy induced by distinct pharmacological mechanisms via 5-HT$_{1A}$ receptor activation in mice. *Prog Neuropsychopharmacol Biol Psychiatry* 46:43–7.

Gomes, F.V., Issy, A.C., Ferreira, F.R., Viveros, M.P., Del Bel, E.A., Guimaraes, F.S. 2014. Cannabidiol attenuates sensorimotor gating disruption and molecular changes induced by chronic antagonism of NMDA receptors in mice. *Int J Neuropsychopharmacol* 18(5).

Gomes, F.V., Llorente, R., Del Bel, E.A., Viveros, M.P., Lopez-Gallardo, M., Guimaraes, F.S. 2015. Decreased glial reactivity could be involved in the antipsychotic-like effect of cannabidiol. *Schizophr Res* 164(1–3):155–63.

Gomes, F.V., Reis, D.G., Alves, F.H., Corrêa, F.M., Guimarães, F.S., Resstel, L.B. 2012. Cannabidiol injected into the bed nucleus of the stria terminalis reduces the expression of contextual fear conditioning via 5-HT$_{1A}$ receptors. *J Psychopharmacol* 26:104–13.

Gomes, F.V., Resstel, L.B., Guimarães, F.S. 2011. The anxiolytic-like effects of cannabidiol injected into the bed nucleus of the stria terminalis are mediated by 5-HT$_{1A}$ receptors. *Psychopharmacology (Berl)* 213(2–3):465–73.

Gonzalez-Cuevas, G., Martin-Fardon, R., Kerr, T.M., Stouffer, D.G., Parsons, L.H., Hammell, D.C., Banks, S.L., Stinchcomb, A.L., Weiss, F. 2018. Unique treatment potential of cannabidiol for the prevention of relapse to drug use: preclinical proof of principle. *Neuropsychopharmacology* 43(10):2036–45.

Grace, A.A., Gomes, F.V. 2019. The circuitry of dopamine system regulation and its disruption in schizophrenia: insights into treatment and prevention. *Schizophr Bull* 45(1):148–57.

Graeff, F.G., Guimarães, F.S., De Andrade, T.G., Deakin, J.F. 1996. Role of 5-HT in stress,anxiety, and depression. *Pharmacol Biochem Behav* 54(1):129–41.

Granjeiro, E.M., Gomes, F.V., Guimaraes, F.S., Correa, F.M., Resstel, L.B. 2011. Effects of intracisternal administration of cannabidiol on the cardiovascular and behavioral responses to acute restraint stress. *Pharmacol Biochem Behav* 99(4):743–8.

Guimarães, F.S., Chiaretti, T.M., Graeff, F.G., Zuardi, A.W. 1990. Antianxiety effect of cannabidiol in the elevated plus-maze. *Psychopharmacology (Berl)* 100(4):558–9.

Guimarães, F.S., Carobrez, A.P., De Aguiar, J.C., Graeff, F.G. 1991. Anxiolytic effect in the elevated plus-maze of the NMDA receptor antagonist AP7 microinjected into the dorsal periaqueductal grey. *Psychopharmacology (Berl)* 103(1):91–4.

Guimaraes, V.M., Zuardi, A.W., Del Bel, E.A., Guimaraes, F.S. 2004. Cannabidiol increases Fos expression in the nucleus accumbens but not in the dorsal striatum. *Life Sci* 75(5):633–8.

Gururajan, A., Taylor, D.A., Malone, D.T. 2011. Effect of cannabidiol in a MK-801-rodent model of aspects of schizophrenia. *Behav Brain Res* 222(2):299–308.

Hallak, J.E., Dursun, S.M., Bosi, D.C., de Macedo, L.R., Machado-de-Sousa, J.P., Abrao, J., Crippa, J.A., McGuire, P., Krystal, J.H., Baker, G.B., Zuardi, A.W. 2011. The interplay of cannabinoid and NMDA glutamate receptor systems in humans: preliminary evidence of interactive effects of cannabidiol and ketamine in healthy human subjects. *Prog Neuropsychopharmacol Biol Psychiatry* 35(1):198–202.

Hallak, J.E., Machado-de-Sousa, J.P., Crippa, J.A., Sanches, R.F., Trzesniak, C., Chaves, C., Bernardo, S.A., Regalo, S.C., Zuardi, A.W. 2010. Performance of schizophrenic patients in the Stroop Color Word Test and electrodermal responsiveness after acute administration of cannabidiol (CBD). *Braz J Psychiatry* 32(1):56–61.

Hammell, D.C., Zhang, L.P., Ma, F., Abshire, S.M., McIlwrath, S.L., Stinchcomb, A.L., Westlund, K.N. 2016. Transdermal cannabidiol reduces inflammation and pain-related behaviours in a rat model of arthritis. *Eur J Pain* 20(6):936–48.

Häring, M., Grieb, M., Monory, K., Lutz, B., Moreira, F. 2013. Cannabinoid CB_1 receptor in the modulation of stress coping behavior in mice: the role of serotonin and different forebrain neuronal subpopulations. *Neuropharmacology* 65:83–89.

Hassan, S., Eldeeb, K., Millns, P.J., Bennett, A.J., Alexander, S.P., Kendall, D.A. 2014. Cannabidiol enhances microglial phagocytosis via transient receptor potential (TRP) channel activation. *Br J Pharmacol* 171(9):2426–39.

Hind, W.H., England, T.J., O'Sullivan, S.E. 2016. Cannabidiol protects an in vitro model of the blood-brain barrier from oxygen-glucose deprivation via PPARγ and 5-HT_{1A} receptors. *Br J Pharmacol* 173(5):815–25.

Hine, B., Torrelio, M., Gershon, S. 1975a. Differential effect of cannabinol and cannabidiol on THC-induced responses during abstinence in morphine-dependent rats. *Res Commun Chem Pathol Pharmacol* 12(1):185–8.

Hine, B., Torrelio, M., Gershon, S. 1975b. Interactions between cannabidiol and delta9-THC during abstinence in morphine-dependent rats. *Life Sci* 17:851–857.

Howlett, A.C. 1985. Cannabinoid inhibition of adenylate cyclase. Biochemistry of the response in neuroblastoma cell membranes. *Mol Pharmacol* 27(4):429–36.

Hsiao, Y.T., Yi, P.L., Li, C.L., Chang, F.C. 2012. Effect of cannabidiol on sleep disruption induced by the repeated combination tests consisting of open field and elevated plus-maze in rats. *Neuropharmacology* 62(1):373–84.

Hunt C.A., Jones, R.T., Herning, R.I., Bachman J. 1981. Evidence that cannabidiol does not significantly alter the pharmacokinetics of tetrahydrocannabinol in man. *J Pharmacokinet Biopharm* 9, 245–60.

Hurd, Y.L. 2017. Cannabidiol: swinging the marijuana pendulum from 'weed' to medication to treat the opioid epidemic. *Trends Neurosci* 40(3):124–127.

Hurd, Y.L., Yoon, M., Manini, A.F., Hernandez, S., Olmedo, R., Ostman, M., Jutras-Aswad, D. 2015. Early phase in the development of cannabidiol as a treatment for addiction: opioid relapse takes initial center stage. *Neurotherapeutics* 12(4):807–15.

Ibeas Bih, C., Chen, T., Nunn, A.V., Bazelot, M., Dallas, M., Whalley, B.J. 2015. Molecular targets of cannabidiol in neurological disorders. *Neurotherapeutics* 12(4):699–730.

Katsidoni, V., Anagnostou, I., Panagis, G. 2013. Cannabidiol inhibits the reward-facilitating effect of morphine: involvement of 5-HT_{1A} receptors in the dorsal raphe nucleus. *Addict Biol* 18(2):286–96.

Kaufman, J., DeLorenzo, C., Choudhury, S., Parsey, R. 2016. The 5-HT_{1A} receptor in major depressive disorder. *Eur Neuropsychopharmacol* 26:397–410.

Kia, H.K., Miquel, M.C., Brisorgueil, M.J., Daval, G., Riad, M., El Mestikawy, S., Hamon, M., Vergé, D. 1996. Immunocytochemical localization of serotonin1A receptors in the rat central nervous system. *J Comp Neurol* 365(2):289–305.

Koob, G.F. 2006. The neurobiology of addiction: a neuroadaptational view relevant for diagnosis. *Addiction* 101(Suppl 1):23–30.

Laprairie, R.B., Bagher, A.M., Kelly, M.E.M., Denovan-Wright, E.M. 2015. Cannabidiol is a negative allosteric modulator of the cannabinoid CB_1 receptor. *Br J Pharmacol* 172:4790–805.

Lattanzi, S., Brigo, F., Trinka, E., Zaccara, G., Cagnetti, C., Del Giovane, C., Silvestrini, M. 2018. Efficacy and safety of cannabidiol in epilepsy: a systematic review and meta-analysis. *Drugs* 78(17):1791–804.

Lemos, J.I., Resstel, L.B., Guimaraes, F.S. 2010. Involvement of the prelimbic prefrontal cortex on cannabidiol-induced attenuation of contextual conditioned fear in rats. *Behav Brain Res* 207(1):105–111.

Leshner, A.I. 1997. Addiction is a brain disease, and it matters. *Science* 278:45–7.

Levin, R., Peres, F.F., Almeida, V., Calzavara, M.B., Zuardi, A.W., Hallak, J.E., Crippa, J.A., Abilio, V.C. 2014. Effects of cannabinoid drugs on the deficit of prepulse inhibition of startle in an animal model of schizophrenia: the SHR strain. *Front Pharmacol* 5:10.

Leweke, F.M., Piomelli, D., Pahlisch, F., Muhl, D., Gerth, C.W., Hoyer, C., Klosterkotter, J., Hellmich, M., Koethe, D. 2012. Cannabidiol enhances anandamide signaling and alleviates psychotic symptoms of schizophrenia. *Transl Psychiatry* 2:e94.

Lewis, D.A., Hashimoto, T., Volk, D.W. 2005. Cortical inhibitory neurons and schizophrenia. *Nat Rev Neurosci* 6(4):312–24.

Li, N., Lee, B., Liu, R.-J., Banasr, M., Dwyer, J.M., Iwata, M., Li, X.-Y., Aghajanian, G., Duman, R.S. 2010. mTOR-dependent synapse formation underlies the rapid antidepressant effects of NMDA antagonists. *Science* 329:959–964.

Linares, I.M., Zuardi, A.W., Pereira, L.C., Queiroz, R.H., Mechoulam, R., Guimarães, F.S., Crippa, J.A. 2018. Cannabidiol presents an inverted U-shaped dose-response curve in a simulated public speaking test. *Braz J Psychiatry*:S1516-44462018005007102.

Linge, R., Jiménez-Sánchez, L., Campa, L., Pilar-Cuéllar, F., Vidal, R., Pazos, A., Adell, A., Díaz, Á. 2016. Cannabidiol induces rapid-acting antidepressant-like effects and enhances cortical 5-HT/glutamate neurotransmission: role of 5-HT$_{1A}$ receptors. *Neuropharmacology* 103:16–26.

Long, L.E., Chesworth, R., Huang, X.F., Wong, A., Spiro, A., McGregor, I.S., Arnold, J.C., Karl, T. 2012. Distinct neurobehavioural effects of cannabidiol in transmembrane domain neuregulin 1 mutant mice. *PLoS One* 7(4):e34129.

Long, L.E., Chesworth, R., Huang, X.F., McGregor, I.S., Arnold, J.C., Karl, T. 2010. A behavioural comparison of acute and chronic Delta9-tetrahydrocannabinol and cannabidiol in C57BL/6JArc mice. *Int J Neuropsychopharmacol* 13(7): 861–76.

Long, L.E., Malone, D.T., Taylor, D.A. 2006. Cannabidiol reverses MK-801-induced disruption of prepulse inhibition in mice. *Neuropsychopharmacology* 31(4):795–803.

Lujan, M.A., Castro-Zavala, A., Alegre-Zurano, L., Valverde, O. 2018. Repeated Cannabidiol treatment reduces cocaine intake and modulates neural proliferation and CB$_1$R expression in the mouse hippocampus. *Neuropharmacology* 143:163–175.

Makiol, C., Kluge, M. 2018. Remission of severe, treatment-resistant schizophrenia following adjunctive cannabidiol. *Aust N Z J Psychiatry*:4867418815982.

Marinho, A.L., Vila-Verde, C., Fogaça, M.V., Guimarães, F.S. 2015. Effects of intra-infralimbic prefrontal cortex injections of cannabidiol in the modulation of emotional behaviors in rats: contribution of 5-HT$_{1A}$ receptors and stressful experiences. *Behav Brain Res* 286:49–56.

Markos, J.R., Harris, H.M., Gul, W., ElSohly, M.A., Sufka, K.J. 2018. Effects of cannabidiol on morphine conditioned place preference in mice. *Planta Med* 84(4):221–224.

Martín-Moreno, A.M., Reigada, D., Ramírez, B.G., Mechoulam, R., Innamorato, N., Cuadrado, A., de Ceballos, M.L. 2011. Cannabidiol and other cannabinoids reduce microglial activation in vitro and in vivo: relevance to Alzheimer's disease. *Mol Pharmacol* 79(6):964–73.

Matsuda, L.A., Lolait, S.J., Brownstein, M.J., Young, A.C., Bonner, T.I. 1990. Structure of a cannabinoid receptor and functional expression of the cloned cDNA. *Nature* 346(6284):561–4.

McGuire, P., Robson, P., Cubala, W.J., Vasile, D., Morrison, P.D., Barron, R., Taylor, A., Wright, S. 2018. Cannabidiol (CBD) as an adjunctive therapy in schizophrenia: a multicenter randomized controlled trial. *Am J Psychiatry* 175(3):225–231.

McLaughlin, R., Hill, M., Bambico, F., Stuhr, K., Gobbi, G., Hillard, C., Gorzalka, B. 2012. Prefrontal cortical anandamide signaling coordinates coping responses to stress through a serotonergic pathway. *Eur Neuropsychopharmacol* 22:664–671.

Mecha, M., Torrao, A.S., Mestre, L., Carrillo-Salinas, F.J., Mechoulam, R., Guaza, C. 2012. Cannabidiol protects oligodendrocyte progenitor cells from inflammation-induced apoptosis by attenuating endoplasmic reticulum stress. *Cell Death Dis* 3:e331.

Mechoulam, R., Shvo, Y. 1963. The structure of cannabidiol. *Tetrahedron* 19:2073–8.

Michalik, L, Auwerx, J., Berger, J.P., Chatterjee, V.K., Glass, C.K., Gonzalez, F.J., Grimaldi, P.A., Kadowaki, T., Lazar, M.A., O'Rahilly, S., Palmer, C.N., Plutzky, J., Reddy, J.K., Spiegelman, B.M., Staels, B., Wahli, W. 2016. International union of pharmacology. LXI. Peroxisome proliferator-activated receptors. *Pharmacol Rev* 58(4):726–41.

Miller, R. 2009. Mechanisms of action of antipsychotic drugs of different classes, refractoriness to therapeutic effects of classical neuroleptics, and individual variation in sensitivity to their actions: Part I. *Curr Neuropharmacol* 7(4):302–14.

Moreira, F.A., Aguiar, D.C., Guimaraes, F.S. 2006. Anxiolytic- like effect of cannabidiol in the rat Vogel conflict test. *Prog Neuropsy chopharmacol Biol Psychiatry* 30:1466–1471.

Moreira, F.A., Aguiar, D.C., Guimarães, F.S. 2007. Anxiolytic-like effect of cannabinoids injected into the rat dorsolateral periaqueductal gray. *Neuropharmacology* 52(3):958–65.

Moreira, F.A., Guimaraes, F.S. 2005. Cannabidiol inhibits the hyperlocomotion induced by psychotomimetic drugs in mice. *Eur J Pharmacol* 512(2–3):199–205.

Morgan, C.J., Das, R.K., Joye, A., Curran, H.V., Kamboj, S.K. 2013. Cannabidiol reduces cigarette consumption in tobacco smokers: preliminary findings. *Addict Behav* 38(9):2433–6.

Morgan, C.J., Freeman, T.P., Schafer, G.L., Curran, H.V. 2010a. Cannabidiol attenuates the appetitive effects of Delta 9-tetrahydrocannabinol in humans smoking their chosen cannabis. *Neuropsychopharmacology* 35(9):1879–85.

Morgan, C.J., Schafer, G., Freeman, T.P., Curran, H.V. 2010b. Impact of cannabidiol on the acute memory and psychotomimetic effects of smoked cannabis: naturalistic study. *Br J Psychiatry* 197(4):285–90.

Nardo, M., Casarotto, P.C., Gomes, F.V., Guimaraes, F.S. 2014. Cannabidiol reverses the mCPP-induced increase in marble-burying behavior. *Fundam Clin Pharmacol* 28(5):544–50.

Navarro, G., Reyes-Resina, I., Rivas-Santisteban, R., Sánchez de Medina, V., Morales, P., Casano, S., Ferreiro-Vera, C., Lillo, A., Aguinaga, D., Jagerovic, N., Nadal, X., Franco, R. 2018. Cannabidiol skews biased agonism at cannabinoid CB_1 and CB_2 receptors with smaller effect in CB_1-CB_2 heteroreceptor complexes. *Biochem Pharmacol* 157:148–158.

NCT03310593. 2017. Cannabidiol as an adjunctive treatment for bipolar depression (CBDBD) [WWW Document]. https://clinicaltrials.gov/ct2/show/NCT03310593?term=cannabidiol&cond=%22Depression%22&rank=1.

Nestler, E.J., Hyman, S.E. 2010. Animal models of neuropsychiatric disorders. *Nature Neurosci* 13:1161–9.

Onaivi, E.S., Green, M.R., Martin, B.R. 1990. Pharmacological characterization of cannabinoids in the elevated plus maze. *J Pharmacol Exp Ther* 253(3):1002–9.

Osborne, A.L., Solowij, N., Babic, I., Huang, X.F., Weston-Green, K. 2017. Improved social interaction, recognition and working memory with cannabidiol treatment in a prenatal infection (poly I:C) rat model. *Neuropsychopharmacology* 42(7):1447–57.

Parker, L.A., Burton, P., Sorge, R.E., Yakiwchuk, C., Mechoulam, R. 2004. Effect of low doses of delta9-tetrahydrocannabinol and cannabidiol on the extinction of cocaine-induced and amphetamine-induced conditioned place preference learning in rats. *Psychopharmacology (Berl)* 175(3):360–6.

Pedrazzi, J.F., Issy, A.C., Gomes, F.V., Guimaraes, F.S., Del-Bel, E.A. 2015. Cannabidiol effects in the prepulse inhibition disruption induced by amphetamine. *Psychopharmacology (Berl)* 232(16):3057–65.

Pellati, F., Borgonetti, V., Brighenti, V., Biagi, M., Benvenuti, S., Corsi, L. 2018. Cannabis sativa L. and nonpsychoactive cannabinoids: their chemistry and role against oxidative stress, inflammation, and cancer. *Biomed Res Int* 2018:1691428.

Peres, F.F., Diana, M.C., Levin, R., Suiama, M.A., Almeida, V., Vendramini, A.M., Santos, C.M., Zuardi, A.W., Hallak, J.E.C., Crippa, J.A., Abilio, V.C. 2018. Cannabidiol administered during peri-adolescence prevents behavioral abnormalities in an animal model of schizophrenia. *Front Pharmacol* 9:901.

Pertwee, R.G., Ross, R.A., Craib, S.J., Thomas, A. 2002. (-)-Cannabidiol antagonizes cannabinoid receptor agonists and noradrenaline in the mouse vas deferens. *Eur J Pharmacol* 456(1–3):99–106.

Piñeyro, G., Blier, P. 1999. Autoregulation of serotonin neurons: role in antidepressant drug action. *Pharmacol Rev* 51(3):533–91.

Poleg, S., Golubchik, P., Offen, D., Weizman, A. 2018. Cannabidiol as a suggested candidate for treatment of autism spectrum disorder. *Prog Neuropsychopharmacol Biol Psychiatry* 89:90–96.

Radewicz, K., Garey, L.J., Gentleman, S.M., Reynolds, R. 2000. Increase in HLA-DR immunoreactive microglia in frontal and temporal cortex of chronic schizophrenics. *J Neuropathol Exp Neurol* 59(2):137–50.

Ren, Y., Whittard, J., Higuera-Matas, A., Morris, C.V., Hurd, Y.L. 2009. Cannabidiol, a nonpsychotropic component of cannabis, inhibits cue-induced heroin seeking and normalizes discrete mesolimbic neuronal disturbances. *J Neurosci* 29(47):14764–9.

Renard, J., Loureiro, M., Rosen, L.G., Zunder, J., de Oliveira, C., Schmid, S., Rushlow, W.J., Laviolette, S.R. 2016. Cannabidiol counteracts amphetamine-induced neuronal and behavioral sensitization of the mesolimbic dopamine pathway through a novel mTOR/p70S6 kinase signaling pathway. *J Neurosci* 36(18):5160–9.

Resstel, L.B., Joca, S.R., Moreira, F.A., Correa, F.M., Guimaraes, F.S. 2006. Effects of cannabidiol and diazepam on behavioural and cardiovascular responses induced by contextual conditioned fear in rats. *Behav Brain Res* 172:294–298.

Resstel, L.B., Tavares, R.F., Lisboa, S.F., Joca, S.R., Correa, F.M., Guimaraes, F.S. 2009. 5-HT$_{1A}$ receptors are involved in the cannabidiol-induced attenuation of behavioural and cardiovascular responses to acute restraint stress in rats. *Br J Pharmacol* 156(1):181–8.

Réus, G.Z., Stringari, R.B., Ribeiro, K.F., Luft, T., Abelaira, H.M., Fries, G.R., Aguiar, B.W., Kapczinski, F., Hallak, J.E., Zuardi, A.W., Crippa, J.a., Quevedo, J. 2011. Administration of cannabidiol and imipramine induces antidepressant-like effects in the forced swimming test and increases brain-derived neurotrophic factor levels in the rat amygdala. *Acta Neuropsychiatr* 23:241–248.

Rock, E.M., Bolognini, D., Limebeer, C.L., Cascio, M.G., Anavi-Goffer, S., Fletcher, P.J., Mechoulam, R., Pertwee, R.G., Parker, L.A. 2012. Cannabidiol, a non-psychotropic component of cannabis, attenuates vomiting and nausea-like behaviour via indirect agonism of 5-HT(1A) somatodendritic autoreceptors in the dorsal raphe nucleus. *Br J Pharmacol* 165(8):2620–34.

Rock, E.M., Limebeer, C.L., Petrie, G.N., Williams, L.A, Mechoulam, R., Parker, L.A. 2017. Effect of prior foot shock stress and Δ(9)-tetrahydrocannabinol, cannabidiolic acid, and cannabidiol on anxiety-like responding in the light-dark emergence test in rats. *Psychopharmacology (Berl)* 234(14):2207–17.

Rubino, T., Guidali, C., Vigano, D., Realini, N., Valenti, M., Massi, P., Parolaro, D. 2008. CB$_1$ receptor stimulation in specific brain areas differently modulate anxiety-related behaviour. *Neuropharmacology* 54:151–160.

Russo, E.B., Burnett, A., Hall, B., Parker, K.K. 2005. Agonistic properties of cannabidiol at 5-HT$_{1A}$ receptors. *Neurochem Res* 30(8):1037–43.

Ryan, D., Drysdale, A.J., Lafourcade, C., Pertwee, R.G., Platt, B. 2009. Cannabidiol targets mitochondria to regulate intracellular Ca^{2+} levels. *J Neurosci* 29(7):2053–63.

Sales, A.J., Crestani, C.C., Guimarães, F.S., Joca, S.R.L. 2018. Antidepressant-like effect induced by cannabidiol is dependent on brain serotonin levels. *Prog Neuro Psychopharmacol Biol Psychiatry* 86:255–261.

Sales, A.J., Fogaça, M.V., Sartim, A.G., Pereira, V.S., Wegener, G., Guimarães, F.S., Joca, S.R.L. 2019. Cannabidiol induces rapid and sustained antidepressant-like effects through increased BDNF signaling and synaptogenesis in the prefrontal cortex. *Mol Neurobiol* 56(2):1070–1081.

Samuels, B.A., Hen, R. 2011. Neurogenesis and affective disorders. *Eur J Neurosci* 33(6):1152–9.

Santarelli, L., Saxe, M., Gross, C., Surget, A., Battaglia, F., Dulawa, S., Weisstaub, N., Lee, J., Duman, R., Arancio, O., Belzung, C., Hen, R. 2003. Requirement of hippocampal neurogenesis for the behavioral effects of antidepressants. *Science* 301(5634):805–9.

Sartim, A.G., Guimarães, F.S., Joca, S.R.L. 2016. Antidepressant-like effect of cannabidiol injection into the ventral medial prefrontal cortex—possible involvement of 5-HT$_{1A}$ and CB$_1$ receptors. *Behav Brain Res* 303:218–27.

Sartim, A.G., Sales, A.J., Guimarães, F.S., Joca, S.R.L. 2018. Hippocampal mammalian target of rapamycin is implicated in stress-coping behavior induced by cannabidiol in the forced swim test. *J Psychopharmacol* 32:922–931.

Schiavon, A.P., Bonato, J.M., Milani, H., Guimarães, F.S., Weffort de Oliveira, R.M. 2016. Influence of single and repeated cannabidiol administration on emotional behavior and markers of cell proliferation and neurogenesis in non-stressed mice. *Prog Neuro Psychopharmacol Biol Psychiatry* 64:27–34.

Schoedel, K.A., Szeto, I., Setnik, B., Sellers, E.M., Levy-Cooperman, N., Mills, C., Etges, T., Sommerville, K. 2018. Abuse potential assessment of cannabidiol (CBD) in recreational polydrug users: a randomized, double-blind, controlled trial. *Epilepsy Behav* 88:162–71.

Shannon, S., Lewis, N., Lee, H., Hughes, S. 2019. Cannabidiol in anxiety and sleep: a large case series. *Perm J*:18–041.

Shbiro, L., Hen-Shoval, D., Hazut, N., Rapps, K., Dar, S., Zalsman, G., Mechoulam, R., Weller, A., Shoval, G. 2019 Effects of cannabidiol in males and females in two different rat models of depression. *Physiol Behav* 201:59–63.

Shoval, G., Shbiro, L., Hershkovitz, L., Hazut, N., Zalsman, G., Mechoulam, R., Weller, A. 2016. Prohedonic effect of cannabidiol in a rat model of depression. *Neuropsychobiology* 73:123–9.

Silveira Filho, N.G., Tufik, S. 1981. Comparative effects between cannabidiol and diazepam on neo- phobia, food intake and conflict behavior. *Res Commun Psychol Psychiatr Behav* 6:251–266.

Soares, V.d.P., Campos, A.C., Bortoli, V.C., Zangrossi, H., Jr., Guimaraes, F.S., Zuardi, A.W. 2010. Intra-dorsal periaqueductal gray administration of cannabidiol blocks panic-like response by activating 5-HT$_{1A}$ receptors. *Behav Brain Res* 213(2):225–229.

Sonego, A.B., Gomes, F.V., Del Bel, E.A., Guimaraes, F.S. 2016. Cannabidiol attenuates haloperidol-induced catalepsy and c-Fos protein expression in the dorsolateral striatum via 5-HT$_{1A}$ receptors in mice. *Behav Brain Res* 309:22–8.

Sonego, A.B., Prado, D.S., Vale, G.T., Sepulveda-Diaz, J.E., Cunha, T.M., Tirapelli, C.R., Del Bel, E.A., Raisman-Vozari, R., Guimaraes, F.S. 2018. Cannabidiol prevents haloperidol-induced vacuos chewing movements and inflammatory changes in mice via PPARgamma receptors. *Brain Behav Immun* 74:241–51.

Song, C., Stevenson, C.W., Guimaraes, F.S., Lee, J.L. 2016. Bidirectional effects of cannabidiol on contextual fear memory extinction. *Front Pharmacol* 7:493.

Stark, T., Ruda-Kucerova, J., Iannotti, F.A., D'Addario, C., Di Marco, R., Pekarik, V., Drazanova, E., Piscitelli, F., Bari, M., Babinska, Z., Giurdanella, G., Di Bartolomeo, M., Salomone, S., Sulcova, A., Maccarrone, M., Wotjak, C.T., Starcuk Jr., Z., Drago, F., Mechoulam, R., Di Marzo, V., Micale, V. 2019. Peripubertal cannabidiol treatment rescues behavioral and neurochemical abnormalities in the MAM model of schizophrenia. *Neuropharmacology* 146:212–21.

Stern, C.A., da Silva, T.R., Raymundi, A.M., de Souza, C.P., Hiroaki-Sato, V.A., Kato, L., Guimarães, F.S., Andreatini, R., Takahashi, R.N., Bertoglio, L.J. 2017. Cannabidiol disrupts the consolidation of specific and generalized fear memories via dorsal hippocampus CB(1) and CB(2) receptors. *Neuropharmacology* 125:220–30.

Stern, C.A., Gazarini, L., Takahashi, R.N., Guimarães, F.S., Bertoglio, L.J. 2012. On disruption of fear memory by reconsolidation blockade: evidence from cannabidiol treatment. *Neuropsychopharmacology* 37(9):2132–42.

Steullet, P., Cabungcal, J.H., Coyle, J., Didriksen, M., Gill, K., Grace, A.A., Hensch, T.K., LaMantia, A.S., Lindemann, L., Maynard, T.M., Meyer, U., Morishita, H., O'Donnell, P., Puhl, M., Cuenod, M., Do, K.Q. 2017. Oxidative stress-driven parvalbumin interneuron impairment as a common mechanism in models of schizophrenia. *Mol Psychiatry* 22(7):936–943.

Tanti, A., Belzung, C. 2013. Hippocampal neurogenesis: a biomarker for depression or antidepressant effects? methodological considerations and perspectives for future research. *Cell Tissue Res* 354:203–219.

Taylor, L., Gidal, B., Blakey, G., Tayo, B., Morrison, G. 2018. A phase I, randomized, double-blind, placebo-controlled, single ascending dose, multiple dose, and food effect trial of the safety, tolerability and pharmacokinetics of highly purified cannabidiol in healthy subjects. *CNS Drugs* 32(11):1053–67.

Thomas, A., Baillie, G.L., Phillips, A.M., Razdan, R.K., Ross, R.A., Pertwee, R.G. 2007. Cannabidiol displays unexpectedly high potency as an antagonist of CB_1 and CB_2 receptor agonists in vitro. *Br J Pharmacol* 150:613–23.

Todd, A.R. 1946. Hashish. *Experientia* 2:55–60.

Turna, J., Syan, S.K., Frey, B.N., Rush, B., Costello, J., Weiss, M., MacKillop, J. 2019. Cannabidiol as a novel candidate alcohol use disorder pharmacotherapy: a systematic review. *Alcohol Clin Exp Res* 43(4):550–563.

Twardowschy, A., Castiblanco-Urbina, M.A., Uribe-Mariño, A., Biagioni, A.F., Salgado-Rohner, C.J., Crippa, J.A., Coimbra, N.C. 2013. The role of $5-HT_{1A}$ receptors in the anti-aversive effects of cannabidiol on panic attack-like behaviors evoked in the presence of the wild snake Epicrates cenchria crassus (Reptilia, Boidae). *J Psychopharmacol* 27(12):1149–59.

Uribe-Mariño, A., Francisco, A., Castiblanco-Urbina, M.A., Twardowschy, A., Salgado-Rohner, C.J., Crippa, J.A., Hallak, J.E., Zuardi, A.W., Coimbra, N.C. 2012. Anti-aversive effects of cannabidiol on innate fear-induced behaviors evoked by an ethological model of panic attacks based on a prey vs. the wild snake Epicrates cenchria crassus confrontation paradigm. *Neuropsychopharmacology* 37(2):412–21.

Vila-Verde, C., Marinho, A.L., Lisboa, S.F., Guimarães, F.S. 2016. Nitric oxide in the prelimbic medial prefrontal cortex is involved in the anxiogenic-like effect induced by acute restraint stress in rats. *Neuroscience* 320:30–42.

Wolf, S.A., Bick-Sander, A., Fabel, K., Leal-Galicia, P., Tauber, S., Ramirez-Rodriguez, G., Müller, A., Melnik, A., Waltinger, T.P., Ullrich, O., Kempermann, G. 2010. Cannabinoid receptor CB_1 mediates baseline and activity-induced survival of new neurons in adult hippocampal neurogenesis. *Cell Commun Signal* 8:12.

Zanelati, T.V., Biojone, C., Moreira, F.A., Guimaraes, F.S., Joca, S.R. 2010. Antidepressant-like effects of cannabidiol in mice: possible involvement of $5-HT_{1A}$ receptors. *Br J Pharmacol* 159(1):122–8.

Zendulka, O., Dovrtělová, G., Nosková, K., Turjap, M., Šulcová, A., Hanuš, L., Juřica, J. 2016. Cannabinoids and cytochrome P450 interactions. *Curr Drug Metab* 17(3):206–26.

Zhang, Z., Wang, W., Zhong, P., Liu, S., Long, J., Zhao, L., Gao, H., Cravatt, B., Liu, Q. 2015. Blockade of 2-arachidonoylglycerol hydrolysis produces antidepressant-like effects and enhances adult hippocampal neurogenesis and synaptic plasticity. *Hippocampus* 25:16–26.

Zhou, J., Cao, X., Mar, A.C., Ding, Y.Q., Wang, X., Li, Q., Li, L. 2014. Activation of post-synaptic 5-HT$_{1A}$ receptors improve stress adaptation. *Psychopharmacology (Berl)* 231:2067–75.

Zuardi, A.W. 2008. Cannabidiol: from an inactive cannabinoid to a drug with wide spectrum of action. *Rev Bras Psiquiatr* 30:271–80

Zuardi, A.W., Karniol, I.G. 1983. Changes in the conditioned emotional response of rats induced by Δ9-THC, CBD and mixture of the two cannabinoids. *Braz Arch Biol Technol* 26:391–7

Zuardi, A.W., Cosme, R.A., Graeff, F.G., Guimarães, F.S. 1993. Effects of ipsapirone and cannabidiol on human experimental anxiety. *J Psychopharmacol* 7:82–8.

Zuardi, A.W., Crippa, J.A., Hallak, J.E., Pinto, J.P., Chagas, M.H., Rodrigues, G.G., Dursun, S.M., Tumas, V. 2009. Cannabidiol for the treatment of psychosis in Parkinson's disease. *J Psychopharmacol* 23(8):979–83.

Zuardi, A.W., Hallak, J.E., Dursun, S.M., Morais, S.L., Sanches, R.F., Musty, R.E., Crippa, J.A. 2006. Cannabidiol monotherapy for treatment-resistant schizophrenia. *J Psychopharmacol* 20(5):683–6.

Zuardi, A.W., Morais, S.L., Guimaraes, F.S., Mechoulam, R. 1995. Antipsychotic effect of cannabidiol. *J Clin Psychiatry* 56(10):485–6.

Zuardi, A.W., Rodrigues, J.A., Cunha, J.M. 1991. Effects of cannabidiol in animal models predictive of antipsychotic activity. *Psychopharmacology (Berl)* 104(2):260–4.

Zuardi, A.W., Rodrigues, N.P., Silva, A.L., Bernardo, S.A., Hallak, J.E.C., Guimarães, F.S., Crippa, J.A.S. 2017. Inverted U-shaped dose-response curve of the anxiolytic effect of cannabidiol during public speaking in real life. *Front Pharmacol* 11(8):259.

Zuardi, A.W., Shirakawa, I., Finkelfarb, E., Karniol, I.G. 1982. Action of cannabidiol on the anxiety and other effects produced by delta 9-THC in normal subjects. *Psychopharmacology (Berl)* 76(3):245–50.

11 Emerging Clinical and Mechanistic Support for CBD Treatment of Autism Spectrum Disorder

Kaylee Martig, Keelee Reid, and Joshua S. Kaplan
Western Washington University

CONTENTS

INTRODUCTION

Autism spectrum disorder (ASD) is a complex heterogeneous neurodevelopmental disorder characterized by core deficits in social, communication, and motor behaviors.[1] Additional common comorbidities such as anxiety, sleep disturbances, hyperactivity, and self-injurious behavior negatively impact quality of life. As a spectrum, the severity of ASD symptoms ranges across individuals as a function of underlying etiology, but we'd like to note here that the following discussion relates the potential utility of cannabis treatment for individuals on the severe end of the ASD spectrum. Any drug should be used only when empirically supported benefits outweigh the potential risks, and as such conversation surrounding the use of cannabis to treat ASD should be for the treatment of severe symptoms, such as severe feeding disorders and self-harm, rather than to limit neurodivergence. The goal is not to eradicate diversity but to improve functioning and quality of life.

The severity of core and comorbid ASD symptoms is determined by numerous environmental[2] and genetic factors.[3] Together, these factors impact a range of neurochemical signaling mechanisms that have been shown to participate in the development and expression of ASD symptoms.[4] One common underlying neural feature of the ASD brain across different etiologies is an increased ratio of excitation/inhibition

(E/I).[5] The promising therapeutic benefits of cannabis-based treatment strategies for ASD can be conceptualized by considering the neural systems defective in ASD and their utility to restore the brain's excitatory/inhibitory balance.

An elevated E/I ratio could reflect increased excitatory signaling by the neurotransmitter, glutamate, or reduced inhibitory signaling by the neurotransmitter, GABA. Reduced GABAergic signaling is a common neurological substrate of the ASD brain[6] that may reflect various genetic or environmental etiologies and is a marker that predicts symptom severity.[7] Impairments to GABAergic signaling may result from factors that perturb the development of neural circuits,[8] reduce the excitability of GABAergic neurons,[9-11] or impair modulatory neurochemical systems, such as the endocannabinoid system.[12] As discussed in the following section, the resulting elevation in the E/I ratio can drive ASD symptoms and represents a targetable mechanism for pharmacological intervention.

AN ELEVATED E/I RATIO IS A NEURAL SUBSTRATE OF CORE ASD SYMPTOMS

The elevated E/I balance in ASD underlies numerous behavioral phenotypes and provides a neuropathological framework for the *Intense World Theory* of ASD to explain ASD's core features.[13] This theory proposes that hyperexcitability of neural circuits leads to hyper-sensitivity to stimuli, hyper-reactivity, developmental hyper-connectivity, hyper-attention, and hyper-emotionality. Within this framework, social withdrawal and avoidance, for example, stems from hyperexcitability of threat-detection circuitry including the amygdala during fear-conditioning assays in rodents[14] and during emotional face processing in humans.[15] The especially strong reactions to stimuli (including sensory and social) can bias preferences away from novelty in favor of highly secure predictable outcomes that is consistent with social withdrawal. Notably, the hyper-responsive cortical and subcortical brain regions implicated in the Intense World Theory are enriched in cannabinoid type I (CB$_1$) receptor expression,[16-20] making the endocannabinoid system a potential therapeutic target to restore E/I balance.

Substantial elevation in the E/I balance among those on the severe end of the autism spectrum can lead to epilepsy, which is observed in 30% of ASD cases and is associated with increased core and comorbid severity.[21] Comorbid ASD and epilepsy have been modeled in the lab by mice expressing a heterozygous mutation to the *SCN1A* gene.[9,10] These mice have reduced excitatory drive of inhibitory GABAergic interneurons resulting in an elevated E/I balance.[10,22] Acute injections of cannabidiol (CBD) restored the E/I balance in these mice, rescued ASD-like social impairment, and reduced the frequency of spontaneous epileptic seizures.[23] Intriguingly, ASD-like social behaviors were improved by CBD in adult mice even after weeks of frequent spontaneous seizure activity.[23] This proposes that in some cases, behavioral rescue can be achieved by acutely restoring the E/I balance, regardless of developmental seizure experience. Therefore, restoring the E/I balance, either by increasing inhibition or reducing excitation may improve ASD symptoms.

Optogenetic approaches have provided valuable insight into the causal role that the E/I balance plays in social behavior independent of disease-related developmental perturbations. Elevating the E/I ratio in the mouse medial prefrontal cortex, but not reducing it, decreased time spent in social interaction and in social exploration. Further, reducing an already elevated E/I ratio by increasing GABAergic transmission partially improved these social behavioral measures.[24] These findings suggest that acutely restoring the E/I balance can improve crude measures of social behavior. These studies were followed-up in a genetic mouse model of ASD that lacked the *CNTNAP2* gene.[25] Mice lacking this gene have an elevated E/I ratio resulting from reduced GABAergic signaling from prefrontal cortical parvalbumin-positive interneurons. The activity of parvalbumin-positive interneurons increases during social interaction in wild-type mice but not mice with the *CNTNAP2* mutation. However, optogenetic stimulation of parvalbumin neurons in these genetic mice rescued the social deficits. Intriguingly, similar behavioral rescue was observed by reducing the excitability of excitatory cortical pyramidal neurons. These findings are supported by studies in humans with ASD demonstrating that increasing prefrontal GABAergic tone restores cortical functional connectivity within the region,[26] which serves as a likely neural correlate of symptom improvement. Together, these findings provide mechanistic support for pharmacological restoration of the E/I balance in rescuing social deficits.

MECHANISTIC SUPPORT FOR CBD CANNABIS-BASED TREATMENT APPROACHES TO ASD

Cannabis-based medicines represent an uncommon approach in medicinal pharmacology; most pharmaceuticals are developed and optimized in a laboratory setting before being empirically tested in pre-clinical and clinical trials. With cannabis, empirical research designed is often informed first by human use and self-medication strategies. There is amassing anecdotal evidence[27] proposing successful cannabis-based treatments for severe core and comorbid ASD symptoms that have otherwise been ineffectively controlled by current medication strategies. These anecdotal reports are gaining foundational support through understanding CBD's underlying therapeutic mechanisms and are now being corroborated by early-stage clinical trials[28,29] that have effectively reduced comorbid ASD symptoms discussed in the next section.

CBD has over 65 known targets in the brain and body.[30] CBD enhances the synaptic levels of the endocannabinoid, anandamide, by blocking its intracellular transport and competitively inhibiting its hydrolyzing FAAH enzyme, thereby enhancing signaling by cannabinoid receptors. CBD also has extensive pharmacodynamic action beyond the endocannabinoid system. Notably, CBD is a positive allosteric modulator of $GABA_A$ receptors. This action, which occurs through CBD binding at an independent site from benzodiazepines, is thought to contribute to CBD's ability to restore E/I balance without causing heavy sedation associated with benzodiazepine use.[31] Additionally, CBD inhibition of GPR55 activity enhances GABAergic signaling in the dentate gyrus of the hippocampus and is implicated in its antiepileptic effects,[23] but it remains unclear if this same mechanism elevates GABAergic signaling at lower doses relevant to ASD-like social behaviors.

Numerous lines of evidence point to a dysfunction of the endocannabinoid system in individuals with ASD.[32] Given the endocannabinoid system's role in modulating neurotransmission at GABAergic and glutamatergic synapses,[33] it can serve as an important regulator of the E/I balance, and in turn, ASD symptoms. The endocannabinoid system plays a neuromodulatory role in regulating emotional responses and social reward.[34] Furthermore, functional CB_1 receptors are prominently expressed in relevant ASD brain regions. In the amygdala, CB_1 receptors play a role in regulating the emotional response to faces.[35,36] In the prefrontal cortex and amygdala, they play a role in attenuating anxiety-like behaviors[37,38] that may also extend to anxiety-like responses within a social context.[24,25]

CB_1 receptors are also abundantly expressed in the cerebellum.[17] Cerebellar dysfunction is the most common non-genetic risk factor for ASD.[39,40] The rate of ASD-like repetitive motor behaviors is inversely correlated with the GABAergic inhibitory output from the principal output neurons for the cerebellar cortex, the Purkinje cell.[41] Further, mice with genetically reduced Purkinje cell signaling, and therefore reduced GABAergic output from the cerebellar cortex, not only show repetitive motor behaviors but also attenuated social approach and reduced preference for social novelty.[42] Disrupted cerebellar cortical output also contributes to the language deficits in ASD.[43,44] Therefore, several core ASD characteristics are recapitulated by reducing GABAergic output from the cerebellar cortex and posits that restoration of inhibitory function may rescue ASD symptoms. Currently, CBD's impact on Purkinje cell and cerebellar function remains to be elucidated.

Fitting with the important contribution of endocannabinoid signaling core ASD symptoms, plasma levels of the endocannabinoid, anandamide, are lower in children with ASD.[45,46] It's unclear at this point what contribution lower anandamide levels have on ASD symptoms, and if elevating levels with CBD, rescues core symptoms. However, in a pre-clinical experiment in the BTBR mouse model of ASD,[47] pharmacological enhancement of anandamide signaling improved social behaviors.[48] Notably, these actions were blocked by a CB_1 antagonist, supporting the important role of endocannabinoid signaling in core ASD symptoms.

To test how CBD affects the ASD brain, a series of recent studies utilized magnetic resonance spectroscopy to measure CBD's impact on the E/I balance by directly measuring GABA, glutamate, and their metabolites. The responsivity to GABA and glutamatergic modulating drugs, riluzole and CBD, differed between control and ASD subjects in the prefrontal cortex.[26,49] Given the important role of the prefrontal cortex in social behavior,[25] these findings reveal a mechanistic pathway towards CBD treatment of core social symptoms in ASD. Further, they highlight three important points: (1) the GABAergic system is different in the ASD brain; (2) GABA levels can be pharmacologically modulated in ASD by CBD; and (3) the response to CBD is unique in the ASD brain. Based on these findings, we must exhibit caution when interpreting studies of CBD in typically developing control animals or human subjects and generalizing their effects to ASD. Therefore, future studies aimed at identifying and understanding therapeutic mechanisms of ASD must use relevant ASD models or subjects.

Together, CBD has molecular action on numerous endocannabinoid and non-endocannabinoid neural substrates underlying core ASD symptoms. Whether these actions lead to clinical improvement through the proposed mechanisms remains to be empirically tested.

CLINICAL STUDIES OF CBD TREATMENT IN ASD

There are currently no empirically confirmed treatments for the core symptoms of ASD. However, several prevalent comorbidities are targeted by existing medications to varying degrees of success.[50] Common comorbidities in ASD include sleep disorders, attention deficit/hyperactivity disorder, epilepsy, gastrointestinal inflammation, and propensity to engage in self-injurious behavior.[21,50,51] These are often medicated with antidepressants, selective serotonin reuptake inhibitors, and antipsychotics. Stem cell therapies represent an emerging treatment direction[52] to combat the elevated levels of inflammation observed in ASD that are thought to contribute to both core symptoms and comorbidities.[53,54] Each of these treatments only targets one or two of the comorbid symptoms, thereby necessitating a complex treatment regimen that creates compliance and side-effect challenges.

Independent of ASD, CBD has demonstrated anxiolytic effects,[55] improves sleep when hindered by pain or anxiety,[56,57] is an effective antiepileptic in treatment-resistant forms of epilepsy,[23,58,59] has antipsychotic properties,[60–62] and is a potent anti-inflammatory.[63,64] CBD's ability to combat these comorbid symptoms raises interest in its utility as an add-on therapy or a monotherapy in treating both the core and comorbid symptoms in ASD.

To date, there are limited clinical studies of cannabis' ability to treat symptoms of ASD. Two recently published early-stage clinical trials conducted in Israel demonstrated improvement in common comorbid symptoms,[29,65] but unfortunately, cannabis' effects on core ASD symptoms were not been empirically assessed. In both studies, participants consumed a whole-plant extract containing 20:1 CBD:THC sublingually 2–4 times/day at either escalating CBD doses starting at 1 mg/kg/day and uptitrated to a maximum of 10 mg/kg/day,[65] or a consistent 16 mg/kg/day[29] (notably, there was no confirmation that the cannabis was consumed sublingually and not swallowed, which could contribute to different pharmacokinetic and pharmacodynamics properties[66]). In one of the studies, considerable behavioral improvement (i.e., "very much improved" or "much improved" on the Clinical Global Impression of Change scale) was noted in 61% of participants. 39% also reported a considerable reduction in anxiety levels, and 47% reported a considerable improvement in communication problems. Disruptive behaviors also improved by approximately 30%.[65] In the other study, overall improvement was observed in 74.5% of participants, no change in 21.6% and a worsening of symptoms in 3.9%. Among the comorbid symptoms, cannabis treatment symptoms relating to hyperactivity in 68.4%, self-injury and rage attacks in 67.6%, sleep problems in 71.4%, and anxiety in 47.1%.[29] These rates of comorbid symptom improvement are comparable to those of other medications including methylphenidate for the treatment of hyperactivity,[67] aripiprazole and risperidone for self-injurious behavior,[68,69] melatonin for sleep problems,[70] and SSRIs for anxiety.[71] Not only can this range of comorbid symptoms be treated with a single pharmacological strategy, but these benefits from cannabis were accompanied by a limited adverse side-effect profile. In one study, approximately half of the participants experienced at least one adverse effect, but these were varied with the most common being sleep disturbances in 14% of participants[65]. In the other, somnolence in 24% and decreased appetite in 12% (notably 8% showed an increase in appetite) were the most prevalent.[29] The clinical studies on cannabis treatment for ASD are limited by potential bias from parental report measures and the lack of a placebo control group. Nonetheless, they suggest that cannabis may be a safe and effective alternative approach to comorbid symptom control. Given that comorbid symptoms are ineffectively treated by prescription medications in a third of patients, cannabis treatment may be an alternative therapeutic approach when other clinical interventions fail.

These early-stage clinical trials have paved the way for larger clinical trials currently underway using CBD-rich cannabis[72] or another cannabinoid, cannabidivarin,[73] which, like CBD, is gaining recognition for its therapeutic potential in several clinical indications including epilepsy and Rett Syndrome by elevating inhibitory signaling.[74-77]

TREATMENT CHALLENGES AND LIMITATIONS

The diverse range of symptoms in ASD presents a unique treatment challenge. THC and CBD, when used independently in their purified forms, have narrow optimally therapeutic dosing ranges. Unfortunately, there are no clear dosing guidelines for clinical cannabis use. At a minimum, optimally effective dosing depends on the product's cannabinoid and terpene composition,[78] an individual's genetics,[79] and the biological sex of the user.[80,81] The current state of clinically relevant studies are limited. Clinical designs either employ a range of cannabinoid formulas or inconsistent dosing across individuals.[65] This forces patients to experiment with different doses to identify their own optimal dose with only limited guidance.

Some guidance can be provided by available studies from both rodents and humans that have identified inverted-U dose response relationships for a range of therapeutic purposes.[82-84] Overshooting the dosing window with THC carries greater risk of adverse effects than CBD,[59,85-88] so it's best to start with lower doses and titrate up. Low doses of THC can reduce anxiety-like behavior in rodents[38,86,89] and humans,[90] but moderate to high doses can be anxiogenic.[91] CBD, on the other hand, has a wider anxiolytic dose range, but its benefits are still lost at high doses.[83,92,93] The dosing challenge is especially apparent when trying to combat multiple symptoms that have their own therapeutic dosing windows. In a mouse model of Dravet Syndrome, which is characterized by epileptic seizures and ASD behaviors,[10,22,23] acute CBD doses of 10 and 20 mg/kg rescued social interaction deficits, but 100 mg/kg were needed to reduce spontaneous seizure frequency and thermally induced seizure characteristics. The loss of CBD's therapeutic efficacy on social interaction deficits at doses required to suppress epileptic seizures likely results from the activation of less sensitive neural targets whose actions dominate over those of those activated by lower doses[30] and highlight the difficulty of simultaneously treating multiple symptoms.

One strategy to overcome the dosing challenges involves integrating a more whole-plant pharmacological approach that has been used for treating other conditions such as pain[82] and epilepsy.[58,94] Whole-plant extracts have the potential to extend the therapeutic dosing window and prolong its effects over purified CBD extracts.[78,82] Through a better understanding of the complex interactions between multiple cannabinoids and terpenes, optimized cannabinoid and terpene combinations could eventually be developed that would blend the dosing ranges for treating multiple symptoms with a single dosing strategy. Currently however, there are no clear guidelines for this optimized approach.

TREATMENT CONSIDERATIONS

One of the primary factors limiting the use of CBD in pediatric populations is a poor understanding of its long-term consequences on the developing brain as a function of dose and use pattern. CBD's favorable safety profile in adults and pre-clinical rodent models[87] is often generalized to children and adolescents, yet no data exist on the long-term consequences of CBD on brain function and morphology. Clinical trials involving patients with pediatric epilepsies used CBD as an add-on therapy, thereby making it difficult to isolate CBD's contribution to adverse effects when used as a monotherapy.[58,95] The rate of patients experiencing adverse events likely increases as a function of dose.[29,58,65,95] The common adverse events detected in the epilepsy studies that utilized higher CBD doses (20–50 mg/kg/day) were diarrhea, somnolence and pyrexia.[58,59] The prevalence of CBD's side effects were lower in the initial clinical trials in ASD, which utilized lower doses.[29,65] Regardless, these adverse effects may seem favorable when compared to those of alternative pharmacological treatment strategies, or the risks associated with not medicated (e.g., self-injurious behavior).

In many cases, patients may be on additional pharmacotherapies to treat mood-related aspects of ASD. In the[65] clinical trial, 82% of children were concurrently being treated by additional pharmacotherapies, the most prevalent being antipsychotics (72%). When considering integrating CBD as a pharmacotherapy, CBD-drug interactions must be screened for possible safety concerns related to elevated levels of additional medications. CBD is a competitive inhibitor of liver cytochrome P450 enzymes[96] which are responsible for metabolizing 70%–80% of clinical medications.[97] Certain drugs may rise to toxic levels when administered in combination with cannabis as inhibition of P450 enzyme activity prevents the breakdown and removal of the drug in the body. In certain cases, it may be necessary to monitor blood levels of other medications to ensure that they remain within adequate safety margins.[98] More research is required to demonstrate long-term safety of cannabis use as a monotherapy or add-on therapy in ASD, particularly in children.

CONCLUSIONS

Elevation of the E/I balance is a common feature of ASD that can drive its symptoms. The endocannabinoid system plays an important neuromodulatory role in maintaining this balance, but many cases of ASD have reduced endocannabinoid signaling. Additional neural targets of phytocannabinoids like CBD also serve to restore E/I balance and may underlie the positive therapeutic benefits that are emerging in the early stages of pre-clinical and clinical trials. However, the aim of this report is not to make a blanket recommendation for the use or non-use of CBD in ASD.

That decision should be made on a case-by-case basis in consultation with a physician that integrates that patient's symptom profile and severity, genotype if known, successful management of symptoms by alternative approaches, while considering the legal ramifications of its use. Regardless of the decision made, it must be recognized that the reported adverse consequences of CBD use, although generally favorable in magnitude, do not provide insight to the effects on the developing brain, peripheral organ function, and immune system function. Despite this, the amassing anecdotal reports and emerging clinical data are delivering hope and promise to many children and families that have finally found support in CBD-based therapeutic strategies.

REFERENCES

1. American Psychiatric Association. *Diagnostic and Statistical Manual of Mental Disorders*. American Psychiatric Association, 2013. doi:10.1176/appi. books.9780890425596.
2. Happé, F., Ronald, A. & Plomin, R. Time to give up on a single explanation for autism. *Nat. Neurosci.* **9**, 1218–1220 (2006).
3. Gaugler, T. *et al.* Most genetic risk for autism resides with common variation. *Nat. Publ. Gr.* **46**, 881 (2014).
4. Eissa, N. *et al.* Current enlightenment about etiology and pharmacological treatment of autism spectrum disorder. *Front. Neurosci.* **12**, 304 (2018).
5. Rubenstein, J. L. R. & Merzenich, M. M. Model of autism: increased ratio of excitation/ inhibition in key neural systems. *Genes, Brain Behav.* **2**, 255–267 (2003).
6. Hussman, J. P. Letters to the editor: suppressed GABAergic inhibition as a common factor in suspected etiologies of autism. *J. Autism Dev. Disord.* **31**, 247–248 (2001).
7. Robertson, C. E., Ratai, E.-M. & Kanwisher, N. Reduced GABAergic action in the autistic brain. *Curr. Biol.* **26**, 80–85 (2016).
8. Ramamoorthi, K. & Lin, Y. The contribution of GABAergic dysfunction to neurodevelopmental disorders. *Trends Mol. Med.* **17**, 452–462 (2011).
9. Weiss, L. A. *et al.* Sodium channels SCN1A, SCN2A and SCN3A in familial autism. *Mol. Psychiatry* **8**, 186–194 (2003).
10. Han, S. *et al.* Autistic-like behaviour in Scn1a+/- mice and rescue by enhanced GABA-mediated neurotransmission. *Nature* **489**, 385–390 (2012).
11. Kaplan, J. S., Stella, N., Catterall, W. A. & Westenbroek, R. E. Cannabidiol attenuates seizures and social deficits in a mouse model of Dravet syndrome. *Proc. Natl. Acad. Sci.* (2017). doi:10.1073/pnas.1711351114.
12. Földy, C., Malenka, R. C. & Südhof, T. C. Autism-associated neuroligin-3 mutations commonly disrupt tonic endocannabinoid signaling. *Neuron* **78**, 498–509 (2013).
13. Markram, K. & Markram, H. The intense world theory – a unifying theory of the neurobiology of autism. *Front. Hum. Neurosci.* **4**, 224 (2010).
14. Markram, K., Rinaldi, T., Mendola, D. L., Sandi, C. & Markram, H. Abnormal fear conditioning and amygdala processing in an animal model of autism. *Neuropsychopharmacology* **33**, 901–912 (2008).
15. Monk, C. S. *et al.* Neural circuitry of emotional face processing in autism spectrum disorders. *J. Psychiatry Neurosci.* **35**, 105 (2010).
16. Katona, I. *et al.* Distribution of CB1 cannabinoid receptors in the amygdala and their role in the control of GABAergic transmission. *J. Neurosci.* **21**, 9506–9518 (2001).
17. Glass, M., Dragunow, M. & Faull, R. L. Cannabinoid receptors in the human brain: a detailed anatomical and quantitative autoradiographic study in the fetal, neonatal and adult human brain. *Neuroscience* **77**, 299–318 (1997).

18. Pouille, F. & Schoppa, N. E. Cannabinoid receptors modulate excitation of an olfactory bulb local circuit by cortical feedback. *Front. Cell. Neurosci.* **12**, 47 (2018).
19. Yoneda, T. *et al.* Developmental and visual input-dependent regulation of the CB1 cannabinoid receptor in the mouse visual cortex. *PLoS One* **8**, e53082 (2013).
20. Eggan, S. M., Stoyak, S. R., Verrico, C. D. & Lewis, D. A. Cannabinoid CB1 receptor immunoreactivity in the prefrontal cortex: comparison of schizophrenia and major depressive disorder. *Neuropsychopharmacology* **35**, 2060–71 (2010).
21. Gillberg, C. & Billstedt, E. Autism and asperger syndrome: coexistence with other clinical disorders. *Acta Psychiatr. Scand.* **102**, 321–30 (2000).
22. Yu, F. H. *et al.* Reduced sodium current in GABAergic interneurons in a mouse model of severe myoclonic epilepsy in infancy. *Nat. Neurosci.* **9**, 1142–1149 (2006).
23. Kaplan, J. S., Stella, N., Catterall, W. A. & Westenbroek, R. E. Cannabidiol attenuates seizures and social deficits in a mouse model of Dravet syndrome. *Proc. Natl. Acad. Sci. U. S. A.* **114**, 11229–11234 (2017).
24. Yizhar, O. *et al.* Neocortical excitation/inhibition balance in information processing and social dysfunction. (2011). doi:10.1038/nature10360.
25. Selimbeyoglu, A. *et al.* Modulation of prefrontal cortex excitation/inhibition balance rescues social behavior in CNTNAP2-deficient mice. *Sci. Transl. Med.* 9, eaah6733 (2017).
26. Ajram, L. A. *et al.* Shifting brain inhibitory balance and connectivity of the prefrontal cortex of adults with autism spectrum disorder. *Transl. Psychiatry* **7**, e1137 (2017).
27. Grinspoon, L. A novel approach to the symptomatic treatment of autism. (2013).
28. Kuester, G., Vergara, K., Ahumada, A. & Gazmuri, A. M. Oral cannabis extracts as a promising treatment for the core symptoms of autism spectrum disorder: preliminary experience in Chilean patients. *J. Neurol. Sci.* **381**, 932–933 (2017).
29. Barchel, D. *et al.* Oral cannabidiol use in children with autism spectrum disorder to treat related symptoms and co-morbidities. *Front. Pharmacol.* **9**, 1521 (2019).
30. Ibeas Bih, C. *et al.* Molecular Targets of Cannabidiol in Neurological Disorders. *Neurotherapeutics* **12**, 699–730 (2015).
31. Bakas, T. *et al.* The direct actions of cannabidiol and 2-arachidonoyl glycerol at GABA A receptors. *Pharmacol. Res.* **119**, 358–370 (2017).
32. Zamberletti, E., Gabaglio, M. & Parolaro, D. The endocannabinoid system and autism spectrum disorders: insights from animal models. *Int. J. Mol. Sci.* **18**, 1916 (2017).
33. Mechoulam, R. & Parker, L. A. The endocannabinoid system and the brain. *Annu. Rev. Psychol.* **64**, 21–47 (2013).
34. Trezza, V. *et al.* Endocannabinoids in amygdala and nucleus accumbens mediate social play reward in adolescent rats. *J. Neurosci.* **32**, 14899–14908 (2012).
35. Chakrabarti, B., Kent, L., Suckling, J., Bullmore, E. & Baron-Cohen, S. Variations in the human cannabinoid receptor (*CNR1*) gene modulate striatal responses to happy faces. *Eur. J. Neurosci.* **23**, 1944–1948 (2006).
36. Chakrabarti, B. & Baron-Cohen, S. Variation in the human cannabinoid receptor CNR1 gene modulates gaze duration for happy faces. *Mol. Autism* **2**, 10 (2011).
37. Rubino, T. *et al.* Role in anxiety behavior of the endocannabinoid system in the prefrontal cortex. *Cereb. Cortex* **18**, 1292–1301 (2008).
38. Rubino, T. *et al.* CB1 receptor stimulation in specific brain areas differently modulate anxiety-related behaviour. *Neuropharmacology* **54**, 151–160 (2008).
39. Wang, S. S.-H., Kloth, A. D. & Badura, A. The cerebellum, sensitive periods, and autism. *Neuron* **83**, 518–532 (2014).
40. Radulescu, E. *et al.* Gray matter textural heterogeneity as a potential in-vivo biomarker of fine structural abnormalities in Asperger syndrome. *Pharmacogenomics J.* **13**, 70–79 (2013).

41. Martin, L. A., Goldowitz, D. & Mittleman, G. Repetitive behavior and increased activity in mice with Purkinje cell loss: a model for understanding the role of cerebellar pathology in autism. *Eur. J. Neurosci.* **31**, 544–555 (2010).

42. Tsai, P. T. *et al.* Autistic-like behaviour and cerebellar dysfunction in Purkinje cell Tsc1 mutant mice. *Nature* **488**, 647–651 (2012).

43. Hodge, S. M. *et al.* Cerebellum, language, and cognition in autism and specific language impairment. *J. Autism Dev. Disord.* **40**, 300–316 (2010).

44. De Smet, H. J., Paquier, P., Verhoeven, J. & Mariën, P. The cerebellum: its role in language and related cognitive and affective functions. *Brain Lang.* **127**, 334–342 (2013).

45. Karhson, D. S. *et al.* Plasma anandamide concentrations are lower in children with autism spectrum disorder. *Mol. Autism* **9**, 18 (2018).

46. Aran, A. *et al.* Lower circulating endocannabinoid levels in children with autism spectrum disorder. *Mol. Autism* **10**, 2 (2019).

47. McFarlane, H. G. *et al.* Autism-like behavioral phenotypes in BTBR T+tf/J mice. *Genes, Brain Behav.* **7**, 152–163 (2008).

48. Wei, D. *et al.* Enhancement of anandamide-mediated endocannabinoid signaling corrects autism-related social impairment. *Cannabis cannabinoid Res.* **1**, 81–89 (2016).

49. Pretzsch, C. M. *et al.* Effects of cannabidiol on brain excitation and inhibition systems; a randomised placebo-controlled single dose trial during magnetic resonance spectroscopy in adults with and without autism spectrum disorder. *Neuropsychopharmacology* (2019). doi:10.1038/s41386-019-0333-8.

50. Poleg, S., Golubchik, P., Offen, D. & Weizman, A. Cannabidiol as a suggested candidate for treatment of autism spectrum disorder. *Prog. Neuro-Psychopharmacology Biol. Psychiatry* **89**, 90–96 (2019).

51. Minshawi, N. F. *et al.* The association between self-injurious behaviors and autism spectrum disorders. *Psychol. Res. Behav. Manag.* **7**, 125–136 (2014).

52. Siniscalco, D. *et al.* Stem cell therapy in autism: recent insights. *Stem Cells Cloning* **11**, 55–67 (2018).

53. Habib, S. S., Al-Regaiey, K., Bashir, S. & Iqbal, M. Role of endocannabinoids on neuroinflammation in autism spectrum disorder prevention. *J. Clin. Diagn. Res.* **11**, CE01–CE03 (2017).

54. Doenni, V. M. *et al.* Deficient adolescent social behavior following early-life inflammation is ameliorated by augmentation of anandamide signaling. *Brain. Behav. Immun.* **58**, 237–247 (2016).

55. Zuardi, A. W., de Souza Crippa, J. A., Hallak, J. E. C., Campos, A. C. & Guimarães, F. S. The anxiolytic effects of cannabidiol (CBD). *Handb. Cannabis Relat. Pathol.* e131–e139 (2017). doi:10.1016/B978-0-12-800756-3.00097-1.

56. Shannon, S., Lewis, N., Lee, H. & Hughes, S. Cannabidiol in anxiety and sleep: a large case series. *Perm. J.* **23**, (2019).

57. Russo, E. B., Guy, G. W. & Robson, P. J. Cannabis, pain, and sleep: lessons from therapeutic clinical trials of Sativex®, a cannabis-based medicine. *Chem. Biodivers.* **4**, 1729–1743 (2007).

58. Devinsky, O. *et al.* Trial of cannabidiol for drug-resistant seizures in the dravet syndrome. *N. Engl. J. Med.* **376**, 2011–2020 (2017).

59. Szaflarski, J. P. *et al.* Long-term safety and treatment effects of cannabidiol in children and adults with treatment-resistant epilepsies: expanded access program results. *Epilepsia* **59**, 1540–1548 (2018).

60. Iseger, T. A. & Bossong, M. G. A systematic review of the antipsychotic properties of cannabidiol in humans. *Schizophr. Res.* **162**, 153–161 (2015).

61. Guimaraes, F., Rodrigues, N., Silva, N. & Gomes, F. Cannabidiol as an antipsychotic drug. *Schizophr. Bull.* **44**, S21–S22 (2018).

62. Osborne, A. L., Solowij, N., Babic, I., Huang, X.-F. & Weston-Green, K. Improved social interaction, recognition and working memory with cannabidiol treatment in a prenatal infection (poly I:C) Rat model. *Neuropsychopharmacology* **42**, 1447–1457 (2017).

63. Nagarkatti, P., Pandey, R., Rieder, S. A., Hegde, V. L. & Nagarkatti, M. Cannabinoids as novel anti-inflammatory drugs. *Future Med. Chem.* **1**, 1333–1349 (2009).

64. Petrosino, S. *et al.* Anti-inflammatory properties of cannabidiol, a nonpsychotropic cannabinoid, in experimental allergic contact dermatitis. *J. Pharmacol. Exp. Ther.* **365**, 652–663 (2018).

65. Aran, A., Cassuto, H., Lubotzky, A., Wattad, N. & Hazan, E. Brief report: cannabidiol-rich cannabis in children with autism spectrum disorder and severe behavioral problems—a retrospective feasibility study. *Journal of Autism and Developmental Disorders* (2018). doi:10.1007/s10803-018-3808-2.

66. Millar, S. A., Stone, N. L., Yates, A. S. & O'Sullivan, S. E. A systematic review on the pharmacokinetics of cannabidiol in humans. *Front. Pharmacol.* (2018). doi:10.3389/fphar.2018.01365.

67. Sturman, N., Deckx, L. & van Driel, M. L. Methylphenidate for children and adolescents with autism spectrum disorder. *Cochrane Database Syst. Rev.* (2017). doi:10.1002/14651858.CD011144.pub2.

68. Marcus, R. N. *et al.* A placebo-controlled, fixed-dose study of aripiprazole in children and adolescents with irritability associated with autistic disorder. *J. Am. Acad. Child Adolesc. Psychiatry* **48**, 1110–1119 (2009).

69. McCracken, J. T. *et al.* Risperidone in children with autism and serious behavioral problems. *N. Engl. J. Med.* **347**, 314–321 (2002).

70. Rossignol, D. A. & Frye, R. E. Melatonin in autism spectrum disorders. *Curr. Clin. Pharmacol.* **9**, 326–334 (2014).

71. Nadeau, J. *et al.* Treatment of comorbid anxiety and autism spectrum disorders. *Neuropsychiatry* (London). **1**, 567–578 (2011).

72. Aran, A. Cannabinoids for behavioral problems in children with ASD - full text view - ClinicalTrials.gov. Available at: https://clinicaltrials.gov/ct2/show/NCT02956226. Accessed: 28th February 2019.

73. Hollander, E. Cannabidivarin (CBDV) vs. placebo in children with autism spectrum disorder (ASD) - full text view - ClinicalTrials.gov. Available at: https://clinicaltrials.gov/ct2/show/NCT03202303?term=cannabidivarin&cond=Autism&rank=1. Accessed: 28th February 2019.

74. Hill, A. *et al.* Cannabidivarin is anticonvulsant in mouse and rat. *Br. J. Pharmacol.* **167**, 1629–1642 (2012).

75. Vigli, D. *et al.* Chronic treatment with the phytocannabinoid Cannabidivarin (CBDV) rescues behavioural alterations and brain atrophy in a mouse model of Rett syndrome. *Neuropharmacology* **140**, 121–129 (2018).

76. Morano, A. *et al.* Cannabis in epilepsy: from clinical practice to basic research focusing on the possible role of cannabidivarin. *Epilepsia open* **1**, 145–151 (2016).

77. Anavi-Goffer, S. *et al.* Modulation of l-α-lysophosphatidylinositol/GPR55 mitogen-activated protein kinase (MAPK) signaling by cannabinoids. *J. Biol. Chem.* **287**, 91–104 (2012).

78. Russo, E. B. The case for the entourage effect and conventional breeding of clinical cannabis: no "strain," no gain. *Front. Plant Sci.* **9**, 1969 (2019).

79. Hryhorowicz, S., Walczak, M., Zakerska-Banaszak, O., Słomski, R. & Skrzypczak-Zielińska, M. Pharmacogenetics of cannabinoids. *Eur. J. Drug Metab. Pharmacokinet.* **43**, 1–12 (2018).

80. Farquhar, C. E. *et al.* Sex, THC, and hormones: effects on density and sensitivity of CB1 cannabinoid receptors in rats. *Drug Alcohol Depend.* (2019). doi:10.1016/j.drugalcdep.2018.09.018.

81. Cuttler, C., Mischley, L. K. & Sexton, M. Sex differences in cannabis use and effects: a cross-sectional survey of cannabis users. *Cannabis cannabinoid Res.* **1**, 166–175 (2016).

82. Gallily, R., Yekhtin, Z. & Ondřej Hanuš, L. Overcoming the bell-shaped dose-response of cannabidiol by using cannabis extract enriched in cannabidiol. *Pharmacol. Pharm.* **6**, 75–85 (2015).

83. Linares, I. *et al.* Cannabidiol presents an inverted U-shaped dose-response curve in the simulated public speaking test. *Eur. Neuropsychopharmacol.* (2016). doi:10.1016/S0924-977X(16)31702-3.

84. Zuardi, A. W. *et al.* Inverted U-shaped dose-response curve of the anxiolytic effect of cannabidiol during public speaking in real life. *Front. Pharmacol.* **8**, 259 (2017).

85. Bhattacharyya, S. *et al.* Acute induction of anxiety in humans by delta-9-tetrahydrocannabinol related to amygdalar cannabinoid-1 (CB1) receptors. *Sci. Rep.* **7**, 15025 (2017).

86. Rey, A. A., Purrio, M., Viveros, M.-P. & Lutz, B. Biphasic effects of cannabinoids in anxiety responses: CB1 and GABAB receptors in the balance of GABAergic and glutamatergic neurotransmission. *Neuropsychopharmacology* **37**, 2624–2634 (2012).

87. Iffland, K. & Grotenhermen, F. An update on safety and side effects of cannabidiol: a review of clinical data and relevant animal studies. *Cannabis cannabinoid Res.* **2**, 139–154 (2017).

88. Niesink, R. J. M. & van Laar, M. W. Does cannabidiol protect against adverse psychological effects of THC? *Front. Psychiatry* **4**, 130 (2013).

89. Fokos, S. & Panagis, G. Effects of Δ9-tetrahydrocannabinol on reward and anxiety in rats exposed to chronic unpredictable stress. *J. Psychopharmacol.* **24**, 767–777 (2010).

90. Gorka, S. M., Fitzgerald, D. A., de Wit, H. & Phan, K. L. Cannabinoid modulation of amygdala subregion functional connectivity to social signals of threat. *Int. J. Neuropsychopharmacol.* **18**, pyu104–pyu104 (2015).

91. Onaivi, E. S., Green, M. R. & Martin, B. R. Pharmacological characterization of cannabinoids in the elevated plus maze. *J. Pharmacol. Exp. Ther.* **253**, 1002–1009 (1990).

92. Zuardi, A. W. *et al.* Inverted U-shaped dose-response curve of the anxiolytic effect of cannabidiol during public speaking in real life. *Front. Pharmacol.* **8**, 259 (2017).

93. Guimarães, F. S., Chiaretti, T. M., Graeff, F. G. & Zuardi, A. W. Antianxiety effect of cannabidiol in the elevated plus-maze. *Psychopharmacology* (Berl). **100**, 558–559 (1990).

94. Berman, P. *et al.* A new ESI-LC/MS approach for comprehensive metabolic profiling of phytocannabinoids in Cannabis. *Sci. Rep.* **8**, 14280 (2018).

95. American Academy of Neurology, J. *et al.* Neurology. *Neurology* **88**, (Advanstar Communications, 2017).

96. Bornheim, L. M. & Correia, M. A. Effect of cannabidiol on cytochrome P-450 isozymes. *Biochem. Pharmacol.* **38**, 2789–2794 (1989).

97. Zanger, U. M. & Schwab, M. Cytochrome P450 enzymes in drug metabolism: regulation of gene expression, enzyme activities, and impact of genetic variation. *Pharmacol. Ther.* **138**, 103–141 (2013).

98. Geffrey, A. L., Pollack, S. F., Bruno, P. L. & Thiele, E. A. Drug-drug interaction between clobazam and cannabidiol in children with refractory epilepsy. *Epilepsia* **56**, 1246–1251 (2015).

12 Recent Cannabinoid Delivery Systems

Natascia Bruni
Istituto Farmaceutico Candioli Srl

*Carlo Della Pepa, Simonetta Oliaro-Bosso,
Daniela Gastaldi, and Franco Dosio*
University of Turin

Enrica Pessione
University of Torino

CONTENTS

INTRODUCTION

Cannabis (cannabis sativa) is a dioic plant that belongs to the Cannabaceae family (Magnoliopsida, Urticales). Knowledge of the medical and psychoactive properties of cannabis dates back to 4000 B.C. All of the different varieties of cannabis, including the one known as cannabis indica, belong to the same species. All C. sativa plants produce active compounds, but each variety produces these compounds in different concentrations and proportions, which do not only depend on genomic background, but also on growing conditions and climate, meaning that they can be referred to as chemical varieties or chemovars, rather than strains [1]. Each chemovar contains varying concentrations of cannabinoids, a class of mono- to tetracyclic C21 (or C22) meroterpenoids. While more than 100 different cannabinoids can be isolated from C. sativa, the primary psychoactive compound is Δ^9-tetrahydrocannabinol (THC), which was first isolated in its pure form by Gaoni & Mechoulam in 1964 [2]. Other pharmacologically important analogues are: cannabidiol (CBD), cannabinol, cannabinoid acids, cannabigerol, and cannabivarins. In addition to cannabinoids, other components, such as monoterpenoids myrcene, limonene, pinene, and sesquiterpenoid beta-caryophyllene, can also mediate the pharmacological effects of C. sativa [3].

Although phytocannabinoids have similar chemical structures, they can elicit different pharmacological action. The identification of THC paved the way for the discovery, in 1988, of cannabinoid receptor type 1 (CB_1) [4], and, later, of cannabinoid receptor type 2 (CB_2) [5]. CB_1 and CB_2, belong to a family of seven transmembrane guanosine binding protein-coupled receptors, are widely expressed and distinguished by their specific functions, localization, and signaling mechanisms. They are one of the important endogenous lipid signaling pathways, named the "endocannabinoid system," which consists of cannabinoid receptors, the endogenous ligands of cannabinoid receptors (endocannabinoids), and the enzymes that regulate the biosynthesis and inactivation of endocannabinoids. This lipid signaling system is involved in many important physiological functions in the central and peripheral nervous system and in the endocrine and immune systems [6,7].

The psychotropic effects of cannabis are principally mediated by CB_1, which is widely distributed throughout the brain, but mainly in the frontal cortex, basal ganglia, and cerebellum. CB_1 is also present in several tissues and organs, including adipose tissue, the gastrointestinal tract, the spinal cord, the adrenal and thyroid glands, liver, reproductive organs, and immune cells. The presence of CB_1 receptors on chondrocytes and osteocytes, as well as evidence for their presence on fibroblast-like synoviocytes, makes CB_1 particularly interesting in the study of rheumatic diseases [8]. CB_1 activation inhibits adenylate cyclase and reduces cAMP levels and protein kinase A (PKA) activity, resulting in the activation of the A-type potassium channels and decreased cellular potassium levels [9].

CB_2 is principally expressed in immune cells, but can also be found in various other cell types, including chondrocytes, osteocytes, and fibroblasts, meaning that it can be considered the peripheral cannabinoid receptor. It is also present in some nervous tissues, such as dorsal root ganglia and microglial cells. CB_2 shows 44% amino acid similarity with CB_1, and similarly inhibits adenylate cyclase as well as activating mitogen-activated protein kinase. Moreover, CB_2 activation can increase intracellular calcium levels via phospholipase C. While both CB_1 and CB_2 are coupled to G-proteins, the transduction pathways that they activate can be different, for example, in their interactions with ion channels [10]. The association of a particular variant of CB_2, known as Q63R, with celiac disease, immune thrombocytopenic purpura, and juvenile idiopathic arthritis is particularly interesting for the field of autoimmune and rheumatic diseases [11].

Overall, seven different endogenous ligands have been identified as acting within the endocannabinoid system to date. The first two endocannabinoids are the derivatives of arachidonic acid N-arachidonoyl ethanolamide (anandamide) and

2-arachidonoylglycerol [12]. A third endocannabinoid, 2-arachidonoyl glyceryl ether (noladin ether), was discovered in 2001. N-arachidonoyl dopamine, O-arachidonoyl-ethanolamide (virodhamine), docosatetraenoylethanolamide, lysophosphatidylinositol, and oleoylethanolamide have since been described as ligands of endocannabinoid receptors [7].

The endocannabinoid system's contribution to the regulation of such a variety of processes makes phytocannabinoid pharmacological modulation a promising therapeutic strategy for many medical fields, including the studies of analgesic, neuroprotective, anti-inflammatory, and antibacterial activity [13,14].

THC is the primary psychoactive component of cannabis and works primarily as a partial agonist of CB_1 (Ki = 53nM) and CB_2 (Ki = 40nM) receptors [15] and has well-known effects on pain, appetite enhancement, digestion, emotions, and processes that are mediated through the endocannabinoid system [7]. Adverse psychoactive events can be caused by THC, depending on dose and previous patient tolerance. By contrast, CBD, which is the major non-psychoactive phytocannabinoid component of C. sativa, has little affinity for these receptors (Ki for human CB_1 and CB_2 of 1.5 and 0.37 µM, respectively) and acts as a partial antagonist CB_1 and as a weak inverse CB_2 agonist (Ki as antagonist of CP55940 from 4.2 ± 2.4 to 0.75 ± 0.3 µM in different human cell lines) [16].

In a recent paper, experiments based on the functional effects of CBD on PLCβ3, ERK, arrestin2 recruitment, and CB_1 internalization, show a negative allosteric modulation of CB_1 at concentration below 1 µM [17].

Additionally, other non-CB_1 receptor mechanisms of CBD have been proposed, among them its agonism at serotonin 1A receptor (or 5-TH1A), vanilloid receptor 1 (TRPV1) and adenosine A2A receptors [18,19]. The complex physiological and pharmacological mechanisms and interaction of CBD with the endocannabinoid system and other molecular targets are extensively reviewed by McPartland et al. [20]. These data may help explain some of the observed CBD effects including analgesic, anti-inflammatory, anti-anxiety, and anti-psychotic activity [21]. The combination of THC and CBD with other phytocannabinoids and other components, such as terpenoids and flavonoids, in cannabis may have a synergistic effect on pain treatment [22,23].

ROLE OF CANNABINOIDS IN INFLAMMATION AND PAIN

Pain and inflammation are the body's physiological responses to tissue injury, infection, and genetic changes [24]. These responses can be divided into two phases: acute and chronic. The acute phase is the early, non-specific phase and is characterized by local vasodilatation, increased capillary permeability, the accumulation of fluid and blood proteins in the interstitial spaces, the migration of neutrophils out of the capillaries, and the release of inflammatory mediators (e.g. cytokines, lymphokines, and histamine). Pain is produced by all these pro-inflammatory agents, that also lead to hyperalgesia through the activation of the corresponding receptors, which are expressed by nociceptive terminals (Figure 12.1). If the condition that causes the damage is not resolved, the inflammatory process progresses towards subacute/chronic inflammation, which is characterized by immunopathological changes, such

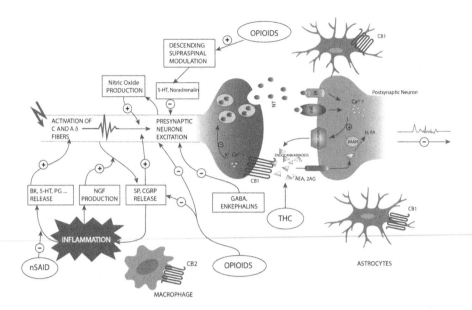

FIGURE 12.1 Simplified scheme representing the pathogenesis of pain following inflammatory disease or nociceptive stimulus, the cytokines involved in the process, the descending supraspinal modulation and the relive neurotransmitters, and endocannabinoid retrograde signaling mediated synaptic transmission. Endocannabinoids are produced from postsynaptic terminals upon neuronal activation. Natural and synthetic cannabinoids act like the two major endocannabinoids shown in the scheme: 2-arachidonoylglycerol (2-AG) and anandamide (AEA). Endocannabinoids readily cross the membrane and travel in a retrograde fashion to activate CB_1 located in the presynaptic terminals. Activated CB_1 will then inhibit neurotransmitter (NT) release through the suppression of calcium influx. NT can bind to ionotropic (iR) or metabotropic (mR) receptors. 2-AG is also able to activate CB_1 located in astrocytes. Although endocannabinoid retrograde signaling is mainly mediated by 2-AG, AEA can activate presynaptic CB_1 as well. Fatty acid amide hydrolase (FAAH) found in postsynaptic terminals is responsible for degrading AEA to AA and ethanolamine (Et). Inflammation leads to release of biochemical mediators (bradykinin (BK), serotonin (5-HT), prostaglandins, etc.) and the up-regulation of pain mediator nerve growth factor (NGF). The substance P (SP) and calcitonin gene-related peptide (CGRP) vasoactive neuropeptides, released from sensory nerve, have also role in inflammation. The interaction with opioids, THC, and non-steroidal anti-inflammatory drugs is also represented.

as the infiltration of inflammatory cells, the overexpression of pro-inflammatory genes, the dysregulation of cellular signaling, and the loss of barrier function.

Chronic state of inflammation plays an important role in the onset of classic inflammatory diseases (e.g. arthritis) but also of various diseases, including cardiovascular and neurodegenerative diseases, diabetes, cancer, asthma. The suppression or inhibition of inflammatory/pro-inflammatory mediators using synthetic anti-inflammatory compounds (both steroidal and non-steroidal) is one of the major routes for the treatment of inflammatory disorders. However, several common side effects, including gastric irritation and ulceration, renal and hepatic failure, hemolytic anemia, asthma exacerbation, skin rashes, are often associated with the use of synthetic anti-inflammatory drugs [25]. Increasing amounts of evidence demonstrate that the endocannabinoid system actively participates in the pathophysiology of osteoarthritis-associated joint pain. Production and release of endocannabinoids are mediated, during inflammatory-joint disease, by the generation of pro-inflammatory cytokines (interferon [IFN]-c), interleukin (IL-12, IL-15, IL-17, IL-18), chemokines, chemical mediators, such as nitric oxide synthetase (NOS)-2, cyclooxygenase-2 (COX-2), matrix metalloproteinases (MMPs) and various other arachidonic acid metabolic by-products [7]. Overall, preclinical and clinical data support the potentially effective anti-inflammatory properties of endocannabinoid agonists that target CB_2 receptors.

The chronic pathological pain state, including neuropathic pain, is a leading health problems worldwide as they endure beyond the resolution of the pain source and can deeply impact quality of life [26]. Unlike physiological pain, in which tissue injury and/or inflammation can induce reversible adaptive changes in the sensory nervous system leading to protective sensitization, changes in sensitivity become persistent or chronic in neuropathic pain. Furthermore, the nervous system, peripheral or central, is injured in neuropathic pain. It is characterized by pain in the absence of a noxious stimulus and may be spontaneous in its temporal characteristics or be evoked by sensory stimuli (hyperalgesia and dynamic mechanical allodynia). For example, neuropathy is still among the most common diabetes complications, affecting up to 50% of patients, despite recent advances in treatment. There is no effective treatment with which to prevent or reverse neuropathic pain [27], thus current treatment is only directed at reducing symptoms. The treatment of chronic pain is still an unmet clinical need, where adequate pain relief is obtained using drugs with adverse effects on central nervous system side [28]. The quality of life of neuropathic pain patients is often aggravated by comorbidities such as sleep disorders, depression, and anxiety compromise.

The finding of the endocannabinoid-mediated retrograde synaptic signaling pathway has opened up a new era, for cannabinoid research, including evaluations of their therapeutic use [29]. Selective CB_2 agonists have shown considerable efficiency in a variety of neuropathic pain preclinical models, while increasing amounts of evidence, derived from clinical studies, have confirmed the potential of the cannabinoid system in affording benefits for patients with chronic pain and chronic inflammatory diseases (arthritis). Currently, patients with chronic arthritic and musculoskeletal pain are the most prevalent users of therapeutic cannabis products [30].

Preclinical studies have shown that cannabinoid receptor agonists block pain in various acute and chronic pain models and that inflammation is attenuated [31–33]. Both CB_1 and CB_2 receptor agonists demonstrate anti-nociceptive activity, whether used singly or in combination, with CB_2 activity believed to affect microglial cells and thereby reduce neuro-inflammatory mechanisms [34, 35]. The CB_2 receptor is thought to be particularly important in central neuronal pain circuits, as agonist activity induces dopamine release in mid-brain areas, contributing to descending pain control and the placebo effect [36]. Inflammatory effects can either be modulated via the upregulation of cannabinoid receptor activity or increased production of endocannabinoids, providing an attenuation in joint destruction in preclinical models of inflammatory arthritis that mimic human rheumatoid arthritis [30,32]. Similarly, CB_1

and CB_2 receptor proteins and endocannabinoids are found in the human synovial tissue of patients with both rheumatoid arthritis and osteoarthritis [37].

Data from clinical trials on synthetic and plant-derived cannabis-based medicines have suggested that they are a promising approach for the management of chronic neuropathic pain of different origins [38–40]. It is also hypothesized that cannabis reduces the alterations in cognitive and autonomic processing that are present in chronic pain states [41]. The frontal-limbic distribution of CB receptors in the brain suggests that cannabis may preferentially target the affective qualities of pain [42]. Furthermore, cannabis may improve neuropathic pain reducing the low-grade inflammation consistent in the pathology [43]. Considering as a whole the problems of chronic neuropathic pain syndromes, which has a poorly understood pathogenesis, a complexity of symptoms and the lack of an optimal treatment, the potential of a therapeutic strategy centered on cannabinoid system appears really quite attractive. However, a range of adverse events (particularly somnolence or sedation, confusion, psychosis) may limit the clinical applications of therapeutics based on cannabis. Some current clinical guidelines and systematic reviews consider cannabis-based medicines as third- or fourth-line therapies for chronic neuropathic pain syndromes, for use when established therapies (e.g. anticonvulsants, antidepressants) have failed [44,45].

Beyond its effects on the inflammatory pathway, the endocannabinoid system also plays a fundamental role in neuronal development affecting axon and dendrite growth [46], and preclinical models have demonstrated that cannabinoid administration alters brain maturation in young animals and leads to neuropsychiatric consequences in adults [47]. Moreover, endocannabinoid system has also been accepted to play a significant role in the maintenance of gut homeostasis, and this is therefore, of particular interest in the management of inflammatory bowel diseases (i.e. Crohn's disease and ulcerative colitis) that show increasing prevalence in westernized countries [48].

CURRENT DRUG DOSAGE FORMS AND NOVEL DELIVERY SYSTEMS

A modern pharmaceutical approach to administration may start from the use of the cannabis plant for medical use, and then move on to the development of quality controlled extracts, the complete evaluation of their analytical profiles, and studies to assess the delivery of the correct dosage for optimal therapeutic effect. Cannabinoids are highly lipophilic molecules (logP 6–7) with very low aqueous solubility (2–10 µg/ml) [49], that are susceptible to degradation, especially in solution, via the action of light and temperature as well as via auto-oxidation [50,51]. Formulation can thus play a crucial role in increasing the solubility and physicochemical stability of the drugs. Commonly used strategies in marketed products include salt formation (i.e. pH adjustment), cosolvency (e.g. ethanol, propylene glycol, PEG400, etc.), micellization (e.g. polysorbate 80, cremophor ELP, etc.), (nano)- (micro)-emulsification, complexation (e.g. cyclodextrins), and encapsulation in lipid-based formulations (e.g. liposomes) and nanoparticles [52–55].

Various administration and delivery forms have been tested for therapeutic use. Cannabis products are commonly either inhaled by smoking/vaporization, or taken orally. The oromucosal, topical transdermal, and rectal routes are minor, but interesting, administration routes. The pharmacokinetics and dynamics of cannabinoids vary as a function of the route of administration with absorption showing the most variability of the principal pharmacokinetic steps. Absorption is affected both by intrinsic product lipophilicity and by inherent organ tissue differences (i.e. alveolar, dermal vs. gastric). A variety of factors, such as recent eating (for oral), depth of inhalation, how long breath is held for, and vaporizer temperature (for inhalation), all affect cannabinoid absorption, which can vary from 20%–30% for oral administration and up to 10%–60% for inhalation. A reference review detailing the pharmacokinetic and pharmacodynamic aspects of cannabinoids has been written by Grotenhermen [49]. The following sections explore the principal administration routes for cannabinoids, available products and the principal strategies (extracted from scientific literature and patents) that can be applied to improve cannabinoid efficacy and stability. Treatment indications and their level of evidence are also reported while the principal characteristics of the formulations have been summarized in Table 12.1.

ORAL ROUTE

The primary advantages displayed by the oral administration of cannabinoids include the existence of pharmaceutical-grade compounds, standardized concentrations/doses and a non-complicated administration route. Oils and capsules currently allow for more convenient and accurate dosing than juices or teas from the raw plant. Nevertheless, absorption is slow, erratic, and variable. Maximal plasma concentrations are usually achieved after 60–120 minutes, although this can take even longer (up to 6 hours) and can be delayed. Furthermore, metabolism produces psychoactive metabolites. Extensive first-pass liver metabolism further reduces the oral bioavailability of THC, while effect duration varies from 8 to 20 hours. Numerous (nearly 100) metabolites have been identified as being produced, primarily in the liver and, to a lesser degree, in other tissues, such as the heart and lungs [49].

There are three oral, and one oromucosal, cannabinoid pharmaceutical preparations that are currently available.

Dronabinol (Marinol® from Abbvie Inc, US) is a semi-synthetic form of THC, which is available in capsule form and as a solution, that has been approved by the FDA for appetite stimulation and the treatment of chemotherapy-induced nausea in patients with AIDS. Oh *et al.* have published a PK study that compares the oral solution and capsule forms of dronabinol under fasting and fed conditions. The solution formulation showed lower inter-individual absorption variability than the capsule formulation, especially in fed conditions, and this fact may be an important consideration in the selection of an appropriate dronabinol product for patients [56]. Dronabinol exerted a modest, but clinically relevant, analgesic effect on central pain in the pain treatment of patients with multiple sclerosis. Although the proportion of patients that showed adverse reactions was higher in dronabinol-treated than in placebo-treated patients, it decreased over the drug's long-term use [57,58].

Nabilone (Cesamet™ from Valeant Pharmaceuticals Int., Canada) is a synthetic cannabinoid derivative that differs structurally from THC as its C-ring is

TABLE 12.1

Currently Available Dosage Forms for Cannabinoids and Their Innovative Delivery Systems

Administration Route	Name	Drug	Delivery System/ Dosage Form	Disease	Application	Development Stage	References
Oral	Dronabinol	THC	Solid	HIV, chemotherapy	Anorexia, nausea	Market	[56]
Oral	Nabilone	THC analogue	Solid	Chemotherapy, chronic pain	Nausea, pain	Market	[59,60]
Oral	Epidiolex	CBD	Liquid	Lennox-Gastaud and Dravet syndromes	Epilepsy	Market	[62–64]
Oral		CBD	Solid	Crohn's disease, GVHD		Clinical trials	[66]
Oral		THC	SEDDS		Improving dissolution, stability	Preclinical	[69–71]
Oral		THC-glycosides	Prodrugs	Drug-resistant inflammatory bowel disease	Inflammation	Clinical trials	[72,73]
Oromucosal	Nabiximols	THC CBD 1:1	Spray	Multiple sclerosis	Spasticity	Market	[75,78]
Oromucosal		CBD	Powder	Cancer	Pain	Clinical trials	[77]
Oromucosal						Formulation study	[79]
Oromucosal		THC CBD 1:1	Chewing gum	Several potential diseases	Pain, spasticity, dementia etc.	Preclinical	[80]
Intranasal		CBD	Liquid formulations		Bioavailability study	Preclinical	[82]
Pulmonary		CBD	Solid/liquid			Formulation study	[86]

(Continued)

TABLE 12.1 (*Continued*)
Currently Available Dosage Forms for Cannabinoids and Their Innovative Delivery Systems

Administration Route	Name	Drug	Delivery System/ Dosage Form	Disease	Application	Development Stage	References
Pulmonary		Phytocannabinoids	Powder metered-dose inhaler		Bioavailability study	Clinical trials	[87]
Transdermal				Induced dermatitis	Inflammation	Preclinical	[92]
Transdermal		CBD	Gel	Arthritis	Inflammation	Preclinical	[93]
Transdermal		CBD	Ethosomes	Oedema	Inflammation	Preclinical	[95]
Transdermal		CBD	Gel	Epilepsy, osteoarthritis, fragile-X syndrome		Clinical trials	[96–98]
Transdermal		CBD	Oil, spray, cream	Epidermolysis bullosa	Pain, blistering	Clinical treatment	[100]
Transdermal		CBD	Patch			Formulation study	[112]
Transdermal		CBD + hyaluronic acid	Gel	Pain, wound management		Formulation study	[105]
Transdermal		CBD + argan oil		Rheumatic diseases	Inflammation	Formulation study	[107]
Transdermal		CBD + boswellic acid			Inflammation	Formulation study	[108]
Topical ocular		THC analogue	Prodrugs	Glaucoma	Reduce intraocular pressure	Formulation study	[111]

THC, Δ^9-tetrahydrocannabinol; CBD, cannabidiol; GVHD, graft-versus-host disease; SEDDS, self-emulsifying drug delivery system.

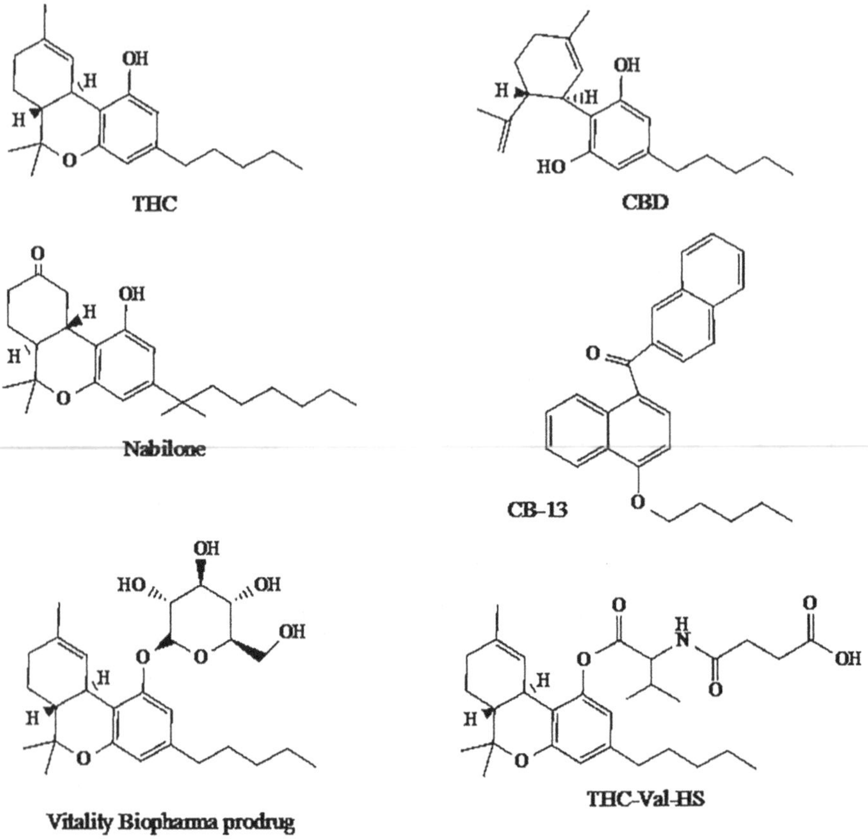

THC

CBD

Nabilone

CB-13

Vitality Biopharma prodrug

THC-Val-HS

FIGURE 12.2 The structures of principal cannabinoids described in the text.

saturated and contains a C-9 ketone group (Figure 12.2). Nabilone is available, in a polyvinylpyrrolidone carrier, as a capsule (1 mg of drug). It displays antiemetic properties and is used for the control of the nausea and vomiting associated with cancer chemotherapy in patients who have failed to respond adequately to conventional antiemetics [59].

Nabilone has higher bioavailability than dronabinol (95% vs. 10%–20%) and presents a higher duration of action. Nabilone has recently proven itself to be a suitable and safe therapeutic option with which to aid in the treatment of cancer patients diagnosed with anorexia. An enriched enrollment, randomized withdrawal design trial (26 patients) assessed the efficacy of nabilone, in the treatment of diabetic peripheral neuropathic pain [60]. Nabilone has an interesting range of applications (e.g. quality of life in lung cancer patients) although larger trials are still necessary if more robust conclusions are to be drawn [61].

Epidiolex (from GW Pharmaceuticals plc, UK) is a liquid formulation of a CBD solution that has recently been approved in the US as an adjuvant treatment in Dravet syndrome, Lennox-Gastaut syndrome, and severe myoclonic epilepsy in infancy.

Results from double-blind, placebo controlled trials have recently been published [62–64].

Furthermore, other improved oral-dosage formulations and therapeutic applications have been presented in a number of patents.

Clinical considerations of the oral administration of a solid-dosage, CBD-containing form for the treatment of inflammatory bowel disease have been published in a patent by Robson (GW patent) [65]. A small cohort of patients (eight patients) reported an improvement in Crohn's disease. Furthermore, oral administration also led to another small cohort of patients being able to reduce steroid dose when treating inflammatory and autoimmune diseases [66]. Based on this research, a CBD therapeutic formulation is being developed by Kalytera Therapeutics (US) for the prevention and treatment of graft-versus-host disease. Kalytera initiated a randomized, open-label, dose-response and comparator-controlled phase IIb trial in December 2017 to evaluate the pharmacokinetic profile, safety, and efficacy of multiple doses of CBD for the prevention of graft-versus-host disease following allergenic hematopoietic cell transplantation (NCT02478424).

The manufacture, specifications, pharmaceutical tests, and preliminary pharmacokinetics of CBD-containing, compressed tablets and granulates for peroral delivery have been reported in a patent by De Vries *et al.* [67].

Self-emulsifying drug delivery systems (SEDDS) can be significant in improving the dissolution, stability, and bioavailability of THC and other cannabinoids. SEDDS, which are isotropic mixtures of oils, surfactants, solvents, and co-solvents/surfactants, can be used in the design of formulations to improve the oral absorption of highly lipophilic drug compounds [68]. Murty *et al.* have described self-emulsifying drug delivery systems for *per os* administration in a number of patents, with the aim of improving the dissolution, stability, and bioavailability of THC and other cannabinoids [69–71]. The solubility of the selected drug, in oils (soybean and sesame oils, oleic acid) and surfactants (oleoyl polyoxyl-6 glycerides, medium-chain mono- and di-glycerides and propylene glycol esters, PEG hydrogenated castor oil) was assessed.

Vitality Biopharma (US) has proposed an invention that has led to several cannabinoid glycoside prodrugs (cannabosides) being obtained and characterized [72,73] (Figure 12.2). This method grants the gastro-intestinal targeting of THC, while avoiding narcotic effects. Vitality Biopharma has released data from independent clinical trial case studies, which demonstrate that cannabinoids induced the remission of drug-resistant inflammatory bowel disease after 8 weeks of treatment (Vitality Biopharma web site).

Administration Through Mucosa

Drugs, such as cannabinoids, that are metabolized by liver and gut enzymes (first-pass hepatic metabolism), have specific pharmacokinetic requirements, demonstrate poor gastrointestinal permeability and cause irritation and therefore require alternatives to systemic oral delivery. Transdermal, nasal, inhaled-pulmonary, and oral transmucosal delivery formulations enable drug uptake directly into the blood, thereby eliminating first-pass metabolism.

The development of the transmucosal dosage form has provided a non-invasive method of administration that has proven itself to be significantly superior to oral dosage in the relief of pain (e.g. oral morphine vs. transmucosal fentanyl) [74].

Nabiximols (Sativex® from GW Pharmaceuticals plc, UK), is an oromucosal spray that contains a roughly 1:1 ratio of THC and CBD, as well as specific minor cannabinoids and other non-cannabinoid components (β-caryophyllene). It is administered at a dose that is equivalent to 2.7 mg THC and 2.5 mg CBD in each 100 µl ethanol spray. THC and CBD may reciprocally interact either by interfering with each other's pharmacokinetics, or, at the cellular level, within the complex endocannabinoid signaling network. However, a study involving nine cannabis smokers reported that no significant pharmacokinetic differences were found in the similar oral THC and Sativex® doses that were administered [75]. Furthermore, studies have suggested that the adverse effects of THC can be antagonized by CBD [76]. Nabiximols is used as an adjunctive treatment for the symptomatic relief of moderate to severe multiple sclerosis-caused spasticity in adults who have not responded adequately to other therapies, and who show clinically significant improvements in spasticity-related symptoms during an initial therapy trial. It may also be of benefit as an adjunctive analgesic treatment for the symptomatic relief of neuropathic pain in adult patients with multiple sclerosis. This same preparation is also used as an adjunctive analgesic treatment in adult patients with advanced cancer who have moderate to severe pain during the highest tolerated dose of strong opioid therapy for persistent background pain [77]. Although not superior to placebo in terms of the primary efficacy endpoint, nabiximols provided multiple secondary endpoint benefits, particularly in patients with advanced cancer who receive a lower opioid dose, such as individuals with early intolerance to opioid therapy. Nabiximols has now received marketing authorization in EU countries for the treatment of spasticity and FDA investigational new drug (IND) status for the treatment of cancer pain. Some clinical trials into the use of Sativex for the treatment of neuropathic pain in multiple sclerosis patients have been successful [78], leading to the drug gaining approval in Israel and Canada. However, further work is still required to define the best responder profile for nabiximols and to explore its full potential in this field is still required.

Transmucosal formulations of CBD with Poloxamer 407, carboxymethyl cellulose and starch have been reported by Temtsin-Krayz et al. Nanoscale-range powders have been produced using the spray drier technique. Crossover bioavailability comparisons of this formulation and Sativex have also been reported [79].

A controlled-release chewing gum, made up of a (1:1) combination of CBD and THC, which provides oromucosal adsorption is being developed by Axim Biotech. Inc (US). The product is currently in clinical trials for the treatment of several diseases (pain, multiple sclerosis-associated spasticity, Parkinson's disease, post-herpetic neuralgia, dementia, etc.) [80]. More recently, Axim have also proposed chewing gums that are formulated to provide the controlled release of microencapsulated cannabinoids, opioid agonists, and/or opioid antagonists during mastication [81].

The intranasal mode of administration (in which drugs are insufflated through the nose) has several advantages; the nasal cavity is covered by a thin mucosa that is well vascularized, meaning that a drug can be transferred quickly across the single epithelial cell layer directly into systemic blood circulation and avoid first-pass hepatic and intestinal metabolism, producing a fast effect. Bypassing the oral route may be more acceptable for patients who experience nausea, vomiting, oral mucositis, and impaired gastrointestinal function. Furthermore, intranasal delivery is superior to iv injection because it is a non-invasive pain-free treatment that can improve patient compliance. The development of a nasal formulation of CBD could potentially aid in the treatment possible breakthrough pain and nausea attacks.

Paudel *et al.* have prepared a variety of formulations (CBD in PEG 400 alone and CBD in a 50:35:15 (v/v) PEG:saline:ethanol solvent system both with and without the following permeation enhancers: 1% sodium glycocholate or 1% dimethyl-beta-cyclodextrin) for the investigation of the intranasal permeation of CBD in an anesthetized rat nasal absorption model [82]. The intranasal application of CBD formulations resulted in the significant and relatively rapid absorption of CBD from the nasal cavity. The nasal absorption of CBD from all the formulations was rapid (Tmax ≤ 10 minutes), while the absolute CBD bioavailability achieved by the different nasal formulations was in the 34%–46% range. Bioavailability decreased when the PEG content of the formulation was lowered from 100% to 50%, while the addition of permeation enhancers did not lead to AUC enhancements.

Bryson has described both semi-solid and liquid nasally administered cannabinoid compositions and a device to provide precise nasal administration [83]. A range of different formulations were described in the patent.

PULMONARY ADMINISTRATION

The intrapulmonary administration of cannabinoids is regarded as an effective mode of delivery as it results in the fast onset of action and high systemic bioavailability. Cannabis-related effects generally begin within a few minutes of the first inhalation (smoked or vaporized) and these effects can increase [84]. A peak value is reached after 10 minutes and is maintained at a steady state for 3–5 hours, which is in accordance with the plasma levels of THC [85]. Interestingly, the PK profile of inhaled cannabis is similar to that of intravenously administered THC, although it displays a lower AUC. The PK profile of CBD is very similar to that of THC, whether it is administered orally, intravenously, or inhaled. These pharmacokinetics (rapid onset, short time peak effect, and intermediate lasting effects) occur because first passage metabolism is avoided and are thus virtually impossible to replicate with the oral administration of cannabis or cannabinoids. The major limitation of inhaling is the variability in inter-patient efficiency that is caused by differences in inhalation techniques, respiratory tract irritation during inhalation, etc. In fact, improved methods with which to standardize dosage have been proposed for these very reasons.

A protocol to deliver CBD and THC via vaporization has been described by Solowij *et al.* Crystalline-form CBD (preliminary experiments), and ethanol solutions of CBD (4 or 200 mg) and THC (4 or 8 mg) were separately loaded onto a vaporizer filling chamber via a liquid pad (a removable disc made of tightly packed stainless steel wire mesh) as supplied by the manufacturer of the Volcano® vaporizer device [86].

A system, which combines method, devices, and systems, for the controlled pulmonary delivery of active agents has also been reported; a metered-dose inhaler to vaporize precise amount of agent (cannabinoids or other plant oils), a system for the evaluation of the PK value obtained after one or two puffs, and an interface for the control of the profile of the drug administered have been provided by Davidson *et al.* [87].

Several patents have presented systems for vaporization and nebulization, from a variety of containers [88], at a selected temperature to form a precise amount of vapor with THC and CBD [89]. Improved drug-delivery devices that can separate and release active cannabis substances have been disclosed in another patent [90]; drug delivery cartridges, which include a substrate coated with at least one of either THC or CBD, are configured to allow for the passage of air through the cartridge to volatilize the agent for inhalation by a user.

TOPICAL AND TRANSDERMAL ROUTE

Transdermal administration delivers drugs through the skin via patches or other delivery systems. Although comparable to oral-dosage forms in term of efficacy, transdermal patches provide numerous advantages. Transdermal administration avoids the first-pass metabolism effect that is associated with the oral route and thus improves drug bioavailability. Furthermore, transdermal administration allows a steady infusion of a drug to be delivered over a prolonged period of time, while also minimizing the adverse effects of higher drug peak concentrations, which can improve patient adherence. Topical administration is potentially ideal for localized symptoms, such as those found in dermatological conditions and arthritis but also in peripheral neuropathic pain for which capsaicin patches have been proposed as a second line treatment after high quality of evidence was provided [91]. However, there are some disadvantages to consider, such as the possibility of local irritation and the low skin penetration of drugs with a hydrophilic structure. Indeed, drugs that are slightly lipophilic (logP 1–4) have a molecular mass of less than 500 Da and that show efficacy at low dosage (less than 10 mg/day for transdermal administration) are ideal for administration via this route. Enhancers may also be added to transdermal formulations to increase the penetration of permeants by disrupting the structure of the skin's outer layer, *i.e.* the stratum corneum, and increasing penetrant solubility.

The evaluation stages for the transdermal administration of cannabinoids range from early preclinical phases and mouse models, to self-initiated topical use and randomized, double-blind controlled studies.

The topical anti-inflammatory activity of phytocannabinoids in a Croton oil mouse ear dermatitis assay has been described by Tubaro *et al.* [92], while preclinical evaluations of the transdermal administration of CBD, via gel application, have been further tested on a rat complete Freund's adjuvant-induced monoarthritic knee joint model [93]. In this latter study, CBD was found to demonstrate therapeutic potential for the relief of arthritic pain-related behavior and to exert an anti-inflammation effect without any evident high-brain-center psychoactive effects. Results showed that a dose of 6.2 mg/day reduced knee joint swelling and that increasing the dose to 62 mg/day failed to yield additional improvements. The transdermal administration of CBD has also been observed to provide better absorption than the oral administration route in same arthritic model [30].

Ethosomal carriers are mainly composed of phospholipids (phosphatidylcholine, phosphatidylserine, phosphatidic acid) with a high concentration of ethanol and water [94]. An ethosomal formulation for CBD, which consisted of 3% CBD and ethanol in a carbomer gel, has been prepared by Lodzki *et al.* [95], and its anti-inflammatory effect was tested on carrageenan-induced aseptic paw edema in a mouse model. The results demonstrated that the carrageenan-induced development of an edema was only prevented in its entirety in the CBD-pre-treated group of mice. The *in vivo* occluded application of CBD ethosomes to the abdominal skin of nude mice resulted in high accumulation of the drug in the skin and the underlying muscle.

A topical transdermal gel containing a proprietary and patent-protected CBD formulation is being developed by Zynerba Pharmaceuticals (US) and is currently in clinical development for the treatment of epilepsy, developmental and epileptic encephalopathy, fragile-X syndrome, and osteoarthritis [96–98]. The gel is designed to be applied once or twice daily. Permeation profiles of a range of formulations have also been reported [99].

A particularly interesting, although anecdotal, result has recently been published by Chelliah *et al.*, who described the benefits that CBD provided as anti-inflammatory agent in three patients affected by epidermolysis bullosa. Pediatric patients benefited from the use of topical CBD (applied as an oil, cream, and spray by their parents) leading to a reduction in pain and blistering as well as rapid wound healing [100]. There were no adverse effects reported, either by the patients or their families, of this topical use of CBD.

The release of cannabinoids from a microneedle formulation that is administered transdermally has been reported by Brooke [101], while a patent by Weimann has more recently focused on CBD delivery [102]. In this latter work, a solution of CBD 10% in ethanol with modified cellulose gave a thixotropic preparation that was placed in a reservoir. Diffusion through the skin occurs and is measured using hydrophilic and hydrophobic membranes. A monolithic version, also containing penetration enhancers (oleic acid and propylene glycol), was also prepared for comparison purposes. Linear release was observed for 24 hours and cumulative amounts exceeded 200 µg/cm^2.

A range of patents for the topical administration of CBD, mixed with other well-known anti-inflammatory phyto-derived products, will also be summarized here, as will their adsorption and effect on pain relief.

Siukus has presented an oleo gel composition made up of non-psychoactive C. sativa components for the treatment and/or reduction of deep tissue joint and muscle inflammation caused by mechanical skeletal muscle trauma and arthritis/osteoarthritis. The oleo gel composition is based on phytocannabinoids (2% of total mass) mixed with an extract of *Olea europaea* (Olive) (82%), *Mentha arvensis* leaf oil (0.5%), and anhydrous colloidal silica (8.2%) [103]. Preclinical evidence was reported.

The same author has more recently published a patent that describes a topical composition made up of an essential combination of synergistically acting phyto-active materials and non-psychotropic phytocannabinoids in combination with a

Calendula flower extract (*Calendula officinalis L.*) and the base formulation to provide anti-inflammation, anti-oxidation, emollient and bactericidal activity [104].

Jackson *et al.* [105] have proposed a topical administration of CBD with silicon fluids, coupled with hyaluronic acid. This system is claimed to enhance application methods and improve absorption into the skin to help ease pain.

The use of cannabinoids, in combination with odorous volatile compounds and emu oil, has also been proposed as a method to improve the effectiveness of cannabinoid transdermal delivery to areas in the hypodermis [106].

The application of CBD with argan oil for the treatment of the pain and swelling associated with inflammation, in arthritic and rheumatic diseases, has been described by Shemanky *et al.* [107]. Gel, cream, and emulsion formulations were tested.

Improved anti-inflammatory effects can be obtained from a composition containing boswellic acids, either isolated from Boswellia family plants (Burseraceae) or in the form of an extract, and either CBD or a C. sativa extract [108].

In order to complete this overview of topical CBD, we should note that CBD exerts interesting sebostatic and anti-inflammatory effects on human sebocytes [109], (data obtained from *in vitro* evaluations). Indeed, CBD has been shown to inhibit the proliferation of hyperproliferative keratinocytes (54), and to possess remarkable antibacterial activity (55). The authors also demonstrated the potent local activity of CBD as an anti-acne agent. Furthermore, its high lipophilicity means that CBD is expected to preferentially enter the skin via the transfollicular route and to accumulate in the sebaceous gland.

Finally, the topical (ocular) administration of THC prodrugs has been proposed as a treatment to reduce intraocular pressure in glaucoma [110]. THC appears to be especially attractive in this case as, in addition to its intraocular lowering activity, the presence of cannabinoid receptors in ocular tissues has recently been confirmed [111]. Hydrophilic THC prodrugs have been obtained by linkage with valine, with dipeptides, and amino acid–dicarboxylic acid (Figure 12.2). Among them the best corneal permeability and intraocular pressure-lowering activity shown by these prodrugs were observed in the THC-Val-HS emulsion and micellar solution formulations.

NANOTECHNOLOGICAL APPROACHES

Pharmaceutical nanotechnology is widely used in drug delivery as it can develop devices that are specifically adapted to improving the therapeutic efficacy of bioactive molecules. Indeed, nanocarriers, such as nanoemulsions, dendrimers, micelles, liposomes, solid lipid nanoparticles, and nanoparticles of biodegradable polymers for controlled, sustained, and targeted drug delivery, are popular and present possible alternatives to traditional formulation approaches. Nanovectors for drug delivery potentially offer a number of advantages: more efficient delivery of highly lipophilic drugs at high doses, protection from aggressive environments (e.g. acidic pH in the digestive tract), as well as targeted and controlled delivery to achieve precise administration to a specific tissue over a determined period of time (e.g. pegylation [113], coating with polysaccharides [114], etc.). Even though the use of nanocarriers as drug-delivery systems offers many advantages, there are still some drawbacks that need to be addressed: instability during blood circulation, low renal clearance, limited accumulation in specific tissues, and low uptake by target cells. Physico-chemical aspects, such as surface charge, size, shape, and deformability, modulate uptake and interactions with host cells as well as influencing uptake by immune cells, the subsequent immune responses, and nanovector biodegradation [115]. An interesting work on the limitations, opportunities, and concerns in this field has recently been published by Park [116]. Significant research effort has been dedicated to the development of nanocarriers for the treatment of cancer, neurological diseases, cardiovascular diseases, and use as antimicrobial agents, for which the principal route is systemic administration.

Their high lipophilicity and low stability (degradation via the effects of tempera-ture, light, and auto-oxidation can occur) mean that cannabinoids benefit greatly from nanotechnology approaches [51]. Indeed, recent years have seen micellar, lipo-somal, and nanosized formulations being proposed for use in topical and systemic preparations. A brief description of the approaches presented in patents and in the literature, follows, while principal formulation data are reported in Table 12.2.

Lipid Carriers

Although liposomes are one of the most frequently studied and used market-approved drug delivery systems [55], only a few patents involving cannabinoids have been published. The main disadvantage for liposomes in the encapsulation of lipophilic compounds is their reduced ability to locate such compounds in their phospholipid bilayer. Low encapsulation efficiency, or drug loading (ratio of encapsulated drug/ sum of all components), is normally obtained for this reason. Rapid bioavailabil-ity and onset in the pulmonary administration of loaded-THC liposomes have been reported by Hung [117]. The formulation was composed of dipalmitoylphosphati-dylcholine and cholesterol, giving liposomes with an average size of 300–500 nm containing 0.3 mg/ml THC. Pharmacokinetic data described slow and prolonged release that continued for more than 5 hours after administration.

Micellar and liposomal preparations have also been proposed by Winniki et al. [118]. Micelles of 1 µm diameter were obtained via solvent injection in water and rapid solvent removal, while liposomes were produced using phosphatidylcholine ~52%, phosphatidylethanolamine 20%, phospholipids 26%, and other compounds in a 2% mixture, via film hydration and solvent injection, ultrasonication, and cal-cium alginate encapsulated liposomal suspension. Stability ranged from a few days (micelles) to several months (liposomes).

A nanotechnology platform proposed by Medlab Clinical (US), named NanoCelle™, that is made up of micelles obtained by mixing oils, glycerol, and non-ionic surfactants is currently undergoing advanced trails. Micelles of nanome-ter size (less than 100 nm) and positive average Z potential have been observed to deliver lipophilic molecules (vitamin D3, statins, testosterone propionate, CBD) for absorption across the oral buccal mucosa, bypassing the gastrointestinal tract. Early research into their use in the treatment of pain is underway in Australia [119,120].

Lipid nanoparticles in a solid particle matrix are produced from oil/water emul-sions by simply replacing the liquid lipid (oil) with a solid lipid, i.e. one that is solid at body temperature. First generation analogues, produced from a solid lipid only, are named solid lipid nanoparticles. The second generation of nanostructured lipid

TABLE 12.2

Nanosized Cannabinoid Delivery Systems

Type	Constituents	Drug	Size (nm)	Encapsulation Efficiency	Application	Development Stage	References
			Lipid-Based				
Liposomes	DPPC, cholesterol	THC	300–500	0.3 mg/ml	i.v.	Pharmacokinetics	[117]
Micelles	PC, PE plus phospholipids	Terpenes, hemp oil				Stability evaluations	[118]
Micelles	Polyethoxylated castor oil, glycerol	Cannabis oil	100	n.d.	Oromucosal	Clinical trials	[119,120]
NCL	Tristearin/tricaprylin 2:1	Cannabinoids	100	High		Formulation study	[122]
NCL	Cetyl palmitate or glyceryl dibehenate	THC	200		Nasal	Preclinical studies	[123]
NCL	Glyceryl dibehenate or glyceryl palmitostearate	CB-13	120	99%	Oral	Preclinical studies	[125]
PNL	PTL401*	THC CBD 1:1	<50	99%	Oral	Preclinical studies	[130]
	PTL401*	Plus piperine			Oral	Clinical trials	[132,133]
Nanoemulsions					Rectal/vaginal	n.d.	[134]
			Polymeric-Based				
PLGA	Plus coating agents	CB-13	253–344	85%	Oral	Preclinical studies	[138]
PLGA	Plus coating agents	THC	290–800	96%	Oral	Preclinical studies	[139]
PCL		CBD	2,000–5,000	100%	Locoregional	Preclinical studies	[140]

NCL, nanostructured lipid carrier; PNL, pro-nano-liposphere; PLGA, poly(lactic-co-glycolic acid); PCL, poly-ε-caprolactone; PC, phosphatidylcholine; PE, phosphatidylethanolamine; EE, encapsulation efficiency calculated as (total drug added—free non-entrapped drug) divided by the total drug added; PLT401 is a proprietary formulation containing polysorbate 20, sorbitan monooleate 80, polyoxyethylene hydrogenated castor oil 40, glyceryl tridecanoate, lecithin, and ethyl lactate; n.d., not defined.

carrier (NLC) particles are produced from a blend of a solid lipid and a liquid lipid, in which the partially crystallized lipid particles, with mean radii $\leq$ 100 nm, are dispersed in an aqueous phase containing one or more emulsifiers [121]. NLC can be considered suitable carrier systems for THC and CBD because they make use of solid particle matrices instead of fluid matrices, such as emulsions and liposomes, meaning that NLC can better host substances and protect them from degradation. The solid particle matrix is also able to slow the diffusion of THC from inside the particle to the particle surface.

Esposito *et al.* have described the development of a method to encapsulate cannabinoid drugs (precisely the inverse agonist of the CB_1 receptor (AM251 and Rimonabant) and the URB597 fatty acid amide hydrolase inhibitor) in NLC [122]. In this circumstance, the lipid phase was composed of tristearin/tricaprylin 2:1 while Poloxamer 188 was added to the water phase. Nanoparticles of around 100 nm with high encapsulation efficiency were obtained.

NLC have recently been proposed for administration as a dosage form for nasal delivery. Nanospheres of 200 nm diameter, composed of either cetyl palmitate or glyceryl dibehenate and loaded with THC, were obtained. *In vitro* mucoadhesion evaluations have revealed that cationic NLC formulations (obtained via the addition of cetylpyridinium chloride) should have high mucoadhesiveness properties [123]. The solid matrix of the NLC was found to have a stabilizing effect on THC. Indeed, 91% of the THC was unaltered after 6 months storage at 4°C. About 1.7 mg THC is administered with one spray of the 0.25% THC-loaded NLC formulation in each nostril. This amount was close to the THC amounts obtained from the oromucosal formulation in a study by Johnson *et al.* [124].

Lipid nanoparticle formulations have been also reported, by Duran-Lobato *et al.* [125], to incorporate and deliver CB-13, a cannabinoid drug that acts as a potent CB_1/CB_2 receptor agonist, and show therapeutic potential. Nanoparticles composed of either glyceryl dibehenate or glyceryl palmitostearate and stabilized with two different surfactants (polysorbate 20 and sodium deoxycholate) were produced using the emulsification-solvent evaporation method. The best formulation in terms of size (120 nm) and polydispersity was obtained using glyceryl palmitostearate as the lipid matrix, which was effective, in the presence of lecithin, in the preparation of cannabinoid-loaded particles with high EE (around 99%) and stability upon storage at 4°C. *In vitro* biocompatibility was assessed and demonstrated that this type of formulation is safe. Furthermore, neither free CB-13 nor LNP produced cytotoxic effects in three cell lines at the tested dose (250 μg/mL of each LNP formulation for 24 hours). This formulation was also stable under intestinal conditions, seemingly making it suitable for the oral delivery of CB-13.

Formulations that are based on self-(nano)emulsifying drug delivery technology (SEDDS) have been proposed as a means of improving the oral bioavailability of drugs that show poor aqueous solubility [126]. The base formulation, which is an isotropic mixture of an active compound in combination with lipids, surfactants, and a co-solvent, has been called a pro-nano-liposphere (PNL) pre-concentrate and is ingested as a soft gelatin capsule. When it reaches the aqueous phase of the gastrointestinal tract, the PNL spontaneously forms a drug-encapsulated oil/water microemulsion with a particle diameter of less than 60 nm. The clinical usefulness of SEDDS, which stems from their ability to increase the solubility and oral bioavailability of poorly soluble drugs, have led to them attracting considerable interest [127]. Products, such as Sandimmune® Neoral (Cyclosporin A), Fortovase® (Saquinavir) and Norvir® (Ritonavir), have confirmed the value of this approach [128]. PTL401 is the proprietary PNL-based formulation of THC and CBD (PhytoTech Therapeutics (Israel)). The PTL401 formulation is composed of THC-CBD (1:1) in a formulation with polysorbate 20, sorbitan monooleate 80, polyoxyethylene hydrogenated castor oil 40, glyceryl tridecanoate, lecithin, and ethyl lactate [129–131]. The CBD-THC PNL formulation also allows absorption enhancers, such as curcumin, resveratrol, and piperine, to be incorporated. PK evaluations in a rat model have indicated that only piperine enhanced the oral bioavailability of CBD *in-vivo* [130]. Moreover, the enhanced oral bioavailability can be attributed to the inhibition of intestinal processes, rather than those of hepatic first-pass metabolism, while additional increases in the AUC of CBD prove that piperine-PNL also has an effect on phase II, and not on just phase I, metabolism. THC-CBD-piperine-PNL demonstrated higher absorption rates than Sativex® in human volunteers, with peak values of 1 hour for both THC and CBD, versus 3 hours for THC and 2 hours for CBD, respectively. Furthermore, the incidence and severity of reported adverse events were similar in both groups [132,133]. Nevertheless, regarding the role of piperine, it is important to remember that it is able to alter the metabolism of many drugs, being a cytochrome and glucuronyl transferase inhibitor. In addition, piperine demonstrates non-negligible toxicity (it is Generally Recognized As Safe only up to 10 mg/day).

Micro and nanoemulsions of active cannabis ingredients (cannabinoids and terpenes) have also been presented in a patent [134], which proposes rectal-vaginal and solid oral-dosage forms.

A proprietary CBD nanotherapeutic formulation (CTX01) for subcutaneous administration is being developed by Cardiol Therapeutics (Canada) for the treatment of heart failure with preserved ejection fraction. Preclinical studies are currently under way (Cardiol website) [135].

Polymeric Carriers

Polymers have played an integral role in the advancement of drug delivery technology and this field has grown tremendously. Polymers are currently used in pharmaceutical formulations and show a wide range of safety and biodegradation variables. Developments in responsive polymers, polymer therapeutics, and advanced systems for molecular recognition or for the intracellular delivery of novel therapeutics have more recently appeared [136,137]. Polymeric drug delivery systems are able to protect drugs from degradation and control drug release.

The poly(lactic-co-glycolic acid) (PLGA) polymer is one of the most commonly used materials for the encapsulation of drugs, as it is mechanically strong, hydrophobic, biocompatible and degrades into toxicologically acceptable products that are eliminated from the body.

PLGA nanoparticles, loaded with CB-13 for oral delivery, have been coated with a variety of agents (chitosan, Eudragit RS, vitamin E, and lecithin) [138]. The nanoparticles exhibited particle sizes of 253–344 nm and high entrapment efficiency values (around 85%). Higher release rates were obtained with vitamin E and lecithin surface modification. Biodistribution evaluations revealed that none of the proposed surface modifications prevented the opsonization process (liver and spleen uptake). Nonetheless, CB-13, which is highly lipophilic and displays low water solubility, can be absorbed well when it is included in these surface-modified polymeric carriers.

Biocompatible polymer PLGA was preferred by Martin-Banderas for the preparation of THC—loaded nanoparticles for use as an anticancer agent [139]. Nanoparticles, with sizes ranging from 290–800 nm, were obtained with PEG, chitosan, and PEG-chitosan being used as coating agents. Encapsulation efficiency and drug loading (around 96% and 4.8%, respectively) were not affected by the type of coating used and sustained drug release, of up to 10 days, was obtained. Surface modification with PEG reduced protein adsorption and thus, most likely, the *in vivo* opsonisation processes.

Poly-ε-caprolactone (PCL) is another polymer that is widely used in drug delivery systems. This is a biocompatible, biodegradable, FDA-approved, semi-crystalline aliphatic polyester that degrades slowly. Hernán Pérez de la Ossa has developed a formulation in which CBD is loaded into PCL particles. Spherical microparticles, with a size range of 20–50 μm and high entrapment efficiency (around 100%), were obtained. CBD was slowly released over within ten days when dissolved in the polymeric matrix of the microspheres in an *in vitro* test [140].

CRITICAL OVERVIEW OF CLINICAL STUDIES

Contrasting the abundance of public domain comment on the therapeutic effects of cannabinoids is the fact that there has only been a limited number of rigorous clinical studies on the topic, due to the illegal status of cannabinoids in most countries. Nevertheless, the licensing of cannabis-based medicines, including herbal cannabis for people with chronic (neuropathic) pain, is scheduled to occur in some countries and has already happened in Canada, Germany, and Israel. Heated debate as to the true efficacy and side effects of cannabis products and derivatives is therefore ongoing. In 2017, the Health and Medicine Division of the US National Academies concluded that there is substantial evidence to support the claim that cannabis is effective for the treatment of chronic pain (cannabis), especially neuropathic pain in adults, for use as antiemetic in the treatment of chemotherapy-induced nausea and vomiting (oral cannabinoids), and as a means to improve patient-reported multiple sclerosis spasticity symptoms (oral cannabinoids) [141]. Nevertheless, only in recent years have a significant number of systematic reviews and meta-analyses evaluated the effects of all cannabinoids in all diseases and focused on cannabinoid use for chronic pain. Whiting *et al.* selected 79 trials and concluded that there was moderate-quality evidence to support the use of cannabinoids for the treatment of chronic pain and spasticity, while there was low-quality evidence for improvements in nausea and vomiting due to chemotherapy, weight gain in HIV, sleep disorders, and Tourette syndrome. Cannabinoids were also associated with an increased risk of short-term side effects [142]. Nugent *et al.* selected 29 chronic pain trials and suggested that there is some, limited evidence to indicate that cannabis is able to alleviate neuropathic pain in some patients, but also that insufficient evidence exists in other types of chronic pain [143]. Furthermore, Mücke *et al.* have also declined to share in the optimistic conclusions that cannabis-based medicines are effective, well-tolerated, and safe in the treatment of chronic neuropathic pain, due to a lack of high-quality evidence for their efficacy [144]. Moreover, there is some evidence to support the idea that cannabis is associated with an increased risk of adverse mental health effects. However, that evidence is generally quite weak as the studies are of low quality, have limited participant numbers, short study durations, a wide variety of cannabinoid preparations and doses, and a frequently, a high rate of bias.

Conclusions in studies into reducing opioid doses in the management of chronic pain, where some trials have shown clinical benefits, are sometimes not completely reliable as they inadequately report dose changes and have mixed results in analgesic effects [145]. Recent analysis has found no evidence to suggest that cannabis can exert an opioid-sparing effect [146].

Concerning the treatment of inflammatory bowel diseases with cannabinoids, preclinical evidence has indicated that CBD protects against intestinal inflammation (reviewed in [147]). However, GW Pharmaceuticals, who completed a phase IIa pilot study in 2014 did not list CBD for the treatment of ulcerative colitis on its development pipeline [148]. Only products from Vitality Biopharma (cannabinoid prodrugs) seem to be designed for a targeted approach to the gut. Nevertheless, there is global demand for larger clinical trials to be conducted to reveal whether treatment with cannabinoids or their derivatives can provide benefits to inflammatory bowel disease patients.

The impact of cannabinoids on patient-reported outcomes, such as health-related quality of life, has recently been analyzed by Goldenberg in a systematic review [149]. Once again, results were disappointing, although there were some small improvements in health-related quality of life for some patients with pain, multiple sclerosis, and inflammatory bowel disease. However, reduced effects were observed in some patients with HIV, leading the authors to conclude that the evidence for the effects of cannabinoids on health-related quality of life is inconclusive. The information that is currently available in the reports of reliable randomized controlled trials is clearly limited, although there are increasing reports of considerable subjective effects (pain treatment).

Other systematic reviews have also described harm caused and some commonly reported adverse effects. Cannabis seems to be associated with harm to the central nervous system and the gastro-intestinal system [143,150].

It would therefore appear that the clinical evidence collated to date is confounded by a number of factors, including studies with mixed patient populations, use of different cannabinoid preparations and in various formulations, and wide dosing ranges.

Cannabis-derivative-based medicines may be able to enrich the drug treatment arsenal for chronic pain and inflammation conditions, although this is very much open to debate at the moment. CBD, unlike THC, is not considered an abused drug and several industries are involved in the production of CBD as an active pharmaceutical ingredient with the highest quality standard. It is relevant, and expected, that regulatory agencies, other than the Medications Health Care Products Regulation Agency, will evaluate and approve CBD as a medicine after a careful study of quality, safety, and efficacy data [13]. While medicinal cannabis has already entered mainstream medicine in many countries, particular care should be taken in a period in which the online availability of a variety of CBD-based products for therapeutic purposes, such as oils, tinctures, and vapors, has rapidly expanded and, along with it, an increase in potential health risks for patients/consumers may be expected.

CONCLUDING REMARKS

Cannabinoids and endocannabinoids are a hot topic in the fields of chemical and biomedical research with more than 1,000 articles being published per year and the trend is for that to increase. Furthermore, research into cannabinoid delivery systems is growing and a plethora of patents have shown interest in the companies working in this field, especially when it comes to local/transdermal administration. Combining formulations may provide an opportunity to produce rapid systemic effects and long-term outcomes (e.g. analgesia). This could be achieved with intranasal cannabinoid sprays used as a low-dose adjuvant to patches in order to aid rapid absorption for systemic effects. Interesting and promising transdermal administration results can also be found in the use of terpenes (from the same source) as CBD and THC penetration enhancers, and thus improve the effectiveness of the therapeutic components. This, once again, highlights the role that quality plays in defining the composition, dosage, and related safety of the components extracted from cannabis.

It is expected that recent developments in pharmacological, pharmaceutical, and technological sciences will result in new therapeutic strategies using both known cannabinoids for new therapeutic strategies as well as cannabinoid synthetic derivatives.

Nanotechnology is indeed a promising approach that may bring cannabinoids closer to clinical use (the SEDDS approach is a fine example), and administration via both the oral and pulmonary routes. Furthermore, it is at an early stage the use of well-known advanced nanomaterials in cannabinoid delivery (e.g. carbon nanotubes). Nevertheless, additional evaluation is required if the cost effectiveness and long-term safety of nano-delivery systems is to be improved.

ACKNOWLEDGMENTS

The work was partially funded by MIUR-University of Torino "Fondi Ricerca Locale (ex-60%)." The authors are grateful to Prof. Franca Viola for fruitful discussions. Dale James Matthew Lawson is gratefully thanked for correcting English of the manuscript.

CONFLICTS OF INTEREST

Istituto Farmaceutico Candioli Srl is the funding sponsor in writing this chapter.

REFERENCES

1. Lewis, M. A.; Russo, E. B.; Smith, K. M., Pharmacological foundations of cannabis chemovars. *Planta Med.* **2018**, 84, (4), 225–233.
2. Gaoni, Y.; Mechoulam, R.; Isolation, Structure, and partial synthesis of an active constituent of hashish. *J. Am. Chem. Soc.* **1964**, 86, (8), 1646–1647.

3. ElSohly, M. A.; Slade, D., Chemical constituents of marijuana: The complex mixture of natural cannabinoids. *Life Sci.* **2005**, 78, (5), 539–548.

4. Matsuda, L. A.; Lolait, S. J.; Brownstein, M. J.; Young, A. C.; Bonner, T. I., Structure of a cannabinoid receptor and functional expression of the cloned cDNA. *Nature* **1990**, 346, (6284), 561–564.

5. Munro, S.; Thomas, K. L.; Abu-Shaar, M., Molecular characterization of a peripheral receptor for cannabinoids. *Nature* **1993**, 365, (6441), 61–65.

6. Svíženská, I.; Dubový, P.; Šulcová, A., Cannabinoid receptors 1 and 2 (CB1 and CB2), their distribution, ligands and functional involvement in nervous system structures - A short review. *Pharmacol. Biochem. Behav.* **2008**, 90, (4), 501–511.

7. Di Marzo, V.; Bifulco, M.; De Petrocellis, L., The endocannabinoid system and its therapeutic exploitation. *Nat. Rev. Drug Discovery* **2004**, 3, (9), 771–784.

8. Fukuda, S.; Kohsaka, H.; Takayasu, A.; Yokoyama, W.; Miyabe, C.; Miyabe, Y.; Harigai, M.; Miyasaka, N.; Nanki, T., Cannabinoid receptor 2 as a potential therapeutic target in rheumatoid arthritis. *BMC Musculoskelet. Disord.* **2014**, 15, (1), 275.

9. Turu, G.; Hunyady, L., Signal transduction of the CB1 cannabinoid receptor. *J. Mol. Endocrinol.* **2010**, 44, (2), 75–85.

10. McAllister, S. D.; Glass, M., CB1 and CB2 receptor-mediated signalling: A focus on endocannabinoids. *Prostaglandins, Leukotrienes and Essent. Fatty Acids (PLEFA)* **2002**, 66, (2), 161–171.

11. Rossi, F.; Mancusi, S.; Bellini, G.; Roberti, D.; Punzo, F.; Vetrella, S.; Matarese, S. M. R.; Nobili, B.; Maione, S.; Perrotta, S., CNR2 functional variant (Q63R) influences childhood immune thrombocytopenic purpura. *Haematologica* **2011**, 96, (12), 1883–1885.

12. Piomelli, D.; Beltramo, M.; Giuffrida, A.; Stella, N., Endogenous cannabinoid signaling. *Neurobiol. Dis.* **1998**, 5, (6), 462–473.

13. Pisanti, S.; Malfitano, A. M.; Ciaglia, E.; Lamberti, A.; Ranieri, R.; Cuomo, G.; Abate, M.; Faggiana, G.; Proto, M. C.; Fiore, D.; Laezza, C.; Bifulco, M., Cannabidiol: State of the art and new challenges for therapeutic applications. *Pharmacol. Ther.* **2017**, 175, 133–150.

14. Appendino, G.; Taglialatela-Scafati, O., Cannabinoids: Chemistry and medicine. In *Natural Products: Phytochemistry, Botany and Metabolism of Alkaloids, Phenolics and Terpenes*, 2013; pp. 3415–3435.

15. Howlett, A. C.; Barth, F.; Bonner, T. I.; Cabral, G.; Casellas, P.; Devane, W. A.; Felder, C. C.; Herkenham, M.; Mackie, K.; Martin, B. R.; Mechoulam, R.; Pertwee, R. G., International Union of Pharmacology. XXVII. Classification of cannabinoid receptors. *Pharmacol. Rev.* **2002**, 54, (2), 161–202.

16. Ligresti, A.; De Petrocellis, L.; Di Marzo, V., From phytocannabinoids to cannabinoid receptors and endocannabinoids: Pleiotropic physiological and pathological roles through complex pharmacology. *Physiol. Rev.* **2016**, 96, (4), 1593–1659.

17. Laprairie, R. B.; Bagher, A. M.; Kelly, M. E. M.; Denovan-Wright, E. M., Cannabidiol is a negative allosteric modulator of the cannabinoid CB1 receptor. *Br. J. Pharmacol.* **2015**, 172, (20), 4790–4805.

18. Russo, E. B.; Burnett, A.; Hall, B.; Parker, K. K., Agonistic properties of cannabidiol at 5-HT1a receptors. *Neurochem. Res.* **2005**, 30, (8), 1037–1043.

19. Costa, B.; Giagnoni, G.; Franke, C.; Trovato, A. E.; Colleoni, M., Vanilloid TRPV1 receptor mediates the antihyperalgesic effect of the nonpsychoactive cannabinoid, cannabidiol, in a rat model of acute inflammation. *Br. J. Pharmacol.* **2004**, 143, (2), 247–250.

20. McPartland, J. M.; Duncan, M.; Di Marzo, V.; Pertwee, R. G., Are cannabidiol and Δ9-tetrahydrocannabivarin negative modulators of the endocannabinoid system? A systematic review. *Br. J. Pharmacol.* **2015**, 172, (3), 737–753.

21. Romero-Sandoval, E. A.; Kolano, A. L.; Alvarado-Vázquez, P. A., Cannabis and cannabinoids for chronic pain. *Curr. Rheumatol. Rep.* **2017**, 19, (11).
22. Russo, E.; Guy, G. W., A tale of two cannabinoids: The therapeutic rationale for combining tetrahydrocannabinol and cannabidiol. *Med. Hypotheses* **2005**, 66, (2), 234–246.
23. Russo, E. B., Taming THC: Potential cannabis synergy and phytocannabinoid-terpenoid entourage effects. *Br. J. Pharmacol.* **2011**, 163, (7), 1344–1364.
24. Stucky, C. L.; Gold, M. S.; Zhang, X., Mechanisms of pain. *Proc. Natl. Acad. Sci.* **2001**, 98, (21), 11845–11846.
25. Pountos, I.; Georgouli, T.; Bird, H.; Giannoudis, P. V., Nonsteroidal anti-inflammatory drugs: Prostaglandins, indications, and side effects. *Int. J. Interferon, Cytokine Mediator Res.*, 2011, 3, 19–27.
26. Jensen, M. P.; Chodroff, M. J.; Dworkin, R. H., The impact of neuropathic pain on health-related quality of life: Review and implications. *Neurology* **2007**, 68, (15), 1178–1182.
27. Finnerup, N. B.; Sindrup, S. H.; Jensen, T. S., The evidence for pharmacological treatment of neuropathic pain. *Pain* **2010**, 150, (3), 573–581.
28. Finnerup, N. B.; Attal, N.; Haroutounian, S.; McNicol, E.; Baron, R.; Dworkin, R. H.; Gilron, I.; Haanpää, M.; Hansson, P.; Jensen, T. S.; Kamerman, P. R.; Lund, K.; Moore, A.; Raja, S. N.; Rice, A. S. C.; Rowbotham, M.; Sena, E.; Siddall, P.; Smith, B. H.; Wallace, M., Pharmacotherapy for neuropathic pain in adults: A systematic review and meta-analysis. *The Lancet Neurology* **2015**, 14, (2), 162–173.
29. Ohno-Shosaku, T.; Kano, M., Endocannabinoid-mediated retrograde modulation of synaptic transmission. *Curr. Opin. Neurobiol.* **2014**, 29, 1–8.
30. Malfait, A. M.; Gallily, R.; Sumariwalla, P. F.; Malik, A. S.; Andreakos, E.; Mechoulam, R.; Feldmann, M., The nonpsychoactive cannabis constituent cannabidiol is an oral anti-arthritic therapeutic in murine collagen-induced arthritis. *Proc. Natl. Acad. Sci. U. S. A.* **2000**, 97, (17), 9561–9566.
31. Akopian, A. N.; Ruparel, N. B.; Patwardhan, A.; Hargreaves, K. M., Cannabinoids desensitize capsaicin and mustard oil responses in sensory neurons via TRPA1 activation. *J. Neurosci.* **2008**, 28, (5), 1064–1075.
32. Schuelert, N.; McDougall, J. J., Cannabinoid-mediated antinociception is enhanced in rat osteoarthritic knees. *Arthritis Rheum.* **2008**, 58, (1), 145–153.
33. Sánchez Robles, E. M.; Bagües Arias, A.; Martín Fontelles, M. I., Cannabinoids and muscular pain. Effectiveness of the local administration in rat. *Eur J Pain* **2012**, 16, (8), 1116–1127.
34. Cheng, Y.; Hitchcock, S. A., Targeting cannabinoid agonists for inflammatory and neuropathic pain. *Expert Opin. Invest. Drugs* **2007**, 16, (7), 951–965.
35. Correa, F.; Docagne, F.; Mestre, L.; Clemente, D.; Hernangómez, M.; Loría, F.; Guaza, C., A role for CB2 receptors in anandamide signalling pathways involved in the regulation of IL-12 and IL-23 in microglial cells. *Biochem. Pharmacol.* **2009**, 77, (1), 86–100.
36. Shang, Y.; Tang, Y., The central cannabinoid receptor type-2 (CB2) and chronic pain. *Int. J. Neurosci.* **2017**, 127, (9), 812–823.
37. Richardson, D.; Pearson, R. G.; Kurian, N.; Latif, M. L.; Garle, M. J.; Barrett, D. A.; Kendall, D. A.; Scammell, B. E.; Reeve, A. J.; Chapman, V., Characterisation of the cannabinoid receptor system in synovial tissue and fluid in patients with osteoarthritis and rheumatoid arthritis. *Arthritis Res. Ther.* **2008**, 10, (2).
38. De Vries, M.; Van Rijckevorsel, D. C.; Wilder-Smith, O. H.; Van Goor, H., Dronabinol and chronic pain: Importance of mechanistic considerations. *Expert Opin. Pharmacother.* **2014**, 15, (11), 1525–1534.
39. Jensen, B.; Chen, J.; Furnish, T.; Wallace, M., Medical marijuana and chronic pain: A review of basic science and clinical evidence. *Curr. Pain Headache Rep.* **2015**, 19, (10), 50.

40. Lötsch, J.; Weyer-Menkhoff, I.; Tegeder, I., Current evidence of cannabinoid-based analgesia obtained in preclinical and human experimental settings. *Eur. J. Pain* **2018**, 22, (3), 471–484.

41. Guindon, J.; Hohmann, A. G., The endocannabinoid system and pain. *CNS Neurol. Disord. Drug Targets* **2009**, 8, (6), 403–421.

42. Lee, M. C.; Ploner, M.; Wiech, K.; Bingel, U.; Wanigasekera, V.; Brooks, J.; Menon, D. K.; Tracey, I., Amygdala activity contributes to the dissociative effect of cannabis on pain perception. *Pain* **2013**, 154, (1), 124–134.

43. Zhang, J.; Echeverry, S.; Lim, T. K.; Lee, S. H.; Shi, X. Q.; Huang, H., Can modulating inflammatory response be a good strategy to treat neuropathic pain? *Curr. Pharm. Des.* **2015**, 21, (7), 831–839.

44. De Moulin, D.; Boulanger, A.; Clark, A. J.; Clarke, H.; Dao, T.; Finley, G. A.; Furlan, A.; Gilron, I.; Gordon, A.; Morley-Forster, P. K.; Sessle, B. J.; Squire, P.; Stinson, J.; Taenzer, P.; Velly, A.; Ware, M. A.; Weinberg, E. L.; Williamson, O. D., Pharmacological management of chronic neuropathic pain: Revised consensus statement from the Canadian Pain Society. *Pain Res. Manag.* **2014**, 19, (6), 328–335.

45. Baron, E. P.; Lucas, P.; Eades, J.; Hogue, O., Patterns of medicinal cannabis use, strain analysis, and substitution effect among patients with migraine, headache, arthritis, and chronic pain in a medicinal cannabis cohort. *J. Headache Pain* **2018**, 19, (1), 37.

46. Njoo, C.; Agarwal, N.; Lutz, B.; Kuner, R., The cannabinoid receptor CB1 interacts with the WAVE1 complex and plays a role in actin dynamics and structural plasticity in neurons. *PLoS Biol.* **2015**, 13, (10), 1–36.

47. Schoch, H.; Huerta, M. Y.; Ruiz, C. M.; Farrell, M. R.; Jung, K. M.; Huang, J. J.; Campbell, R. R.; Piomelli, D.; Mahler, S. V., Adolescent cannabinoid exposure effects on natural reward seeking and learning in rats. *Psychopharmacology* **2018**, 235, (1), 121–134.

48. Ananthakrishnan, A. N., Epidemiology and risk factors for IBD. *Nat. Rev. Gastroenterol. Hepatol.* **2015**, 12, (4), 205–217.

49. Grotenhermen, F., Pharmacokinetics and pharmacodynamics of cannabinoids. *Clin. Pharmacokinet.* **2003**, 42, (4), 327–360.

50. Pacifici, R.; Marchei, E.; Salvatore, F.; Guandalini, L.; Busardò, F. P.; Pichini, S., Evaluation of long-term stability of cannabinoids in standardized preparations of cannabis flowering tops and cannabis oil by ultra-high-performance liquid chromatography tandem mass spectrometry. *Clin. Chem. Lab. Med.* **2018**, 56, (4), e94–e96.

51. Fairbairn, J. W.; Liebmann, J. A.; Rowan, M. G., The stability of cannabis and its preparations on storage. *J. Pharm. Pharmacol.* **1976**, 28, (1), 1–7.

52. Kumari, A.; Yadav, S. K.; Yadav, S. C., Biodegradable polymeric nanoparticles based drug delivery systems. *Colloids Surf. B. Biointerfaces* **2010**, 75, (1), 1–18.

53. Lawrence, M. J.; Rees, G. D., Microemulsion-based media as novel drug delivery systems. *Adv. Drug Del. Rev.* **2000**, 45, (1), 89–121.

54. Allen, T. M.; Cullis, P. R., Drug delivery systems: Entering the mainstream. *Science* **2004**, 303, (5665), 1818–1822.

55. Allen, T. M.; Cullis, P. R., Liposomal drug delivery systems: From concept to clinical applications. *Adv. Drug Del. Rev.* **2013**, 65, (1), 36–48.

56. Oh, D. A.; Parikh, N.; Khurana, V.; Smith, C. C.; Vetticaden, S., Effect of food on the pharmacokinetics of dronabinol oral solution versus dronabinol capsules in healthy volunteers. *Clin. Pharmacol.* **2017**, 9, 9–17.

57. Schimrigk, S.; Marziniak, M.; Neubauer, C.; Kugler, E. M.; Werner, G.; Abramov-Sommariva, D., Dronabinol is a safe long-term treatment option for neuropathic pain patients. *Eur. Neurol.* 2017, 78, (5–6), 320–329.

58. Svendsen, K. B.; Jensen, T. S.; Bach, F. W., Does the cannabinoid dronabinol reduce central pain in multiple sclerosis? Randomised double blind placebo controlled crossover trial. *BMJ* **2004**, 329, (7460), 253.

59. Schussel, V.; Kenzo, L.; Santos, A.; Bueno, J.; Yoshimura, E.; de Oliveira Cruz Latorraca, C.; Pachito, D. V.; Riera, R., Cannabinoids for nausea and vomiting related to chemotherapy: Overview of systematic reviews. *Phytother. Res.* **2018**, 32, (4), 567–576.

60. Toth, C.; Mawani, S.; Brady, S.; Chan, C.; Liu, C.; Mehina, E.; Garven, A.; Bestard, J.; Korngut, L., An enriched-enrolment, randomized withdrawal, flexible-dose, double-blind, placebo-controlled, parallel assignment efficacy study of nabilone as adjuvant in the treatment of diabetic peripheral neuropathic pain. *Pain* **2012**, 153, (10), 2073–2082.

61. Turcott, J. G.; Del Rocío Guillen Núñez, M.; Flores-Estrada, D.; Oñate-Ocaña, L. F.; Zatarain-Barrón, Z. L.; Barrón, F.; Arrieta, O., The effect of nabilone on appetite, nutritional status, and quality of life in lung cancer patients: A randomized, double-blind clinical trial. *Support. Care Cancer* **2018**, 1–10.

62. Devinsky, O.; Cross, J. H.; Laux, L.; Marsh, E.; Miller, I.; Nabbout, R.; Scheffer, I. E.; Thiele, E. A.; Wright, S., Trial of cannabidiol for drug-resistant seizures in the dravet syndrome. *N. Engl. J. Med.* **2017**, 376, (21), 2011–2020.

63. Devinsky, O.; Patel, A. D.; Cross, J. H.; Villanueva, V.; Wirrell, E. C.; Privitera, M.; Greenwood, S. M.; Roberts, C.; Checketts, D.; VanLandingham, K. E.; Zuberi, S. M., Effect of cannabidiol on drop seizures in the lennox–gastaut syndrome. *N. Engl. J. Med.* **2018**, 378, (20), 1888–1897.

64. Thiele, E. A.; Marsh, E. D.; French, J. A.; Mazurkiewicz-Beldzinska, M.; Benbadis, S. R.; Joshi, C.; Lyons, P. D.; Taylor, A.; Roberts, C.; Sommerville, K.; Gunning, B.; Gawlowicz, J.; Lisewski, P.; Mazurkiewicz Beldzinska, M.; Mitosek Szewczyk, K.; Steinborn, B.; Zolnowska, M.; Hughes, E.; McLellan, A.; Benbadis, S.; Ciliberto, M.; Clark, G.; Dlugos, D.; Filloux, F.; Flamini, R.; French, J.; Frost, M.; Haut, S.; Joshi, C.; Kapoor, S.; Kessler, S.; Laux, L.; Lyons, P.; Marsh, E.; Moore, D.; Morse, R.; Nagaraddi, V.; Rosenfeld, W.; Seltzer, L.; Shellhaas, R.; Sullivan, J.; Thiele, E.; Thio, L. L.; Wang, D.; Wilfong, A., Cannabidiol in patients with seizures associated with Lennox-Gastaut syndrome (GWPCARE4): A randomised, double-blind, placebo-controlled phase 3 trial. *The Lancet* **2018**, 391, (10125), 1085–1096.

65. Robson, P.; Guy, G.; Pertwee, R.; Jamontt, J. Use of tetrahydrocannabinol and/or cannabidiol for the treatment of inflammatory bowel disease. WO2009004302A1, **2009**.

66. Yeshurun, M.; Sagiv, S. P. Cannabidiol for reducing a steroid dose and treating inflammatory and autoimmune diseases. WO2017191630A1, **2017**.

67. De Vries, J. A.; Fernandez Cid, M. V.; Heredia Lopez, A. M.; Eiroa Martinez, C. M. Compressed tablet containing cannabidiol, method for its manufacture and use of such tablet in oral treatment of psychosis or anxiety disorders. WO2015065179A1, **2015**.

68. Gursoy, R. N.; Benita, S., Self-emulsifying drug delivery systems (SEDDS) for improved oral delivery of lipophilic drugs. *Biomed. Pharmacother.* **2004**, 58, (3), 173–182.

69. Murty, R. B.; Murty, S. B. An improved oral dosage form of tetrahydrocannabinol and a method of avoiding and/or suppressing hepatic first pass metabolism via targeted chylomicron/lipoprotein delivery. WO2012033478A1, **2012**.

70. Murty, R. B.; Murty, S. B. Oral dosage form of tetrahydrocannabinol and a method of avoiding and/or suppressing hepatic first pass metabolism via targeted chylomicron/lipoprotein delivery. US20110092583A1, **2011**.

71. Murty, S. B.; Murty, R. B. An improved oral gastrointestinal delivery system of cannabinoids and/or standardized marijuana extracts. US20160184258A1, **2016**.

72. Zipp, B. J.; Hardman, J. M.; Brooke, R. T. Methods for production of cannabinoid glycoside prodrugs by glycosyltransferase-mediated glycosylation of cannabinoids. *WO2017053574A1,* **2017**.

73. Hardman, J. M.; Brooke, R. T.; Zipp, B. J., Cannabinoid glycosides: In vitro production of a new class of cannabinoids with improved physicochemical properties. *bioRxiv, Biochem.* **2017**, 1–37.

74. Mercadante, S.; Radbruch, L.; Davies, A.; Poulain, P.; Sitte, T.; Perkins, P.; Colberg, T.; Camba, M. A., A comparison of intranasal fentanyl spray with oral transmucosal fentanyl citrate for the treatment of breakthrough cancer pain: An open-label, randomised, crossover trial. *Curr. Med. Res. Opin.* **2009**, 25, (11), 2805–2815.

75. Karschner, E. L.; Darwin, W. D.; Goodwin, R. S.; Wright, S.; Huestis, M. A., Plasma Cannabinoid Pharmacokinetics following Controlled Oral Δ^9-Tetrahydrocannabinol and Oromucosal Cannabis Extract Administration. *Clin. Chem.* **2011**, 57, (1), 66–75.

76. Tanasescu, R.; Constantinescu, C. S., Pharmacokinetic evaluation of nabiximols for the treatment of multiple sclerosis pain. *Expert Opin. Drug Metab. Toxicol.* **2013**, 9, (9), 1219–1228.

77. Lichtman, A. H.; Lux, E. A.; McQuade, R.; Rossetti, S.; Sanchez, R.; Sun, W.; Wright, S.; Kornyeyeva, E.; Fallon, M. T., Results of a double-blind, randomized, placebo-controlled study of nabiximols oromucosal spray as a adjunctive therapy in advanced cancer patients with chronic uncontrolled pain. *J. Pain Symptom Manage.* **2017**.

78. Nurmikko, T. J.; Serpell, M. G.; Hoggart, B.; Toomey, P. J.; Morlion, B. J.; Haines, D., Sativex successfully treats neuropathic pain characterised by allodynia: A randomised, double-blind, placebo-controlled clinical trial. *Pain* **2007**, 133, (1–3), 210–220.

79. Temtsin-Krayz, G.; Glozman, S.; Kazhdan, P. Pharmaceutical compositions comprising lipophilic compd. and water-sol. polymers for transmucosal delivery. WO2017072774A1, **2017**.

80. Van Damme, P. A.; Anastassov, G. E. Chewing gum compositions comprising cannabinoids. WO2009120080A1, **2009**.

81. Anastassov, G.; Changoer, L. Chewing gum composition comprising cannabinoids and opioid agonists and/or antagonists. WO2018075665A1, **2018**.

82. Paudel, K. S.; Hammell, D. C.; Agu, R. U.; Valiveti, S.; Stinchcomb, A. L., Cannabidiol bioavailability after nasal and transdermal application: Effect of permeation enhancers. *Drug Dev. Ind. Pharm.* **2010**, 36, (9), 1088–1097.

83. Bryson, N.; Sharma, A. C. Nasal cannabidiol compositions. WO2017208072A2, **2017**.

84. Huestis Marilyn, A., Human cannabinoid pharmacokinetics. *Chem. Biodivers.* **2007**, 4, (8), 1770–1804.

85. Hartman, R. L.; Brown, T. L.; Milavetz, G.; Spurgin, A.; Gorelick, D. A.; Gaffney, G.; Huestis, M. A., Controlled cannabis vaporizer administration: Blood and plasma cannabinoids with and without alcohol. *Clin. Chem.* **2015**, 61, (6), 850–869.

86. Solowij, N.; Broyd, S. J.; van Hell, H. H.; Hazekamp, A., A protocol for the delivery of cannabidiol (CBD) and combined CBD and Δ9-tetrahydrocannabinol (THC) by vaporisation. *BMC Pharmacol. Toxicol.* **2014**, 15, (1), 58.

87. Davidson, P.; Almog, S.; Kindler, S. Methods, devices and systems for pulmonary delivery of active agents. WO2016001922A1, **2016**.

88. Cameron, J. Hybrid vapor delivery system utilizing nebulized and non-nebulized elements. WO2016187115A1, **2016**.

89. Raichman, Y. Vaporizing devices and methods for delivering a compound using the same. US20180104214A1, **2018**.

90. McCullough, T. Methods and devices using cannabis vapors. US20150223515A1, **2015**.

91. Mason, L.; Moore, R. A.; Derry, S.; Edwards, J. E.; McQuay, H. J., Systematic review of topical capsaicin for the treatment of chronic pain. *Br. Med. J.* **2004**, 328, (7446), 991–994.

92. Tubaro, A.; Giangaspero, A.; Sosa, S.; Negri, R.; Grassi, G.; Casano, S.; Loggia, R. D.; Appendino, G., Comparative topical anti-inflammatory activity of cannabinoids and cannabivarins. *Fitoterapia* **2010**, 81, (7), 816–819.

93. Hammell, D. C.; Zhang, L. P.; Ma, F.; Abshire, S. M.; McIlwrath, S. L.; Stinchcomb, A. L.; Westlund, K. N., Transdermal cannabidiol reduces inflammation and pain-related behaviours in a rat model of arthritis. *Eur. J. Pain* **2016**, 20, (6), 936–948.

94. Touitou, E.; Dayan, N.; Bergelson, L.; Godin, B.; Eliaz, M., Ethosomes - Novel vesicular carriers for enhanced delivery: Characterization and skin penetration properties. *J. Control. Release* **2000**, 65, (3), 403–418.

95. Lodzki, M.; Godin, B.; Rakou, L.; Mechoulam, R.; Gallily, R.; Touitou, E., Cannabidiol - Transdermal delivery and anti-inflammatory effect in a murine model. *J. Control. Release* **2003**, 93, (3), 377–387.

96. Stinchcomb, A. L. Transdermal delivery of cannabinoids. US20020111377A1, **2002**.

97. Stinchcomb, A. L.; Nalluri, B. N. Transdermal delivery of cannabinoids. US20050266061A1, **2005**.

98. Stinchcomb, A. L.; Banks, S. L.; Golinski, M. J.; Howard, J. L.; Hammell, D. C. Cannabidiol prodrugs in topical and transdermal administration with microneedles. WO2011026144A1, **2011**.

99. Stinchcomb, A. L.; Valiveti, S.; Hammell, D. C.; Ramsey, D. R., Human skin permeation of Δ8-tetrahydrocannabinol, cannabidiol and cannabinol. *J. Pharm. Pharmacol.* **2004**, 56, (3), 291–297.

100. Chelliah, M. P.; Zinn, Z.; Khuu, P.; Teng, J. M. C., Self-initiated use of topical cannabidiol oil for epidermolysis bullosa. *Pediatr. Dermatol.* **2018**.

101. Brooke, L. L.; Herrmann, C. C.; Yum, S. I. Cannabinoid patch for Cannabis transdermal delivery. US6328992B1, **2001**.

102. Wallace, W. H. Method for relieving analgesia and reducing inflamation using a cannabinoid delivery topical liniment. US6949582B1, **2005**.

103. Siurkus, J. The oleo gel composition and delivery system with active compounds from Cannabis sativa and Mentha arvensis for reduction of inflammation and pain in deep tissues. WO2017178937A1, **2017**.

104. Siurkus, J.; Peciura, R. The topical composition with active compounds from Cannabis sativa and Calendula officinalis for reduction of skin lesions. WO2017175126A1, **2017**.

105. Jackson, D. K.; Hyatt, K. Silicone and hyaluronic acid (HLA) delivery systems for products by sustainable processes for medical uses including wound management. US20130184354A1, **2013**.

106. Lowe, G. A.; Lowe, V. Composition of cannabinoids, odorous volatile compounds, and emu oil for topical application and transdermal delivery to hypodermis. US9526752B1, **2016**.

107. Shemanski, M. E. Formulations of argan oil and cannabidiol for treating inflammatory disorders including arthritis. WO2017160923A1, **2017**.

108. Skalicky, J.; Husek, J.; Hofbauerova, J.; Dittrich, M. A composition for the treatment of inflammatory diseases comprising boswellic acids and cannabidiol. EP2444081A1, **2012**.

109. Oláh, A.; Tóth, B. I.; Borbíró, I.; Sugawara, K.; Szöllõsi, A. G.; Czifra, G.; Pál, B.; Ambrus, L.; Kloepper, J.; Camera, E.; Ludovici, M.; Picardo, M.; Voets, T.; Zouboulis, C. C.; Paus, R.; Bíró, T., Cannabidiol exerts sebostatic and antiinflammatory effects on human sebocytes. *J. Clin. Invest.* **2014**, 124, (9), 3713–3724.

110. Adelli, G. R.; Bhagav, P.; Taskar, P.; Hingorani, T.; Pettaway, S.; Gul, W.; Elsohly, M. A.; Repka, M. A.; Majumdar, S., Development of a Δ9-tetrahydrocannabinol amino acid-dicarboxylate prodrug with improved ocular bioavailability. *Invest. Ophthalmol. Vis. Sci.* **2017**, 58, (4), 2167–2179.

111. Cairns, E. A.; Baldridge, W. H.; Kelly, M. E. M., The endocannabinoid system as a therapeutic target in glaucoma. *Neural Plast.* **2016**, 2016, 10.

112. Weimann, L. J. Device and method for the transdermal delivery of cannabidiol. US20160361271A1, **2016**.

113. Immordino, M. L.; Dosio, F.; Cattel, L., Stealth liposomes: Review of the basic science, rationale, and clinical applications, existing and potential. *Int. J. Nanomed.* **2006**, 1, (3), 297–315.

114. Dosio, F.; Arpicco, S.; Stella, B.; Fattal, E., Hyaluronic acid for anticancer drug and nucleic acid delivery. *Adv. Drug Del. Rev.* **2016**, 97, 204–236.
115. Boraschi, D.; Italiani, P.; Palomba, R.; Decuzzi, P.; Duschl, A.; Fadeel, B.; Moghimi, S. M., Nanoparticles and innate immunity: New perspectives on host defence. *Semin. Immunol.* **2017**, 34, 33–51.
116. Park, K., Facing the truth about nanotechnology in drug delivery. *ACS Nano* **2013**, 7, (9), 7442–7447.
117. Hung, O.; Zamecnik, J.; Shek, P. N.; Tikuisis, P. Pulmonary delivery of liposome-encapsulated cannabinoids. WO2001003668A1, **2001**.
118. Donsky, M.; Winnicki, R. Terpene and cannabinoid liposome and micelle formulations. WO2015068052A2, **2015**.
119. Vitetta, L.; Hall, S. Protection of plant extracts and compounds from degradation. WO2017193169A1, **2017**.
120. Hall, S. M.; Vitetta, L.; Zhou, Y.; Rutolo, D. A., Jr.; Coulson, S. M. Transmucosal and transdermal delivery systems comprising non-ionic surfactant and polyol. WO2016141069A1, **2016**.
121. Pardeike, J.; Hommoss, A.; Müller, R. H., Lipid nanoparticles (SLN, NLC) in cosmetic and pharmaceutical dermal products. *Int. J. Pharm.* 2009, 366, (1–2), 170–184.
122. Esposito, E.; Drechsler, M.; Cortesi, R.; Nastruzzi, C., Encapsulation of cannabinoid drugs in nanostructured lipid carriers. *Eur. J. Pharm. Biopharm.* **2016**, 102, 87–91.
123. Hommoss, G.; Pyo, S. M.; Müller, R. H., Mucoadhesive tetrahydrocannabinol-loaded NLC – Formulation optimization and long-term physicochemical stability. *Eur. J. Pharm. Biopharm.* **2017**, 117, 408–417.
124. Johnson, J. R.; Burnell-Nugent, M.; Lossignol, D.; Ganae-Motan, E. D.; Potts, R.; Fallon, M. T., Multicenter, double-blind, randomized, placebo-controlled, parallel-group study of the efficacy, safety, and tolerability of THC:CBD extract and THC extract in patients with intractable cancer-related pain. *J. Pain Symptom Manage.* **2010**, 39, (2), 167–179.
125. Durán-Lobato, M.; Martín-Banderas, L.; Lopes, R.; Gonçalves, L. M. D.; Fernández-Arévalo, M.; Almeida, A. J., Lipid nanoparticles as an emerging platform for cannabinoid delivery: Physicochemical optimization and biocompatibility. *Drug Dev. Ind. Pharm.* **2016**, 42, (2), 190–198.
126. Elgart, A.; Cherniakov, I.; Aldouby, Y.; Domb, A. J.; Hoffman, A., Improved oral bioavailability of BCS class 2 compounds by self nano-emulsifying drug delivery systems (SNEDDS): The underlying mechanisms for amiodarone and talinolol. *Pharm. Res.* **2013**, 30, (12), 3029–3044.
127. Mistry, R. B.; Sheth, N. S., A review: Self emulsifying drug delivery system. *Int. J. Pharm. Pharm. Sci.* 2011, 3, (Suppl. 2), 23–28.
128. Avramoff, A.; Khan, W.; Ezra, A.; Elgart, A.; Hoffman, A.; Domb, A. J., Cyclosporin pro-dispersion liposphere formulation. *J. Control. Release* 2012, 160, (2), 401–406.
129. Atsmon, J.; Cherniakov, I.; Izgelov, D.; Hoffman, A.; Domb, A. J.; Deutsch, L.; Deutsch, F.; Heffetz, D.; Sacks, H., PTL401, a new formulation based on pro-nano dispersion technology, improves oral cannabinoids bioavailability in healthy volunteers. *J. Pharm. Sci.* **2018**, 107, (5), 1423–1429.
130. Cherniakov, I.; Izgelov, D.; Domb, A. J.; Hoffman, A., The effect of Pro NanoLipospheres (PNL) formulation containing natural absorption enhancers on the oral bioavailability of delta-9-tetrahydrocannabinol (THC) and cannabidiol (CBD) in a rat model. *Eur. J. Pharm. Sci.* **2017**, 109, 21–30.
131. Hoffman, A.; Domb, A. J.; Elgart, A.; Cherniakov, I. Formulation and method for increasing oral bioavailability of drugs. US20140348926A1, **2014**.

132. Cherniakov, I.; Izgelov, D.; Barasch, D.; Davidson, E.; Domb, A. J.; Hoffman, A., Piperine-pro-nanolipospheres as a novel oral delivery system of cannabinoids: Pharmacokinetic evaluation in healthy volunteers in comparison to buccal spray administration. *J. Control. Release* **2017**, 266, 1–7.

133. Hoffman, A.; Domb, A. J.; Elgart, A.; Cherniakov, I. Formulation and method for increasing oral bioavailability of drugs by utilizing pro-nano lipospheres incorporating piperine. WO2013108254A1, **2013**.

134. Wallis, S. W. Therapeutic delivery formulations and systems comprising cannabinoids and terpenes. CA2952335A1, **2017**.

135. Cardiol, T. Cannabidiol nanotherapeutic. http://adisinsight.springer.com/drugs/800052179.

136. Liechty, W. B.; Kryscio, D. R.; Slaughter, B. V.; Peppas, N. A., Polymers for drug delivery systems. *Annu. Rev. Chem. Biomol. Eng.* **2010**, 1, 149–173.

137. Mitragotri, S.; Burke, P. A.; Langer, R., Overcoming the challenges in administering biopharmaceuticals: Formulation and delivery strategies. *Nat. Rev. Drug Discovery* **2014**, 13, (9), 655–672.

138. Durán-Lobato, M.; Muñoz-Rubio, I.; Holgado, M. Á.; Álvarez-Fuentes, J.; Fernández-Arévalo, M.; Martín-Banderas, L., Enhanced cellular uptake and biodistribution of a synthetic cannabinoid loaded in surface-modified poly(lactic-co-glycolic acid) nanoparticles. *J. Biomed. Nanotechnol.* **2014**, 10, (6), 1068–1079.

139. Martín-Banderas, L.; Muñoz-Rubio, I.; Prados, J.; Álvarez-Fuentes, J.; Calderón-Montaño, J. M.; López-Lázaro, M.; Arias, J. L.; Leiva, M. C.; Holgado, M. A.; Fernández-Arévalo, M., In vitro and in vivo evaluation of Δ9-tetrahidrocannabinol/PLGA nanoparticles for cancer chemotherapy. *Int. J. Pharm.* 2015, 487, (1–2), 205–212.

140. Hernan Perez De La Ossa, D.; Ligresti, A.; Gil-Alegre, M. E.; Aberturas, M. R.; Molpeceres, J.; Di Marzo, V.; Torres Suárez, A. I., Poly-ε-caprolactone microspheres as a drug delivery system for cannabinoid administration: Development, characterization and in vitro evaluation of their antitumoral efficacy. *J. Control. Release* 2012, 161, (3), 927–932.

141. National Academies of Sciences, E., and Medicine The Health Effects of Cannabis and Cannabinoids: The Current State of Evidence and Recommendations for Research. http://nationalacademies.org/hmd/reports/2017/health-effects-of-Cannabis-and-cannabinoids.aspx (01/2019).

142. Whiting, P. F.; Wolff, R. F.; Deshpande, S.; Di Nisio, M.; Duffy, S.; Hernandez, A. V.; Keurentjes, J. C.; Lang, S.; Misso, K.; Ryder, S.; Schmidlkofer, S.; Westwood, M.; Kleijnen, J., Cannabinoids for medical use: A systematic review and meta-analysis. *J Am. Med. Assoc.* **2015**, 313, (24), 2456–2473.

143. Nugent, S. M.; Morasco, B. J.; O'Neil, M. E.; Freeman, M.; Low, A.; Kondo, K.; Elven, C.; Zakher, B.; Motu'apuaka, M.; Paynter, R.; Kansagara, D., The effects of cannabis among adults with chronic pain and an overview of general harms a systematic review. *Ann. Intern. Med.* **2017**, 167, (5), 319–331.

144. Mücke, M.; Phillips, T.; Radbruch, L.; Petzke, F.; Häuser, W., Cannabis-based medicines for chronic neuropathic pain in adults. *Cochrane Database of Systematic Reviews* **2018**, 2018, (3).

145. Nielsen, S.; Sabioni, P.; Trigo, J. M.; Ware, M. A.; Betz-Stablein, B. D.; Murnion, B.; Lintzeris, N.; Khor, K. E.; Farrell, M.; Smith, A.; Le Foll, B., Opioid-sparing effect of cannabinoids: A systematic review and meta-analysis. *Neuropsychopharmacology* **2017**, 42, (9), 1752–1765.

146. Campbell, G.; Hall, W. D.; Peacock, A.; Lintzeris, N.; Bruno, R.; Larance, B.; Nielsen, S.; Cohen, M.; Chan, G.; Mattick, R. P.; Blyth, F.; Shanahan, M.; Dobbins, T.; Farrell, M.; Degenhardt, L., Effect of cannabis use in people with chronic non-cancer pain prescribed opioids: Findings from a 4-year prospective cohort study. *The Lancet Public Health* **2018**, 3, (7), e341–e350.

147. Esposito, G.; De Filippis, D.; Cirillo, C.; Iuvone, T.; Capoccia, E.; Scuderi, C.; Steardo, A.; Cuomo, R.; Steardo, L., Cannabidiol in inflammatory bowel diseases: A brief overview. *Phytother. Res.* **2013**, 27, (5), 633–636.
148. Hasenoehrl, C.; Storr, M.; Schicho, R., Cannabinoids for treating inflammatory bowel diseases: Where are we and where do we go? *Expert Rev. Gastroenterol. Hepatol.* **2017**, 11, (4), 329–337.
149. Goldenberg, M.; Reid, M. W.; IsHak, W. W.; Danovitch, I., The impact of cannabis and cannabinoids for medical conditions on health-related quality of life: A systematic review and meta-analysis. *Drug Alcohol Depend.* **2017**, 174, 80–90.
150. Aviram, J.; Samuelly-Leichtag, G., Efficacy of cannabis-based medicines for pain management: A systematic review and meta-analysis of randomized controlled trials. *Pain Physician* **2017**, 20, (6), E755–E796.

13 Achieving and Sustaining Precision Effects

Understanding and Prescribing Cannabis Chemotypes

Uwe Blesching

CONTENTS

MOVING BEYOND THE SATIVA/INDICA DISTINCTION

Patients need to know how to achieve desired therapeutic effects and how to sustain them. Much of the current industry-wide system for choosing cannabis or cannabis-based products is still based on the assumed therapeutic qualities of cannabis's main species, sativa and indica, a distinction that has informed choices for decades. Yet it is woefully imprecise.

Consider this: Two people use the same identical seeds or clones to grow a specific cannabis species—but even subtle differences in their growing environments can significantly change the chemical composition of all plant constituents. Environmental

161

(epigenetic) signals such as temperature, nutrition, and quality of light will initiate specific changes in genetic *expressions* without changing the plant's genome or DNA. As such, even though the two cannabis species are genetically identical, the therapeutic (or adverse) effects they engender could be as different as mixing up a Zoloft with a Vicodin. Furthermore, none of the assumed qualities are evidence-based, making any success you may have had a good guess at best, further complicating consistently repeatable results. (The ability to repeat results is a hallmark of effective therapy.) While using the old system may still have value in the general context of breeding or as a means to discuss terpene profiles, for example, relying on it in a medical context makes it nearly impossible to use the abundance of available scientific literature to align types of cannabis with the specific patient populations that would benefit from them most (Graphic 13.1).

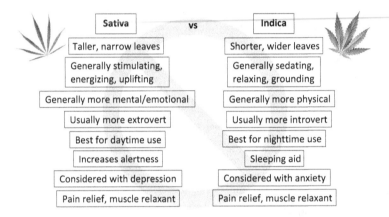

GRAPHIC 13.1 Moving beyond the sativa/indica distinction in prescribing cannabis for medicinal purposes. These generalizations are insufficient and unreliable for prescribing with precision.

In direct contrast, a newer, scientifically informed system has become available that addresses virtually all the shortcomings of the old one. As the last four decades of research discovered, three basic numbers form the key to predicting specific therapeutic effects for any type of cannabis plant, though they are not the only variables. These key numbers are: one, the amount of the primary psychoactive cannabis constituent tetrahydrocannabinol (THC); two, the amount of the non-psychoactive cannabis constituent cannabidiol (CBD); and three, the ratio of THC to CBD. It is these three factors, as expressed by two percentages and a ratio, that allow us to discern three basic types of cannabis, identified by the Roman numerals I, II, and III and called *cannabis chemotypes*.[1] A chemotype I contains more THC than CBD. A chemotype II contains relatively equal amounts of THC and CBD. And, finally, a chemotype III contains more CBD than THC.

This ratio-based system was devised by the researchers E. Small and H.D. Beckstead in 1973,[2,3] and their method of classifying individual cannabis plants by THC and CBD content continues to inform the cannabinoid health sciences today as we learn how to apply this key categorization. Every cannabis plant can be assigned to one of the three chemotypes.

Two additional chemotypes have been proposed in the scientific literature: chemotypes IV and V. Neither contributes unique, practical, or therapeutically significant information not already covered by chemotypes I through III, or by reports on the biological impact of individual cannabinoids. Chemotype IV reported by Fournier et al. in 1987[4] is defined as having CBG as the most abundant cannabinoid. Chemotype V proposed by Mandolino and Carboni in 2004[5] includes strains that are void of any detectable cannabinoids.

In terms of practical significance, these three chemotypes determine not just what kind of cannabis experience you or your patients will have, but also the therapeutic or adverse effects that a particular type of cannabis is likely to produce. Furthermore, it is these numbers that provide you with the basis for using the scientific literature in a practical and meaningful manner, allowing you to produce consistent and precise effects. In other words, awareness of THC:CBD ratio numbers is the first and most significant step in a process that will help you dial in, produce, fine-tune, and sustain the precise effects you seek.

Graphic 13.2 is a visual representation of the emerging science of chemotype-based prescribing. In contrast to the sativa/indica model, each of the effects listed is grounded in evidence. When the scale tips to the left of the center column (as is the case with any chemotype I, which has more THC than CBD), all effects on the left are amplified while those on the right are diminished. In a chemotype II with a ratio of 1:1, both sides express relatively equally. And when the scale tips to the right (as with any chemotype III), all effects to the right of the center column are amplified while those on the left are diminished.

THC		Receptors	CBD		
Pain, itch, ↓obesity[1]	○ Agonist[2]	TRPA1	○ Agonist[4,21]	Pain, itch, inflammation	
N/A		TRPV1	○ Agonist[22,23]	Analgesia[22]	
Heat, pain, inflammation[3]	○ Agonist[4]	TRPV2	○ Agonist[3]	May↓chronic pain[24]	
N/A		TRPV4	○ Agonist[25]	May reduce acne[25]	
Cold sensation, analgesia[5]	◐ Antagonist[6]	TRPM8	◐Antagonist[6]	↓inflammation,[26] ↓prostate ca[27]	
Synergistic analgesia 6 x <CBD[7]	Allo.modulator	Opioid μ/δ	Allo.modulator	Synergistic analgesia[7]	
CNS modulation	○ Agonist	GPCR CB1	○ Agonist[28]	CBD↓effects of THC[29,30]	◐Antagonist*[21]
↓Immune,[8] ↓↑Mood[9]	○ Agonist	GPCR CB2	○Agonist[31]	↓↑Immune[8] ↑Mood[32]	◐Antagonist*[21]
N/A		GPCR 3	Inverse agonist[33]	Alzheimer's[33] neuropathy[34]	
N/A		GPCR 6	Inverse agonist[33]	Parkinson's[33]	
Testes, spleen[10]↓HTN[11]	○ Agonist[12]	GPCR 18	N/A		
Heart funct.,[13] may↑certain ca[14-16]	○ Agonist[17]	GPCR 55	◐ Antagonist[17]	↓Bone loss,[35] may↓certain cancers[14-16]	
	Mod.via CB1&2	NTR	Modulator	↑5HT1A[36]↑$GABA_A$,[37]↓Ade.uptake[38]	
Arterial vasorelaxation,[18] ↓cancer[19]	○Agonist γ[18,20]	PPAR's α/γ	○Agonist α,[39]	↓Lung ca[39]↓ inflammation↓pain[40]	
Selective (allosteric) antagonist of CB1/CB2 receptor agonists[21]	N/A	Enzymes	↓FAAH[41]↑AEA	↑Mood,↓psychosis[41]	

GRAPHIC 13.2 The scientific basis for chemotype-based prescribing. (For sources cited in this graphic, see the "Graphics References" at the end of this chapter.)

Because a chemotype defines the quantities and ratio of cannabis' most potent constituents, THC and CBD, it signals to us what we can expect from ingesting this particular specimen. With this improved understanding of the scientific underpinnings of a chemotype-based approach to using cannabis flower and cannabis-containing products, in just a little while we will try to ground the information in some practical applications.

The **center column** depicts currently known receptor sites (and enzymatic pathways) that are activated by THC and/or CBD (depicted from top to bottom from white to increasing shades of gray).

- **White**: Ionic cannabinoid receptors aka Transient Receptor Potential channels (TRPs) pronounced *Trips* ("V" stands for vanilloid; "M" for melastatin; and "A" for ankyrin).
- **Gray 1**: G-protein-coupled receptors (GPCR) include GPCR CB_1 and CB_2, $GPCR_3$, $GPCR_6$, $GPCR_{18}$, $GPCR_{55}$, and opioid receptor sites (mu/μ and delta/δ).
- **Gray 2**: Various neurotransmitter modulation sites.
- **Gray 3**: Nuclear receptor proteins called Peroxisome Proliferator-Activated Receptors (PPARs).
- **Gray 4**: Enzymatic pathways of endocannabinoid degradation (e.g. anandamide, 2-AG).

Adjacent on the sides of the center column is the type of connection, either THC or CBD, produced at each of them. Generally speaking, these two cannabinoids can behave or act as an agonist, antagonist, inverse agonist, allosteric modulator, or a neurotransmitter modulator.

- **Agonist** (white circle): A compound such as THC, CBD, or any drug that binds to a specific receptor such as CB_1 or CB_2 and produces a specific biological effect. You may want to think of an agonist as a light switch that turns an option on.
- **Antagonist** (gray circle): A compound that binds to the same receptor site as an agonist does but instead blocks or reduces the normal response. Continuing with the switch analogy, an antagonist either dims the light or turns it off.
- **Allosteric modulator**: Allosteric binding sites are indirect binding sites that can influence an agonist and antagonist. In contrast, **orthosteric** binding sites are direct or primary binding sites of a receptor to a compound.
- **Selective (allosteric) antagonist of CB_1/CB_2 receptor agonists**: When you look at the fields on the right side next to CB_1 and CB_2, you will notice that CBD is indicated to be both an agonist (white circle) and an antagonist (gray circle). CBD is a very weak agonist at CB_1 and CB_2 but at the same time functions as a tissue-specific allosteric (indirect) modulator of CB_1 and CB_2 agonists. As such, and practically speaking, CBD can act

differently in different types of tissues, resulting in its capacity to reduce the effects of CB_1 and CB_2 agonists such as THC. In other words, this is the reason why CBD appears to tame some of the psychoactive effects of THC.

- **Neurotransmitter modulation** via the endocannabinoid system inhibits or enhances, either in part or significantly, the release of over 20 diverse communication molecules such as neurotransmitters, hormones, pro- and anti-inflammatory cytokines, endogenous opioids such as dopamine, GABA, glutamate, oxytocin, serotonin, cortisol, epinephrine, and acetylcholine, for example.

And finally, the outer columns provide a few examples of the specific effects that are generated by either THC or CBD (respective side on the left or right of center).

Please note that individual fields include a number of separate note references unique to this chart that allow you to take a deeper look.

CHEMOTYPE I

Usually when people talk about their fears of using cannabis—such as fears of getting "high," losing control, experiencing adverse effects, or fears about its addiction potential—they are referring to the common effects of a chemotype I of cannabis. It's true that with this chemotype and its high THC content, the line between an adverse effect and a therapeutic one can be razor-thin and very individualized. Additionally, any addiction potential is clearly associated with THC most prominently among all cannabinoids.

However, the very abilities of THC to produce these effects, unwanted and feared by some, are integral to the powerful sedative qualities that make this chemotype so therapeutic and practically useful as a medicine.

For instance, CB_1 receptor sites are abundantly present in the central nervous system (CNS). THC binds with these receptor sites to initiate a number of effects that are of particular relevance to patients with pathologies affecting the CNS (that is, the brain and spinal cord). Patients with conditions such as traumatic tears in the CNS (e.g. injuries, stroke), degenerative neurological disorders (e.g. Alzheimer's), or specific types of pain such as pathological pain (e.g. amyotrophic lateral sclerosis), severe pains associated with HIV/AIDS, and nociceptive pain tend to benefit from a chemotype I abundant in THC. The same is true for conditions where an over-excitability of specifically stressed tissues causes tension or spasms (e.g. spinal cord injuries); these patients benefit from the sedative aspect of this chemotype. A carefully dosed chemotype I also has the noteworthy ability to positively improve a number of mood disorders such as depression and various forms of anxiety. However, it can't be said often enough that there is indeed a fine line between a therapeutic effect and an adverse effect when medicating with a chemotype-I strain. A careful and slow approach is required at this stage in our collective knowledge, especially if the patient is new to cannabis in general (Graphic 13.3).

THC		Receptors	CBD		
Pain, itch, ↓obesity[1]	○ Agonist[2]	TRPA1	○Agonist[4,21]	Pain, itch, inflammation	
N/A		TRPV1	○ Agonist[22,23]	Analgesia[22]	
Heat, pain, inflammation[3]	○ Agonist[4]	TRPV2	○ Agonist[3]	May↓chronic pain[24]	
N/A		TRPV4	○ Agonist[25]	May reduce acne[25]	
Cold sensation, analgesia[5]	● Antagonist[6]	TRPM8	●Antagonist[6]	↓Inflammation,[26] ↓prostate ca[27]	
Synergistic analgesia 6 x <CBD[7]	Allo.modulator	Opioid μ/δ	Allo.modulator	Synergistic analgesia[7]	
CNS modulation	○ Agonist	GPCR CB1	○Agonist[28]	CBD↓effects of THC[29,30]	●Antagonist*[21]
↓Immune,[8] ↓↑ Mood[9]	○ Agonist	GPCR CB2	○Agonist[31]	↓↑ Immune[8] ↑Mood[32]	●Antagonist*[21]
N/A		GPCR 3	Inverse agonist[33]	Alzheimer's[33] neuropathy[34]	
N/A		GPCR 6	Inverse agonist[33]	Parkinson's[33]	
Testes, spleen[10]↓HTN[11]	○ Agonist[12]	GPCR 18	N/A		
Heart funct.,[13]may↑certain ca[14-16]	○ Agonist[17]	GPCR 55	● Antagonist[17]	↓Bone loss,[35]may↓certain cancers[14-16]	
	Mod.via CB1&2	NTR	Modulator	↑5HT1A[36]↑GABA$_A$,[37]↓Ade.uptake[38]	
Arterial vasorelaxation,[18]↓cancer[19]	○Agonist γ[18,20]	PPAR's α/γ	○Agonist α,[39]	↓Lung ca[39]↓ inflammation↓pain[40]	
Selective (allosteric) antagonist of CB1/CB2 receptor agonists[21]	N/A	Enzymes	↓FAAH[41]↑AEA	↑Mood,↓psychosis[41]	

GRAPHIC 13.3 Chemotype I (effects on left are amplified while those on the right are diminished). (For sources cited in this graphic, see the "Graphics References" at the end of this chapter.)

Mental and emotional effects from chemotype I range widely—from the positive experiences of euphoria, deep relaxation, new ways of thinking (with "breakthrough" insights), melting away of stress, enhanced creativity, satisfying laugher (sometimes uncontrollable), mirth, improvements in mood, or enhanced libido, for example, to experiences of a negative nature such as tension, anxiety, panic, paranoia, or sense of impending doom.

The reader is reminded that "feeling high"—experiencing altered consciousness or extraordinary states of awareness—can be considered an adverse effect by some. Other people seek out these same effects for therapeutic, creative, or transpersonal purposes. Most adverse effects are easily managed by reassurance and being in a safe, calm, relaxing atmosphere. Play gentle music or nature sounds, hold hands if desired, or just have the comforting presence of another person—it can make a difference.

Another use for THC in conjunction with CB₁ activation is suppression of nausea and vomiting. Relevant patient populations that benefit from a chemotype I include cancer patients, especially those undergoing chemotherapy and experiencing otherwise uncontrollable nausea and vomiting while also suffering from stress, tension, insomnia, pain, nephrotoxicity, cardiotoxicity, and a general loss of quality of life. An appropriately dosed use of a chemotype I can make a significant difference in mitigating all these primary and secondary symptoms.

Further, THC reduces cough responses and functions as a bronchodilator. Through binding with and activating CB₂ receptor sites (which are abundantly present in the body's immune system), THC can down-regulate immune functions. Patients suffering from an overactive immune system (e.g. allergic asthma, chronic coughing) often find relief in strains belonging to this chemotype.

A pharmaceutical version of a chemotype I is the FDA-approved, man-made drug Dronabinol (Marinol, Syndros). It contains a THC:CBD ratio of 1:0. Treatment examples for Dronabinol include appetite stimulation to reduce weight loss in patients with AIDS; and it is used as an anti-emetic in cancer patients experiencing chemotherapy-induced nausea and vomiting. Potential adverse effects of Dronabinol and chemotype I cannabis may include: "feeling high," altered consciousness, paranoia, anxiety, insomnia, pain, or nausea.

The following summary of chemotype-I strains and uses (plus those for chemotypes II and III) is far from exhaustive. Note that if you are not drawn to pharmaceutical cannabis compounds such as Dronabinol, your process of finding a similar ratio and cannabis effect will be more complex, though ideally it leads to a much more personalized form of medicine and you get the added benefits of the other plant constituents that tend to harmonize and even amplify therapeutic effects.

CHEMOTYPE I SUMMARY

Mental/Emotional

Cognition:

- "Feeling high," ranging from a pleasant euphoria to an unpleasant self-consciousness/paranoia/panic attack

Memory:

- Increases the ability to relax and be in the presence of intensely fearful memories, a positive effect in treating certain anxieties or phobias
- Slows habitual memory, helpful in cases of OCD and addiction triggers, for example
- Impairs short-term and long-term memories (normally THC-dose-dependent and temporary)

Mood:

- Deep relaxation and stress reduction
- Conscious sedation (especially therapeutic in overly excited/stressed nervous system-based conditions; see sample conditions below)
- Significant mood improvement is possible, but there is a very narrow line between anxiolytic and anxiogenic effects, ranging from euphoria (joy) to dysphoria (feeling anxious, scared, or panicky)

Physiological
- Bronchodilation (e.g. allergic asthma, cough)
- Appetite stimulation (weight loss, anorexia, cachexia)
- Immune-system modulation (down-regulation is relevant to conditions in which the body's immune system begins to attack itself, e.g. rheumatoid arthritis)

Pain types that may benefit:

- Central pain (e.g. stroke)
- Pathological pain (e.g. amyotrophic lateral sclerosis)
- Nociceptive pain (noxious stimulus from, e.g., chemical, heat, mechanical sources)
- Mental-emotional pains

Sample conditions that may benefit from a chemotype I include:

- HIV/AIDS-based neuropathies
- Severe physical withdrawal symptoms (e.g. heroin, opioids, methamphetamines)
- Chemotherapy-induced nausea and vomiting
- Spinal cord injury-induced chronic muscle spasms
- Alzheimer's disease with nighttime agitation or disturbed behavior
- Autism with agitation with self/other-harming behavior

Addiction potential: Low but there is a potential risk for psychological addiction.

CHEMOTYPE II

One of the general differences between a chemotype-I strain and a chemotype-II strain is that more CBD is introduced into the mix. The synergy of THC and CBD is a factor, because THC tends to support the therapeutic abilities of CBD, while CBD tends to tame the potential adverse effects associated with THC. A chemotype II gives a particular segment of patients their necessary central nervous system or CNS activation, but in a more tempered way than a chemotype I delivers. As such, use of a chemotype II reduces the risk of changes in cognition ("getting high"), reduces the potential for adverse effects, and lowers any risk of developing a psychological addiction.

Mental and emotional effects can differ widely from those of chemotype-I cannabis strains. Many chemotype II-using patients describe the differences in term of medium relaxation with a light sensation of feeling high, accompanied by a sense of uplift in mood, mild euphoria, an easy smile, a calmness of spirit, serenity, or tranquility. Fewer adverse effects occur with chemotype II. Some more sensitive patients, especially when using higher levels of THC concentrations that still fall within the chemotype-II range, may experience adverse effects, but if they do, effects are usually milder and shorter in duration than the effects of a chemotype I.

If you or a patient in your care could benefit from any of the effects or treatment examples listed in the chemotype-I section, but there is concern about the potential risks, then a chemotype II is probably a better choice, especially to start one's regimen. You still get the activation of THC at CB_1 and CB_2 receptor sites, but at a lower potency. In comparison to the use of a chemotype I, the line between a therapeutic and an adverse effect is much wider, providing more of a buffer from any potential ill effects that are dose-dependent on the amount of THC consumed (Graphic 13.4).

THC		Receptors	CBD		
Pain, itch, ↓obesity[1]	○ Agonist[2]	TRPA1	○ Agonist[4,21]	Pain, itch, inflammation	
N/A		TRPV1	○ Agonist[22,23]	Analgesia[22]	
Heat, pain, inflammation[3]	○ Agonist[4]	TRPV2	○ Agonist[3]	May↓chronic pain[24]	
N/A		TRPV4	○ Agonist[25]	May reduce acne[25]	
Cold sensation, analgesia[5]	◉ Antagonist[6]	TRPM8	◉Antagonist[6]	↓Inflammation,[26] ↓prostate ca[27]	
Synergistic analgesia 6 x <CBD[7]	Allo.modulator	Opioid μ/δ	Allo.modulator	Synergistic analgesia[7]	
CNS modulation	○ Agonist	GPCR CB1	○ Agonist[28]	CBD↓effects of THC[29,30]	◉Antagonist*[21]
↓Immune,[8] ↓↑ Mood[9]	○ Agonist	GPCR CB2	◯Agonist[31]	↓↑ Immune[8] ↑Mood[32]	◉Antagonist*[21]
N/A		GPCR 3	Inverse agonist[33]	Alzheimer's[33] neuropathy[34]	
N/A		GPCR 6	Inverse agonist[33]	Parkinson's[33]	
Testes, spleen[10]↓HTN[11]	○ Agonist[12]	GPCR 18	N/A		
Heart funct.,[13]may↑certain ca[14-16]	○ Agonist[17]	GPCR 55	◉ Antagonist[17]	↓Bone loss,[35]may↓certain cancers[14-16]	
	Mod.via CB1&2	NTR	Modulator	↑5HT1A[36]↑$GABA_A$[37]↓Ade.uptake[38]	
Arterial vasorelaxation,[18]↓cancer[19]	○ Agonist γ[18,20]	PPAR's α/γ	◯Agonist α,[55]	↓Lung ca[39]↓ inflammation↓pain[40]	
Selective (allosteric) antagonist of CB1/CB2 receptor agonists[21]	N/A	Enzymes	↓FAAH[41]↑AEA	↑Mood,↓psychosis[41]	

GRAPHIC 13.4 Chemotype II (both sides express relatively equally). (For sources cited in this graphic, see the "Graphics References" at the end of this chapter.)

Let's look at a couple of practical examples of using a chemotype II. A number of clinical trials demonstrated that a chemotype II was effective in the treatment of primary and secondary symptoms of multiple sclerosis, such as reduction of muscle spasms, pains related to spasms, and frequency of bladder incontinence. Similarly, in the treatment of various types of pain, a chemotype-II trend has emerged, suggesting its use in cases of certain peripheral neuropathies associated with cancer, cancer treatments (e.g. cisplatin), or auto-immune disorders (e.g. multiple sclerosis). This is especially important in the context of treating chronic neuropathies where the use of opioids has poor performance results.[6–8]

One of the few double-blind placebo human trials comparing the efficacy of all three pharmaceutical versions of all three cannabis chemotypes side by side in the treatment of a single condition (fibromyalgia) comes to us from the Netherlands, where researchers discovered that a single inhalation (using a vaporizer) of a chemotype II (Bediol® 6.3% THC:8% CBD) with the ratio of ~1:1.3 (THC:CBD) produced a 30% reduction in pain compared to placebo.[9]

The academic world continues to generate excitement with scientific findings suggesting efficacy of cannabis in the treatment of various cancers. The emerging picture is very complex but already suggests some important considerations. Allow me to give one example in the context of choosing the most appropriate chemotype. While THC has been shown to produce a number of pathways by which it creates apoptotic (anti-cancer) effects, various pre-clinical trials have discovered that colon, ovarian, and metastasizing breast cancer cell lines rely, at least in part, on GPCR-55 for proliferation.[10–12] Since THC is an agonist at GPCR-55 and CBD an antagonist at the same receptor, these early study results suggest caution in using a chemotype I for these particular cancers. While it might turn out that THC's positive effects other than GPCR-55-based effects outweigh the potential pitfalls of GPCR-55 activation on possible proliferation, a chemotype II concentrate may be the advisable option until the science is more compelling for this specific situation.

A pharmaceutical example of a chemotype II is a class of drugs called Nabiximols, a common US example being Sativex, a fully FDA-approved drug made from whole-plant cannabis including some other plant constituents (e.g. terpenes). In a number of other countries, it is approved as an additional pain medication for cancer patients who find no relief even with the highest allowable dose of opioids.[13] Adverse effects of Sativex may include: dizziness or fatigue (very common); dry mouth, disorientation, depression (common); and throat irritation/application irritation, feeling very high, rapid heart rate (uncommon).[14]

And, as you might suspect, adverse effects of chemotype-II strains in general mirror those of Sativex and may include dizziness, dry mucous membranes (mouth), and disorientation, for example.

CHEMOTYPE II SUMMARY

Mental/Emotional

Cognition:

- Lower risk of feeling "high" but still some potential for changes in cognition (THC-dose-dependent)

Memory:

- Similar changes to various types of memory functions as when using a chemotype I but much milder in nature
- Increased CBD content reduces THC-induced memory impairments

Mood:

- Moderate relaxation and stress reduction
- Low to moderate sedative affects (therapeutic in moderately over-excited/ stressed nervous system-based conditions)
- Mood improvement (wider line between anxiolytic and anxiogenic effects)
- Moderate effects as anxiolytic or anxiogenic

Physiological

Pain types that may benefit:

- Peripheral neuropathies
- Pain due to muscle spasms (e.g. multiple sclerosis)
- Cancer treatment-induced or cancer-based neuropathies
- Mental-emotional pains

Sample conditions that may benefit from a chemotype II include:

- Multiple sclerosis (calms and reduces pain, spasm, urinary incontinence)
- Fibromyalgia (provides systemic analgesia)

Addiction potential: Very low risk of developing psychological addiction (THC-dose-dependent)

CHEMOTPYE III

If you are a patient or care-giver of someone who wants to make sure there is no risk of getting "high" (experiencing changes in cognition), if you want to avoid any of the adverse effects commonly associated with cannabis use in general, and if you want to be sure there is not even a slight risk of getting psychologically addicted, this chemotype is for you. Mental and emotional effects include a gentle uplift in mood with no effects on cognitive abilities. Thinking, perception, and sensory experiences remain unaltered. However, there is one caveat: In some sensitive patients, a chemotype III that contains a still-significant level of THC (e.g. CBD OG) may result in adverse effects such as anxiety, although in much milder forms compared to high-THC chemotype I. This possibility is easily reduced or eliminated by using strains with no or a very low amount of THC (<0.3%) and tested by a reputable laboratory. Knowing the quantity of THC present in your chemotype III will give you agency and confidence about what kind of cannabis experience you wish to have. Following are THC and CBD percentages in some common chemotype-III strains: Cannatonic, 0.8% THC:20.8% CBD[15]; CBD OG, 9.01% THC:19.5% CBD[16]; AC/DC, 0.8% THC:15.4% CBD.[17]

Strains abundant in CBD with only small or trace amounts of THC carry their own rich abilities to produce a great number of proven therapeutic benefits. For instance, patients in need of a general uplift in mood tend to benefit from a chemotype-III medicine, as do patients with a number of chronic degenerative neurological illnesses with underlying or contributing pathologies such as oxidative stress and neurodegeneration-related seizure disorders (especially pediatric seizures), or drug dependencies (e.g. alcohol, opioid, methamphetamines), as well as those affected by mental conditions such as depression, anxiety, or psychotic disorders. Patients with serious pains who rely on opioid treatment often utilize a chemotype III to create a synergistic effect; it lets them reduce the opioids while achieving the same analgesic effect, with the benefit of lower costs and a reduction in dependence and overdose risks.

A pharmaceutical version of a chemotype III is the FDA-approved drug Epidiolex, a plant-derived cannabidiol-only medication.[18] Treatment examples from various countries where Epidiolex is legal include treatment-resistant epilepsy syndromes such as Dravet syndrome, Lennox-Gastaut syndrome, tuberous sclerosis complex, and infantile spasms.[19] Adverse effects of Epidiolex most commonly reported (from among severely sick patients) include drowsiness (somnolence) and changes in appetite and weight (up or down). A study conducted on pediatric patients suffering from treatment-resistant epilepsy demonstrated that Epidiolex is a promising treatment for these kids, and it is generally well-tolerated in doses up to 25 mg/kg/d (Graphic 13.5).[20]

THC		Receptors	CBD		
Pain, itch, ↓obesity[1]	○ Agonist[2]	TRPA1	○ Agonist[4,21]	Pain, itch, inflammation	
N/A		TRPV1	○ Agonist[22,23]	Analgesia[22]	
Heat, pain, inflammation[3]	○ Agonist[4]	TRPV2	○ Agonist[3]	May↓chronic pain[24]	
N/A		TRPV4	○ Agonist[25]	May reduce acne[25]	
Cold sensation, analgesia[5]	● Antagonist[6]	TRPM8	●Antagonist[6]	↓Inflammation,[26] ↓prostate ca[27]	
Synergistic analgesia 6 x <CBD[7]	Allo.modulator	Opioid μ/δ	Allo.modulator	Synergistic analgesia[7]	
CNS modulation	○ Agonist	GPCR CB1	○ Agonist[28]	CBD↓effects of THC[29,30]	◑Antagonist*[21]
↓Immune,[8] ↓↑ Mood[9]	○ Agonist	GPCR CB2	○Agonist[31]	↓↑ Immune[8] ↑Mood[32]	◑Antagonist*[21]
N/A		GPCR 3	Inverse agonist[33]	Alzheimer's[33] neuropathy[34]	
N/A		GPCR 6	Inverse agonist[33]	Parkinson's[33]	
Testes, spleen[10]↓HTN[11]	○ Agonist[12]	GPCR 18	N/A		
Heart funct.,[13]may↑certain ca[14-16]	○ Agonist[17]	GPCR 55	● Antagonist[17]	↓Bone loss,[35]may↓certain cancers[14-16]	
	Mod.via CB1&2	NTR	Modulator	↑5HT1A[36]↑GABA$_A$,[37]↓Ade.uptake[38]	
Arterial vasorelaxation,[18]↓cancer[19]	○ Agonist γ[18,20]	PPAR's α/γ	○Agonist α,[39]	↓Lung ca[39]↓ inflammation↓pain[40]	
Selective (allosteric) antagonist of CB1/CB2 receptor agonists[21]	N/A	Enzymes	↓FAAH[41]↑AEA	↑Mood,↓psychosis[41]	

GRAPHIC 13.5 Chemotype III (effects on the right are amplified while those on the left are diminished). (For sources cited in this graphic, see the "Graphics References" at the end of this chapter.)

Chemotype-III strains with no or only trace amounts of THC are generally considered safe for humans, including for chronic use and in high doses up to 1,500 mg/day.[21] However, some studies suggest that all chemotypes of cannabis including a chemotype III may interfere with certain pharmaceutical drugs. For instance, the concomitant use of clobazam (a pharmaceutical drug to treat seizures) with CBD makes the pharma drug more potent, leading to a possible increase in its adverse-effect potential such as drowsiness, ataxia, or irritability.[22] However, these adverse effects can be anticipated and avoided by lowering either clobazam or CBD amounts. The same concern applies to all other pharmaceutical drugs that are metabolized (broken down) by the enzymes belonging to the family cytochrome P450. This is due to the fact that CBD inhibits the break-down enzymes.

Furthermore, a chemotype III, in reaching for balance (homeostasis), may produce temporary tissue-specific pro- and/or anti-inflammatory responses, and as such can reduce inflammation in many patients or increase inflammation in certain severely immunocompromised patients such as those suffering from allergic inflammations of the lung, for instance.[23]

The reader may also want to take notice that purified, single-molecule CBD products may have limited therapeutic uses. Research conducted on mice in the context of treating inflammatory or nociceptive types of pain demonstrated superior effects of a full-spectrum (whole plant) CBD-abundant cannabis extract.[24]

The treatment indications as well as adverse effects for the pharmaceutical versions and corresponding strains tend to mirror each other.

CHEMOTYPE III SUMMARY

Mental/Emotional

Cognition:

- No risk of getting "high," and no changes in cognition (unless your strain contains more than 0.3% THC)

Memory:

- Positive neuroprotection in cases of dementia improves memory function

Mood:

- Mild relaxation and stress reduction; gentle uplift in affect (emotions)
- No sedative effects
- Mood improvements (anxiolytic with no anxiogenic effect if THC is less than 0.3%)

Physiological

Pain types that may benefit:

- General analgesic properties—possibly synergistic with opioids
- Inflammatory pain
- Chronic pain
- Mental-emotional pain

Sample conditions that may benefit from a chemotype III include:

- Acne
- Heart disease
- Irritable bowel disease
- Mental or mood disorders
    - Depression
    - Psychosis
    - Addiction
    - Anxieties
        - Post-traumatic stress disorder (PTSD)
        - OCD
- Seizure disorders
    - Epilepsy (pediatric and adult)
    - Dravet syndrome
    - Lennox-Gastaut syndrome
    - Tuberous sclerosis complex
    - Infantile spasms

Addiction potential: None (if THC amount is less than 0.3%)

In summary and in direct contrast to using the sativa and indica distinctions, the complexity of the scientific evidence of chemotype-based prescribing provides the foundation to produce a growing number of specific therapeutic effects in a consistent manner.

This chapter is based on the book entitled *Healing with Cannabis: Dialing in Your Optimal CBD to THC Ratio* (2019) published *by Ed Rosenthal's Quick Trading* and distributed by *Ingram/PGW*. You can also access regularly updated evidence-based trends linking the three cannabis chemotypes with specific conditions, symptoms, effects, and more at our free Cannabinoid Health Sciences Data Bank. Go to *CannaKeys.com* and click on the *Data Bank* link to have instant access.

REFERENCES

1. Hillig K. W. and Mahlberg P. G. A chemotaxonomic analysis of cannabinoid variation in Cannabis (Cannabaceae). *Am. J. Bot.* 2004 June;91(6):966–975.
2. Small E. and Beckstead H. D. Cannabinoid phenotypes in Cannabis sativa. *Nature.* 1973;245:147–148.
3. Small E. and Beckstead H. D. Common cannabinoid phenotypes in 350 stocks of Cannabis. *Lloydia.* 1973;36:144–165.
4. Fournier G., Richez-Dumanois C., Duvezin J., Mathieu J.-P. and Paris M. Identification of a new chemotype in Cannabis sativa: cannabigerol-dominant plants, biogenetic and agronomic prospects. *Plant. Med.* 1987;53:277–280.
5. Mandolino G. and Carboni A. Potential of marker assisted selection in hemp genetic improvement. *Euphytica.* 2004;140:107–120.
6. Sommer C., Peripheral neuropathies: long-term opioid therapy in neuropathy: benefit or harm? *Nat. Rev. Neurol.* 2017;13:516–517.
7. Finnerup N. B., Attal N. and Haroutounian S., *et al.* Pharmacotherapy for neuropathic pain in adults: systematic review, meta-analysis and updated NeuPSIG recommendations. *Lancet Neurol.* 2015;14(2):162–173.
8. Hoffman E. M., Watson J. C., St. Sauver J., Staff N. P. and Klein C. J. Association of long-term opioid therapy with functional status, adverse out- comes, and mortality among patients with polyneuropathy. *JAMA Neurol.* 2017 July 1;74(7):773–779.
9. Kathmann M., Flau K., Redmer A., Tränkle C. and Schlicker E. Cannabidiol is an allosteric modulator at mu- and delta-opioid receptors. *Naunyn Schmiedebergs Arch. Pharmacol.* 2006 Feb;372(5):354–361.
10. Kargl J., Andersen L., Hasenöhrl C., Feuersinger D., Stančić A., Fauland A., Magnes C., El-Heliebi A., Lax S., Uranitsch S., Haybaeck J., Heinemann A. and Schicho R. GPR55 promotes migration and adhesion of colon cancer cells indicating a role in metastasis. *Br. J. Pharmacol.* 2016 Jan;173(1):142–154.
11. Hofmann N. A., Yang J., Trauger S. A., Nakayama H., Huang L., Strunk D., Moses M. A., Klagsbrun M., Bischoff J. and Graier W. F. The GPR 55 agonist, L-α-lysophosphatidylinositol, mediates ovarian carcinoma cell-induced angiogenesis. *Br. J. Pharmacol.* 2015 Aug;172(16):4107–4118.
12. Andradas C., Blasco-Benito S., Castillo-Lluva S., Dillenburg-Pilla P., Diez-Alarcia R., Juanes-García A., García-Taboada E., Hernando-Llorente R., Soriano J., Hamann S., Wenners A., Alkatout I., Klapper W., Rocken C., Bauer M., Arnold N., Quintanilla M., Megías D., Vicente-Manzanares M., Urigüen L., Gutkind J. S., Guzmán M., Pérez-Gómez E. and Sánchez C. Activation of the orphan receptor GPR55

by lysophosphatidylinositol promotes metastasis in triple-negative breast cancer. *Oncotarget.* 2016 Jul 26;7(30):47565–47575.

13. GW Pharmaceuticals. Prescriber Information. www.gwpharm.com/products-pipeline/sativex/prescriber-information-full.

14. Bayer and GW Pharmaceutical Ltd. Sativex Oromucosal Spray, Patient Information Leaflet. Last changes May 20, 2015.

15. Source: High Times. The Strongest Strains on Earth 2016. LA Cup; lab-testing results by CSA Labs, Los Angeles, using gas chromatography–mass spectrometry (GC-MS). Written by Nico Escondido. June 28, 2016.

16. Source: High Times. The Strongest Strains on Earth 2016. LA Cup; lab-testing results by CSA Labs, Los Angeles, using gas chromatography–mass spectrometry (GC-MS). Written by Nico Escondido. June 28, 2016.

17. Source: High Times. The Strongest Strains on Earth 2016. LA Cup; lab-testing results by CSA Labs, Los Angeles, using gas chromatography–mass spectrometry (GC-MS). Written by Nico Escondido. June 28, 2016.

18. GW Pharmaceuticals. Epidiolex. www.gwpharm.com/epilepsy-patients-caregivers/patients.

19. GW Pharmaceuticals. Epidiolex. www.gwpharm.com/epilepsy-patients-caregivers/patients.

20. Devinsky O., Sullivan J., Friedman D., Thiele E., Marsh E., Laux L., Hedlund J., Tilton N., Bluvstein J. and Cilio M. Efficacy and safety of epidiolex (cannabidiol) in children and young adults with treatment-resistant epilepsy: initial data from an expanded access program. American Epilepsy Society. Annual Meeting Abstracts: Views. (Abst. 3.303), 2014.

21. Bergamaschi M. M., Queiroz R. H. C., Crippa J. A. S. and Zuardi A. W. Safety and side effects of cannabidiol, a Cannabis sativa constituent. *Curr. Drug Safety.* 2011;6(4):13 pages.

22. Geffrey A. L., Pollack S. F., Bruno P. L., *et al.* Drug–drug interaction between clobazam and cannabidiol in children with refractory epilepsy. *Epilepsia.* 2015;56:1246–1251.

23. Srivastava M. D., Srivastava B. I. and Brouhard B. D9-Tetrahydrocannabinol and cannabidiol alter cytokine production by human immune cells. *Immunopharmacology.* 1998;40(3):179–185.

24. Gallily, R., Yekhtin, Z. and Hanuš, L. O. overcoming the bell-shaped dose-response of cannabidiol by using cannabis extract enriched in cannabidiol. *Pharmacol. Pharm.* 2015;6:75–85.

GRAPHICS REFERENCES

1. Tamura Y., Iwasaki Y., Narukawa M. and Watanabe T. Ingestion of cinnamaldehyde, a TRPA1 agonist, reduces visceral fats in mice fed a high-fat and high-sucrose diet. *J Nutr Sci Vitaminol.* (Tokyo). 2012;58(1):9–13.

2. Akopian, A. N., Ruparel, N. B., Jeske, N. A., Patwardhan, A. and Hargreaves, K. M. Role of ionotropic cannabinoid receptors in peripheral antinociception and antihyperalgesia. *Trends Pharmacol. Sci.* 2009;30:79–84.

3. Qin N., Neeper Michael P., Liu Y., Hutchinson T. L., Lubin M. L. and Flores C. M. TRPV2 is activated by cannabidiol and mediates CGRP release in cultured rat dorsal root ganglion neurons. *J. Neurosci.* 2008 June 11;28(24):6231–6238.

4. De Petrocellis L., Ligresti A., Moriello A. S., Allarà M., Bisogno T., Petrosino S., Stott C. G. and Di Marzo V. Effects of cannabinoids and cannabinoid-enriched cannabis extracts on TRP channels and endocannabinoid metabolic enzymes. *Br. J. Pharm.* 2011;163:1479–1494.

5. Winchester W. J., Gore K., Glatt S., Petit W., Gardiner J. C., Conlon K., Postlethwaite M., Saintot P. P., Roberts S., Gosset J. R., Matsuura T., Andrews M. D., Glossop P. A., Palmer M. J., Clear N., Collins S., Beaumont K. and Reynolds D. S. Inhibition of TRPM8 channels reduces pain in the cold pressor test in humans. *Pharmacol. Exp. Ther.* 2014 Nov;351(2):259–269.

6. De Petrocellis L., Vellani V., Schiano-Moriello A., Marini P., Magherini P. C. and Orlando P., *et al.* Plant-derived cannabinoids modulate the activity of transient receptor potential channels of ankyrin type-1 and melastatin type-8. *J. Pharmacol. Exp. Ther.* 2008;325:1007–1015.

7. Kathmann M., Flau K., Redmer A., Tränkle C. and Schlicker E. Cannabidiol is an allosteric modulator at mu- and delta-opioid receptors. *Naunyn Schmiedebergs Arch. Pharmacol.* 2006 Feb;372(5):354–361.

8. Basu S. and Dittel B. N. Unraveling the complexities of cannabinoid receptor 2 (CB2) immune regulation in health and disease. *Immunol. Res.* 2011;51(1):26–38.

9. Bahi A., Al Mansouri S., Al Memari E., Al Ameri M., Nurulain S. M. and Ojha S. β-Caryophyllene, a CB2 receptor agonist produces multiple behavioral changes relevant to anxiety and depression in mice. *Physiol. Behav.* 2014 Aug;135:119–124.

10. Gantz I., Muraoka A., Yang Y. K., Samuelson L. C., Zimmerman E. M., Cook H. and Yamada T. Cloning and chromosomal localization of a gene (GPR18) encoding a novel seven transmembrane receptor highly expressed in spleen and testis. *Genomics.* 1997;42:462–466.

11. Penumarti, A. Role of central cannabinoid receptor GPR18 in cardiovascular regulation. Doctoral Dissertation, East Carolina University, January 2014.

12. McHugh, D., Page, J., Dunn, E. and Bradshaw, H. B. Δ9-Tetrahydrocannabinol and N-arachidonyl glycine are full agonists at GPR18 receptors and induce migration in human endometrial HEC-1B cells. *Br. J. Pharm.* April 2012;165(8):2414–2424.

13. Yu, J., Deliu, E. and Zhang. X.-Q., *et al.* Differential activation of cultured neonatal cardiomyocytes by plasmalemmal *versus* intracellular G protein-coupled receptor 55. *J. Biol. Chem.* 2013;288(31):22481–22492.

14. Kargl, J., Andersen, L., Hasenöhrl, C., Feuersinger, D., Stančić, A., Fauland, A., Magnes, C., El-Heliebi, A., Lax, S., Uranitsch, S., Haybaeck, J., Heinemann, A. and Schicho, R. GPR55 promotes migration and adhesion of colon cancer cells indicating a role in metastasis. *Br. J. Pharmacol.* 2016 Jan;173(1):142–154.

15. Hofmann N. A., Yang J., Trauger S. A., Nakayama H., Huang L., Strunk D., Moses M. A., Klagsbrun M., Bischoff J. and Graier W. F. The GPR 55 agonist, L-α-lysophosphatidylinositol, mediates ovarian carcinoma cell-induced angiogenesis. *Br. J. Pharmacol.* 2015 Aug;172(16):4107–4118.

16. Andradas C., Blasco-Benito S., Castillo-Lluva S., Dillenburg-Pilla P., Diez-Alarcia R., Juanes-García A., García-Taboada E., Hernando-Llorente R., Soriano J., Hamann S., Wenners A., Alkatout I., Klapper W., Rocken C., Bauer M., Arnold N., Quintanilla M., Megías D., Vicente-Manzanares M., Urigüen L., Gutkind J. S., Guzmán M., Pérez-Gómez E. and Sánchez C. Activation of the orphan receptor GPR55 by lysophosphatidylinositol promotes metastasis in triple-negative breast cancer. *Oncotarget.* 2016 Jul 26;7(30):47565–47575.

17. Ryberg E., Larsson N., Sjögren S., Hjorth S., Hermansson N.-O., Leonova J., Elebring T., Nilsson K., Drmota T., Greasley P. J. The orphan receptor GPR55 is a novel cannabinoid receptor. *Br. J. Pharm.* 2007;152:1092–1101.

18. O'Sullivan S. E., Tarling E. J., Bennett A. J., Kendall D. A. and Randall M. D. Novel time-dependent vascular actions of Δ9-tetrahydrocannabinol mediated by peroxisome proliferator-activated receptor γ. *Biochem. Biophys. Res. Commun.* 2005;337:824–831.

19. Krishnan A., Nair S. A. and Pillai M. R. Biology of PPAR gamma in cancer: a critical review on existing lacunae. *Curr. Mol. Med.* 2007;7(6):532–540.

20. O'Sullivan S. E., Tarling E. J., Bennett A. J., Kendall D. A., Randall M. D. Novel time-dependent vascular actions of Δ9-tetrahydrocannabinol mediated by peroxisome proliferator-activated receptor γ. *Biochem. Biophys. Res. Commun.* 2005;337:824–831.

21. Bishop-Bailey D. Peroxisome proliferator-activated receptors in the cardiovascular system. *Br. J. Pharmacol.* 2000;129(5):823–834.

22. Thomas A., Baillie G. L., Phillips A. M., Razdan R. K., Ross R. A. and Pertwee R. G. Cannabidiol displays unexpectedly high potency as an antagonist of CB1 and CB2 receptor agonists *in vitro*. *Br. J. Pharmacol.* 2007;150(5):613–623.

22. De Petrocellis L., Ligresti A., Moriello A. S., *et al.* Effects of cannabinoids and cannabinoid-enriched *Cannabis* extracts on TRP channels and endocannabinoid metabolic enzymes. *Br. J. Pharmacol.* 2011;163(7):1479–1494.

23. Costa B., Giagnoni G., Franke C., Trovato A. E. and Colleoni M. Vanilloid TRPV1 receptor mediates the antihyperalgesic effect of the nonpsychoactive cannabinoid, cannabidiol, in a rat model of acute inflammation. *Br. J. Pharmacol.* 2004;143(2):247–250.

24. Bisogno T., Hanus L., De Petrocellis L., Tchilibon S., Ponde D. E., Brandi I., *et al.* Molecular targets for cannabidiol and its synthetic analogues: effect on vanilloid VR1 receptors and on the cellular uptake and enzymatic hydrolysis of anandamide. *Br. J. Pharmacol.* 2001;134:845–852.

25. Costa B., Giagnoni G., Franke C., Trovato A. E., Colleoni M. Vanilloid TRPV1 receptor mediates the antihyperalgesic effect of the nonpsychoactive cannabinoid, cannabidiol, in a rat model of acute inflammation. *Br. J. Pharmacol.* 2004;143(2):247–250.

26. Qin N., Neeper M. P., Liu Y., Hutchinson T. L., Lubin M. L., Flores C. M. TRPV2 is activated by cannabidiol and mediates CGRP release in cultured rat dorsal root ganglion neurons. *J. Neurosci.* 2008;28:6231–6238.

27. Levine J. D. and Alessandri-Haber N. TRP channels: targets for the relief of pain. *Biochim. Biophys. Acta.* 2007;1772:989–1003.

28. Oláh A., Tóth B. I., Borbíró I., *et al.* Cannabidiol exerts sebostatic and antiinflammatory effects on human sebocytes. *J. Clin. Invest.* 2014;124(9):3713–3724.

29. Oláh A., Tóth B. I., Borbíró I., *et al.* Cannabidiol exerts sebostatic and antiinflammatory effects on human sebocytes. *J. Clin. Invest.* 2014;124(9):3713–3724.

30. De Petrocellis L., Vellani V., Schiano-Moriello A., Marini P., Magherini P. C., Orlando P., *et al.* Plant-derived cannabinoids modulate the activity of transient receptor potential channels of ankyrin type-1 and melastatin type-8. *J. Pharmacol. Exp. Ther.* 2008;325:1007–1015.

31. Ramachandran, R., Hyun, E., Zhao, L., Lapointe, T. K., Chapman, K., Hirota, C. L., Ghosh, S., McKemy, D. D., Vergnolle, N., Beck, P. L., Altier, C. and Hollenberg, M. D. TRPM8 activation attenuates inflammatory responses in mouse models of colitis *Proc. Natl. Acad. Sci. U.S.A.* 2013;110:7476–7481.

32. De Petrocellis L., Ligresti A., Schiano Moriello A., *et al.* Non-THC cannabinoids inhibit prostate carcinoma growth in vitro and in vivo: pro-apoptotic effects and underlying mechanisms. *Br. J. Pharmacol.* 2013;168(1):79–102.

33. Kathmann M., Flau K., Redmer A., Tränkle C., Schlicker E. Cannabidiol is an allosteric modulator at mu- and delta-opioid receptors. *Naunyn Schmiedebergs Arch. Pharmacol.* 2006 Feb;372(5):354–361.

34. McPartland J. M., Glass M., Pertwee R. G. Meta-analysis of cannabinoid ligand binding affinity and receptor distribution: interspecies differences. *Br. J. Pharmacol.* 2007;152(5):583–593.

35. Karniol I., Carlini E. Pharmacological interaction between cannabidiol and δ9-tetrahydrocannabinol. *Psychopharmacologia.* 1973;33:53–70.

36. Englund A., Morrison P. D., Nottage J., *et al.* Cannabidiol inhibits THC-elicited paranoid symptoms and hippocampal-dependent memory impairment. *J. Psychopharmacol.* 2013;27:19–27.

37. Thomas A., Baillie G. L., Phillips A. M., Razdan R. K., Ross R. A., Pertwee R. G. Cannabidiol displays unexpectedly high potency as an antagonist of CB1 and CB2 receptor agonists *in vitro*. *Br. J. Pharmacol.* 2007;150(5):613–623.
38. Rosenthaler S., Pöhn B., Kolmanz C., Nguyen Huu C., Krewenka C., Huber A., Kranner B., Rausch W.-D., Moldzio R. Differences in receptor binding affinity of several phytocannabinoids do not explain their effects on neural cell cultures. *Neurotoxicol. Teratol.* 2014;46:49–56.
39. Basu S., Dittel B. N. Unraveling the complexities of cannabinoid receptor 2 (CB2) immune regulation in health and disease. *Immunol. Res.* 2011;51(1):26–38.
40. Bahi A., Al Mansouri S., Al Memari E., Al Ameri M., Nurulain S. M., Ojha S. β-Caryophyllene, a CB2 receptor agonist produces multiple behavioral changes relevant to anxiety and depression in mice. *Physiol. Behav.* 2014 Aug;135:119–124.
41. Thomas A., Baillie G. L., Phillips A. M., Razdan R. K., Ross R. A., Pertwee R. G. Cannabidiol displays unexpectedly high potency as an antagonist of CB1 and CB2 receptor agonists *in vitro*. *Br. J. Pharmacol.* 2007;150(5):613–623.
42. Laun A. S. and Song Z.-H. GPR3 and GPR6, novel molecular targets for cannabidiol. *Biochem. Biophys. Res. Commun.* 2017 August 12;490(1);17–21.
43. Laun A. S. and Song Z.-H. GPR3 and GPR6, novel molecular targets for cannabidiol. *Biochem. Biophys. Res. Commun.* 2017 August 12;490(1);17–21.
44. Ruiz-Medina J., Ledent C. and Valverde O. GPR3 orphan receptor is involved in neuropathic pain after peripheral nerve injury and regulates morphine-induced antinociception. *Neuropharmacology.* 2011 July–August;61(1–2):43–50.
45. Laun A. S. and Song Z.-H. GPR3 and GPR6, novel molecular targets for cannabidiol. *Biochem. Biophys. Res. Commun.* 2017 August 12;490(1);17–21.
46. Laun A. S. and Song Z.-H. GPR3 and GPR6, novel molecular targets for cannabidiol. *Biochem. Biophys. Res. Commun.* 2017 August 12;490(1);17–21.
47. Ryberg E., Larsson N., Sjögren S., Hjorth S., Hermansson N.-O., Leonova J., Elebring T., Nilsson K., Drmota T., Greasley P. J. The orphan receptor GPR55 is a novel cannabinoid receptor. *Br. J. Pharm.* 2007;152:1092–1101.
48. Whytea L. S., Rybergb E., Simsc N. A., Ridgea S. A., Mackied K., Greasleyb P. J., Rossa R. A. and Rogersa M. J. The putative cannabinoid receptor GPR55 affects osteoclast function in vitro and bone mass in vivo. *PNSA* 2009;106(38):16511–16516.
49. Kargl J., Andersen L., Hasenöhrl C., Feuersinger D., Stančić A., Fauland A., Magnes C., El-Heliebi A., Lax S., Uranitsch S., Haybaeck J., Heinemann A. and Schicho R. GPR55 promotes migration and adhesion of colon cancer cells indicating a role in metastasis. *Br. J. Pharmacol.* 2016 Jan;173(1):142–154.
50. Hofmann N. A., Yang J., Trauger S. A., Nakayama H., Huang L., Strunk D., Moses M. A., Klagsbrun M., Bischoff J. and Graier W. F. The GPR 55 agonist, L-α-lysophosphatidylinositol, mediates ovarian carcinoma cell-induced angiogenesis. *Br. J. Pharmacol.* 2015 Aug;172(16):4107–4118.
51. Andradas C., Blasco-Benito S., Castillo-Lluva S., Dillenburg-Pilla P., Diez-Alarcia R., Juanes-García A., García-Taboada E., Hernando-Llorente R., Soriano J., Hamann S., Wenners A., Alkatout I., Klapper W., Rocken C., Bauer M., Arnold N., Quintanilla M., Megías D., Vicente-Manzanares M., Urigüen L., Gutkind J. S., Guzmán M., Pérez-Gómez E. and Sánchez C. Activation of the orphan receptor GPR55 by lysophosphatidylinositol promotes metastasis in triple-negative breast cancer. *Oncotarget.* 2016 Jul 26;7(30):47565–47575.
52. Resstel L. B. M., Tavares R. F., Lisboa S. F. S., Joca S. R. L., Corrêa F. M. A. and Guimarães F. S. 5-HT1A receptors are involved in the cannabidiol-induced attenuation of behavioural and cardiovascular responses to acute restraint stress in rats. *Br. J. Pharmacol.* 2009 Jan;156(1):181–188.

53. Bakas T., van Nieuwenhuijzen P. S., Devenish S. O., McGregor I. S., Arnold J. C. and Chebib M. The direct actions of cannabidiol and 2-arachidonoyl glycerol at GABAA receptor. *Pharmacol. Res.* 2017 May;119:358–370.
54. Carrier E. J., Auchampach J. A. and Hillard C. J. Inhibition of an equilibrative nucleoside transporter by cannabidiol: a mechanism of cannabinoid immunosuppression. *Proc. Natl. Acad. Sci. U. S. A.* 2006 May 16;103(20):7895–7900.
55. Ramer R., Heinemann K., Merkord J., Rohde H., Salamon A., Linnebacher M., Hinz B. COX-2 and PPAR-γ confer cannabidiol-induced apoptosis of human lung cancer cells. *Mol. Cancer. Ther.* 2013 Jan;12(1):69–82.
56. Ramer R., Heinemann K., Merkord J., Rohde H., Salamon A., Linnebacher M., Hinz B. COX-2 and PPAR-γ confer cannabidiol-induced apoptosis of human lung cancer cells. *Mol. Cancer. Ther.* 2013 Jan;12(1):69–82.
57. Maeda T. and Kishioka S. PPAR and pain. *Int. Rev. Neurobiol.* 2009;85:165–177.
58. Maeda T. and Kishioka S. PPAR and Pain. *Int. Rev. Neurobiol.* 2009;85:165–77.
59. Leweke F. M., Piomelli D., Pahlisch F., *et al.* Cannabidiol enhances anandamide signaling and alleviates psychotic symptoms of schizophrenia. *Transl. Psychiatry* 2012;2(3):e94.
60. Leweke F. M., Piomelli D., Pahlisch F., *et al.* Cannabidiol enhances anandamide signaling and alleviates psychotic symptoms of schizophrenia. *Transl. Psychiatry* 2012;2(3):e94.

14 Drug Interactions & Dosing Issues

Betty Wedman-St Louis
Clinical Nutritionist

CONTENTS

Cannabis-based medications exert their effects through the activation of cannabinoid receptors—CB_1, CB_2, GPR_{55}, GPR_{119}, GPR_{18}, and LPI (lysophosphatidylinositol) a possible sixth receptor [1,2]. Medications based on cannabis have been used therapeutically in many cultures for centuries for pain, spasms, asthma, sleep disorders, depression, and loss of appetite [3]. It was only in 1964 that the principle active ingredient in cannabis was defined [4] and the discovery of the body's own cannabinoid system with specific receptors and endogenous ligands followed in 1990.

The active components in cannabis, phytocannabinoids, can influence a wide array of biological processes in the human body through the production of endogenous analogs for arachidonoylethanolamine (anandamide or AEA) and 2-arachidonoylglycerol (2-AG) [5]. Sir William Brooke O'Shaughnessy, a Scottish physician, scientist, and engineer knew nothing about these functions when he reported the use of cannabis tinctures in rheumatism, tetanus, rabies, childhood epilepsy, and delirium tremens, which was learned during his stay in India in 1839. Physicians throughout Europe began to use cannabis tinctures in the second half of the 19th century, and cannabis was an accepted therapeutic agent in Western medicine [6].

DRUG INTERACTIONS

Endogenous and exogenous cannabinoids are substrates of various cytochrome 450 monooxygenases [7]. Zendulka, et al. report that out of 70 known phytocannabinoids, only Δ 9-THC, CBN, and CBD are reviewed in terms of oxidative metabolism due to lack of data found about other phytocannabinoids.

Exogenous cannabinoid interaction with other drugs depends on similar metabolic status since cannabinoids are strongly bound to proteins [8]. They might interact with drugs that are metabolized by enzymes of the CYP complex [9]. Some medicines may enhance or attenuate certain activities of cannabinoids while other activities may be reduced [10]. Of greatest clinical relevance, according to Grotenherman, is the sedating effect of other psychotropic substances—alcohol, benzodiazepines—and the interactions with medications such as amphetamines, adrenaline, atropine, β blockers, diuretics, and tricyclic antidepressants [9,10].

Exogenous cannabinoids that inhibit or induce drug metabolism in humans are an important factor in clinical care according to Stout and Cimino [11]. Cytochrome P-450 (CYP-450) enzymes are significant contributors to the metabolism of several exogenous cannabinoids:

- Tetrahydrocannabinol (THC)—CYP 2C9, 3A4
- Cannabidiol (CBD)—CYP 2C19, 3A4, 2D6, 2C9
- Cannabinol (CBN)—CYP 2C9, 3A4

With over 75 different CYP-450 enzymes essential for the metabolism of many medications—and six of them metabolizing 90% of the drugs—it can seem like a clinical nightmare [12,13]. Several recent studies are beginning to elaborate on how cannabinoids are interacting with liver enzymes.

Jiang, et al. [14] showed that 7 out of 14 recombinant human CYP enzymes may be involved in CBD metabolism: CYP 1A1, CYP 1A2, CYP 2C9, CYP 2C19, CYP 2D6, CYP 3A4, and CYP 3A5. In vitro studies indicate that THC and CBD both inhibit CYP 1A1, CYP 1A2, and CYP 1B1 enzymes [15]. Yamaori, et al. [16] and Watanabe, et al. [17] identify both THC and CBD are metabolized by CYP 3A4 and CYP 2C9 but in different ways:

- CYP 3A4 inhibitors slightly increase CBD levels.
- CYP 3A4 inducers slightly decrease THC and CBD levels.

Tetrahydrocannabinol (THC) can decrease serum concentrations of clozapine, duloxetine, naproxen, cyclobenzaprine, olanzapine, haloperidol, and chlorpromazine [17,18]. Ketoconazole, an inhibitor of CYP 3A4, was reported to increase concentrations with increases in THC concentrations. Clarithromycin, erythromycin, cyclosporine, itraconazole, voriconazole, and boceprevir would be expected to have a similar increase with THC concentrations [19].

Cannabidiol (CBD) is a potent inhibitor of CYP 3A4 and CYP 2D6. Since CYP 3A4 is responsible for metabolizing over 25% of all pharmaceuticals, CBD may increase serum concentrations of cyclosporine, sildenafil, antihistamines, haloperidol, antiretrovials, and some statins (atorvastatin and simvastatin, but not pravastatin or rosuvastatin). CYP 2D6 metabolizes many antidepressants so serum concentrations of SSRIs like tricyclic antidepressants, antipsychotics, beta blockers, and opioids may be increased. CBD can affect metabolism of omeprazole and risperidone by CYP 2D6 interaction [20].

Both THC and CBD increase warfarin levels, and increased INRs have been reported [21]. Geffrey, et al. [22] reported that CBD used for pediatric epilepsy increased clobazam levels but inhibited CYP 2C9 needed for the metabolism of warfarin and diclofenac.

Monoamine oxidase inhibitors (MAOIs) like tranylcypromine (Parnate), phenelzine (Nardil), and isocarboxazid (Marplan) have fallen out of favor for treatment of depression due to the reported side effects and interactions with food and other medications. There is a high risk of similar interactions if used with cannabis [21].

SUMMARY OF CANNABIS DRUG INTERACTIONS

These classifications are a guide for healthcare providers when counseling cannabis users [23].

- **High Clinical Interactions**: morphine, Norco (acetaminophen/hydrocodone), tramadol
- **Moderate Clinical Interactions**: alcohol, amitriptyline, Ativan, Benadryl, Cymbalta, Flexeril, Klonopin, Lamictal, Lexapro, Lyrica, Xanax, Zoloft, Zyrtec

Drugs that can INCREASE the effects of orally administered cannabis include [24]:

- Amiodarone (Cardarone)
- Clarithromycin (Biaxin)
- Diltiazem (Tiazac, Cardizem, Dilacor)
- Erythromycin
- Fluconazole
- Isoniazid
- Itraconazole (Sporanox)
- Ketoconazole
- Miconazole (Monistat)
- Ritonavir (Norvir)
- Verapamil (Calan, Verelan)

Drugs that can DECREASE the effects of oral cannabis are [24]:

- Carbamazepine (Tegretol, Carbatrol)
- Phenobarbital
- Phenytoin (Dilantin)
- Primidone (Mylosine)
- Rifabutin (Mycobutin)
- Rifampicin

CANNABIS DOSING

More than two-thirds of Americans now live in jurisdictions that have legalized either the medical or adult use of cannabis, and states with legalized medical cannabis have a decreased amount of opioid overdose deaths [25]. Since the endocannabinoid system was first described in 1992 [26], ongoing research has focused on the therapeutic benefits of CBD and condition-specific dosing due to its safe use with little or no side effects [27].

- CBD is non-toxic with no adverse changes in appetite, gastrointestinal transit, psychomotor or psychological functions
- Chronic use and high doses up to 1,500 mg/day are well tolerated

The approved use of psychoactive THC continues to evolve. Hemp-based products do not contain high levels of THC and are currently legal throughout the U.S.

DOSE MAKES THE DIFFERENCE

Dosage is the key factor in achieving the most benefits from cannabis. Some individuals can use 1 mg of full spectrum cannabinoids daily and achieve pain reduction or anxiety relief while others require 1,000 to 1,500 mg daily. The proper dose for an individual can be a moving target requiring different doses for different effects or lifestyle situations. Others may see therapeutic benefits diminish as the dose increases. A general rule is start low 5–25 mg CBD per day and gradually increase to 50–75 mg CBD per day with dosing at bedtime to alleviate any anxiety about "reactions to cannabis." An additional dose increase can be added, if needed, during the day.

A high dose of 100+mg CBD from full spectrum products is not frequently needed to achieve the optimal dose range represented in this graphic. An isolate product may be needed at twice the dose of a full spectrum product.

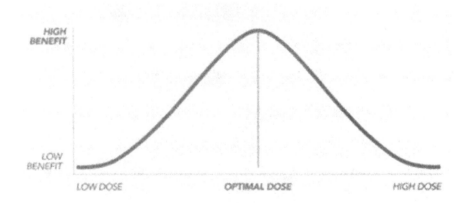

DOSING STRATEGIES CBD + THC

When CBD and THC are combined, they can enhance the benefits of each since they have overlapping therapeutic qualities for pain, anxiety, seizures, and nausea management. Jordan Tishler, M.D., discussed his dosing strategy based on why the person was choosing to use cannabis [28]. The person who elects cannabis for wellness—to improve their balance and sharpen their mind (usually 25–45 years old and an educated professional)—will do well on a 1:1 ratio or 2:1 ratio of CBD:THC but may be more comfortable starting out with a 4 mg CBD to 1 mg THC since less is more when sensitizing the endocannabinoid system for balance and homeostasis [29].

Those needing pain relief and reliable symptom control without intoxication may need 10–15 mg THC with 25–30 mg CBD. Epilepsy and autism dosing may need to be a ratio of 20 CBD to 1 THC or 15 mg CBD: 0.75 mg THC. Asthma relief with vaping can be effective with 3–5 mg THC per puff.

While THC and CBD have different pharmacological properties, they both can have analgesic and anti-inflammatory effects through different mechanisms. So there is no clinical evidence for stating a particular ratio of THC to CBD is recommended for a specific patient. Some trial and error is still needed to find the best solution for each individual. In addition, individual physiologies change over time and so should the dosing. Cannabis is an herbal plant, not a single substance pharmaceutical drug that is easier to standardize and regulate [30].

The psychoactive effects of cannabis depend on THC's ability to activate CB_1 receptors. The presence of CBD changes the THC's ability to activate CB_1 receptors as shown in laboratory studies [31]. Other laboratory studies have shown that CBD alone reduces behavioral measures of anxiety [32]. Cancer and neurological disorders usually benefit from a balanced ratio of CBD and THC for pain [33], so optimizing a therapeutic use of cannabis may entail a careful, step-by-step process which can start with a low dose of non-intoxicating CBD and gradually increase the THC, as needed.

PEDIATRIC DOSING

The use of cannabidiol (CBD) in pediatric patients is preferred by many healthcare professionals because psychoactive and physiological effects of THC do not need to be considered [34]. A general dosing strategy is based on body weight—0.2 mg/kg to 0.5 mg/kg as a starting dose according to Elliot Kane, M.D., professor, Department of Pediatrics & Anesthesiology, Perioperative and Pain Management at Stanford University. "I titrate to an effective dose of a maximum 1 mg/kg. Most dispensaries will carry tinctures" [36].

Bonnie Goldstein, M.D., medical director of Canna-Centers doses pediatric epilepsy with full spectrum CBD with 1 mg/kg every 8 hours as a starting dose with increases of 0.5–1 mg/kg/day every 2 weeks for oral, sublingual, and G-tube administration with an average dose of 5 to 8 mg/kg/day [37]. Dr. Goldstein indicates that PANDAS (Pediatric Autoimmune Neuropsychiatric Disorders) associated with Streptococcal infections responded well to CBD full spectrum oil with a reduction in OCD, tics, anxiety, and aggression.

Autism spectrum disorder showed improved (calmer, less self-injurious behavior) and improved communication skills on lower doses than those used in epilepsy [38]. It was assessed that high CBD was too stimulating and a CBD:THC ratio was more effective.

RAW CANNABINOIDS—ACID FORMS

In raw plant form, cannabis contains acid forms of the cannabinoids: THCA, CBDA, CBGA, etc. [39]. THCA is the non-intoxicating precursor that becomes THC when it is exposed to heat over a period of time called decarboxylation. The same holds true regarding the other cannabinoid acid forms. THCA is a larger molecule than THC (decarboxylation removes the carboxylic acid group), which limits its ability to react in the body with CB_1 receptors. Research is still preliminary about the benefits of raw cannabis but it has been associated with reducing IBS, glaucoma, fibromyalgia, and other inflammatory conditions.

Verhoeckx, et al. showed that THCA inhibited tumor necrosis factor alpha (TNF-α) and has distinct effects on phosphatidylcholine specific phospholipase C activity [40]. Acid forms of cannabinoids may exert immuno-modulating effects via different pathways. Takeda, et al. reported on the down-regulation of breast cancer metastasis by COX-2 expression due to CBDA [41].

Other studies have reviewed the use of acid cannabinoids for anti-convulsant activity [42], headaches [43], and anti-ementic activity [44].

CANNABINOID TOLERANCE

Another dosing challenge is cannabinoid tolerance due to the desensitization of receptors with regular phytocannabinoid stimulation for recreational and medicinal purposes [45]. After chronic cannabinoid consumption of THC, withdrawal signs were noted in the laboratory animal studies [46]. Hsieh, et al. [47] related tolerance to:

- dephosphorylation by phosphatase 1 or phosphatase 2A needed for recycling receptors to the cell surface and
- with prolonged exposure, CB_1 receptors are down-regulated and new protein synthesis is required for receptor recovery

How long it takes to produce a tolerance effect is still unknown but several reports indicate that stopping THC use 1 to 2 days/week or 1–3 weeks every 3 to 4 months can reduce tolerance [48,49]. Other options may be skipping one day each week to reduce tolerance. CBD has different tolerance producing effects than THC. Shirmrit Uliel-Sibony, M.D., lead author of the study and head of the pediatric epilepsy service at Tel Aviv Sourasky Medical Center Dana-Dwek Children's Hospital identified that efficacy may decline in children treated with CBD for extended periods [50].

ROUTE OF ADMINISTRATION

Different routes of administration provide more direct routes to the bloodstream and exert an effect in the brain and other parts of the body in an inconsistent manner. The Giving Tree Wellness Center Product Guidelines are an excellent reference for evaluation cannabis products [51]:

- **Smoking** a joint 0.5 to –1 gram cannabis (containing 10%–20% THC) = 16.3 mg THC in 10% THC. Effects start in 10–20 minutes and last 2–4 hours. Smoking may cause lung/throat irritation but gives a patient better control over managing acute pain. 1 to –2 puffs may be sufficient for many patients to reduce pain.
- **Vaporing** is heating cannabis to 180°C–200°C (356°F–392°F) which releases cannabinoids as a vapor without smoke (terpenes are usually lost from the oil because of the heat). 36%–61% THC of the concentrate is delivered to the body. Effects last 2–4 hours providing less lung/throat irritation than smoking and easier to control dosing.
- **Ingestion** or eating cannabis reduces the onset of effects by 30 to –60 minutes with peak effect in 3 to –6 hours and lasting 6 to –8 hours.
- Capsules may contain 10–50 mg cannabinoids with dosing two to three times per 24 hours. Start with 10–20 mg capsule and wait 30 to –60 minutes before adding a second dose if no symptom effects are experienced.
- Cannabis oil concentrates (provided in syringe) may contain up to 800–1,000 mg/ml cannabinoids and can be cut into small servings.
- Sublingual/oromucosal products like alcohol tinctures and oil extracts are absorbed rapidly and are provided in 1 ounce dropper bottles. Alcohol tinctures are 10–15 mg cannabinoids/ml while oil extracts are 10–20 mg cannabinoids/ml or higher. Cannabis lozenges and lollipops, gum and mouthstrips are also available producing effect in less than 30 minutes and lasting 4–6 hours. Start with low dose, wait 15–30 minutes before increasing dose. Tinctures administered under the tongue will be absorbed faster than when added to tea or juice.
- Edibles come in many forms at any concentration of cannabinoids. They have a longer duration of effects and users should not consume more than 5 mg THC and wait 2–3 hours before consuming an additional dose. Eating cannabis-infused edibles on an empty stomach will produce faster psychoactive effects. The gradual nature of digestion accounts for longer effects.
- **Topicals** are used by applying cannabis preparation to the skin which minimizes psychoactive effects due to no central nervous system receptors. Skin disorders and peripheral pain do well with salves and lotions. Patches are also available and designed for penetration through the skin. The usual dose for a patch is 10–12 mg cannabinoids, and it can be applied 1–4 times daily. Some patches have time-release ingredients to cover 3–6 hour periods. Topicals have no cognitive impairment and are great for joint pain, knees, neck, and stomach or abdominal cramps.

- **Suppositories** for rectal and vaginal use provide cannabis directly to the bloodstream avoiding the first-pass metabolism in the liver. They provide quick acting pain relief without psychoactive effects and long lasting pain control usually within 10–15 minutes and lasting 4 to 8 hours.

Chronic pathological pain, including neuropathic pain is the leading health problem worldwide [52]. Treatment of chronic pain is still an unmet clinical need according to Bruni, et al. [53]. Adequate pain relief is usually obtained by using drugs with adverse effects on the central nervous system. Cannabis-derived products should be considered to enrich the treatment arsenal for chronic pain and inflammatory conditions [54].

REFERENCES

1. Mackie K. Cannabinoid receptors: where they are and what they do. *J Neuroendocrinol* 2008;20(Suppl 1):10–4.
2. Zou S, Kumar U. Cannabinoid receptors and the endocannabinoid system: signaling and function in the central nervous system. *Int J Mol Sci* 2018;19(3):833.
3. Grotenherman F, Muller-Vahl K. The therapeutic potential of cannabis and cannabinoids. *Dt sch Arztebl Int* 2012;109(29–30):495–501.
4. Gaomi Y, Mechoulam R. Isolation, structure, and partial synthesis of an active constituent of hashish. *J Am Chem Soc* 1964;86:1646–47.
5. Olah A, Szekanecz Z, Biro T. Targeting cannabinoid signaling in the immune system: "high"-ly exciting questions, possibilities, and challenges. *Front Immunol* 2017;8:1487.
6. Grotenherman F, Muller-Vahl K. Medical uses of marijuana and cannabinoids. *Crit Rev Plant Sci* 2016;35(5–6):378–405.
7. Zendulka O, Dovrtelova G, Noskova K, et al. Cannabinoids and cytochrome 450 interactions. *Curr Drug Metab* 2016;17:000.
8. Pryor GT, Husain S, Mitoma C. Acute and subacute interactions between delta-9-tetrahydrocannabinol and other drugs in the rat. *Ann NY Acad Sci* 1976;281:171–89.
9. Grotenherman F. Pharmacokinetics and pharmacodynamics of cannabinoids. *Clin Pharmacokinet* 2003;42(4):327–60.
10. Sutin KM, Nahas GG. Physiological and pharmacological interactions of marihuana (Δ9-THC) with drugs and anesthetics. In: Nahas G, Sutin KM, Harvey DJ, et al., eds. *Marihuana and Medicine.* Totowa, NJ: Humana Press, 1999, 253–71.
11. Stout SM, Cimino NM. Exogenous cannabinoids as substrates, inhibitors, and inducers of human drug metabolizing enzymes: a systemic review. *Drug Metab Rev* 2014;446(1):86–95.
12. Danielson PB. The cytochrome 450 super family: biochemistry, evolution and drug metabolism in humans. *Curr Drug Metab* 2002;3(6):561–97.
13. Lynch T, Price A. The effect of cytochrome P 450 metabolism on drug response, interactions, and adverse effects. *Am Fam Physician* 2007;76(3):391–6.
14. Jiang R, Yamaori S, Takeda S, et al. Identification of cytochrome P450 enzymes responsible for metabolism of cannabidiol by human liver microsomes. *Life Sci* 2011;89(5–6):165–70.
15. Arellano AL, Papaseit E, Romaguera A, et al. Neuropsychiatric and general interactions of natural and synthetic cannabinoids with drugs of abuse and medicines. *CNS Neurol Disord Drug Targets* 2017;16(5):554–566.

16. Yamaori S, Koeda K, Kushihara M, et al. Comparison in the in vitro inhibiting effects of major phytocannabinoids and polycyclic aromatic hydrocarbons contained in marijuana smoke on P450 2C9 activity. *Drug Metab Pharmacokinet* 2012;27(3):294–300.
17. Watanabe K, Yamaori S, Funahashi T, et al. Cytochrome P450 enzymes involved in the metabolism of tetrahydrcannabinols and cannabinol by human hepatic microsomes. *Life Sci* 2007;80(15):1415–9.
18. Flockhart DA. Drug interactions: cytochrome P450 Drug Interaction Table. Indiana University School of Medicine, 2007. http://medicine.iupui.edu/clinpharm/ddis.
19. Horn JR, Hansten PD. Drug interactions with marijuana. Pharmacy Times Dec 9, 2014. www.pharmacytimes.com/publications/issue2014/december2014/drug-interactions-with-marijuana.
20. Ujvary I, Hanus L. Human metabolites of cannabidiol: a review on their formation, biological activity, and relevance in therapy. *Cannabis Cannabinoid Res* 2016;1:90–101.
21. Paunescu H, Coman OA, Coman L, et al. Cannabinoid system and cyclooxygenases inhibitors. *J Med Life* 2011;4(1):11–20.
22. Geffrey AL, Pollack SF, Bruno PL. Drug-drug interaction between clobazam and cannabidiol in children with refractory epilepsy. *Epilepsia* 2015;56(8):1246–51.
23. Cannabis drug interactions. Drugs.com. www.drugs.com/drug-interactions/cannabis.
24. Backes M. Cannabis as medicine. *Cannabis Pharmacy*. Black Dog & Leventhal Publishers, 2017, 33.
25. The health effects of cannabis and cannabinoids. The Current State of Evidence and Recommendations for Research. National Academies Press, Washington, D.C, 2017.
26. Devane WA, Hanus L, Breuer A, et al. Isolation and structure of a brain constituent that binds to the cannabinoid receptor. *Science* 1992;258(5090):1946–9.
27. Bergamaschi MM, Queiroz RH, Zuardi AW, et al. Safety and side effects of cannabidiol, a Cannabis sativa constituent. *Curr Drug Saf* 2011;6:237–49.
28. Tishler J. Are low doses of marijuana more effective than high doses? http://inhalemd.com/blog.
29. Tishler J. Microdosing. Medical Marijuana- an educational symposium for Florida physicians, June 3, 2017.
30. Malka D. Delivery and dosage of cannabis medicine. Medical Marijuana- an educational symposium for Florida physicians. June 3, 2017.
31. Russo EB, Guy GW. A tale of two cannabinoids: the therapeutic rationale for combining tetrahydrocannabinol and cannabidiol. *Med Hypotheses* 2006;66(2):234–46.
32. Bergamaschi MM, Queiroz RH, Chagas MHN, et al. Cannabidiol reduces the anxiety induced by simulated public speaking in treatment-naive social phobia patients. *Neuropsychopharmacology* 2011;36(6):1219–26.
33. Grotenherman F, Muller-Vahl K. The therapeutic potential of cannabis and cannabinoids. *Dt sch Arztebl Int* 2012;109(29–30):495–501.
34. Campbell CT, Phillips MS, Manasco K. Cannabinoids in pediatrics. *J Pediatr Pharmacol Ther* 2017;22(3):176–185.
35. Welty TE, Luebke A, Gidal BE. Cannabidiol: promise and pitfalls. *Epilepsy Curr* 2014;14(5):250–252.
36. Melville NA. Medical cannabis for pain may reduce need for opioids. March 8, 2018. www.medscape.com.
37. Goldstein B. Medical Cannabis: practical treatment of pediatric patients for epilepsy, autism, cancer and psychiatric disorders. CannMed 2016.
38. Siniscalco D, Sapone A, Giordano C, et al. Cannabinoid receptor type 2, but not type 1, is upregulated in perpheral blood mononuclear cells of children affected by autism disorders. *J Autism and Developmental Disorders* 2013;43(11):2686–95.
39. Zirpel B, Kayser O, Stehle F. Elucidation of structure-function relationship of THCA and CBDA synthase from Cannabais sativa L. *J Biotechnol* 2018;284:17–26.

40. Verhoeckx KC, Korthout HA, van Meeteran-Kreikamp AP, et al. Unheated Cannabis sativa extracts and its major compound THC-acid have potential immunomodulating properties not mediated by CB1 and CB2 receptor coupled pathways. *Int Immunopharmacol* 2006;6(4):656–65.

41. Takeda S, Okazxaki H, Ikeda E, et al. Down-regulation of cyclooxygenase-2 (COX-2) by cannabidiolic acid in human breast cancer cells. *J Toxicol Sci* 2014;39(5):711.

42. Karler R, Turkanis SA. Cannabis and epilepsy. *Adv Biosci* 1978;22:619–41.

43. Pellesi L, Licata M, Verri P, et al. Pharmacokinetics and tolerability of oral cannabis preparations in patients with medication overuse headaches (MOH)- a pilot study. *Eur J Clin Pharmacol* 2018;74(11):1427–36.

44. Rock EM, Limebeer CL, Navaratnam R, et al. A comparison of cannabidiolic acid with other treatments for anticipatory nausea using a rat model of contextually elicited conditioned gaping. *Psychopharmacology* 2014;231(16):3207–15.

45. Lichtman AH, Martin BR. Cannabinoid tolerance and dependence. *Handbook Exp Pharmacol* 2005;168:691–771.

46. Gonzalez S, Cebeira M, Fernandez-Ruiz J. Cannabinoid tolerance a review of studies in laboratory animals. *Pharmacol Biochem Behav* 2005;81(2):300–18.

47. Hsieh C, Brown S, Derleh C. Internalization and recycling of the CB1 cannabinoid receptor. *J Neurochem* 1999;73(2):493–501.

48. Jones RT. Cannabis tolerance and dependence. In: Fehr KO, Kalant H, eds. *Cannabis and Health Hazards.* Toronto: Toronto Addiction Research Foundation, 1983.

49. Smith DE, Seymour RB. Cannabis and cannabis withdrawl. *J Subs Misuse.* 1996;2:49–53.

50. Uliel-Sibony S. Patients with epilepsy may develop tolerance to CBD enriched oil. *Neurol Rev* 22019;27(1):10.

51. Giving Tree Wellness Center- A Medical Grade Cannabis Company. Product Guidelines. www.givingtreeaz.com.

52. Jensen MP, Chodroff MJ, Dworkin RH. The impact of neuropathy pain on health-related quality of life: review and implications. *Neurology* 2007; 68:1178–82.

53. Bruni N, Pepa CD, Oliaro-Bosso S, et al. Cannabinoid delivery systems for pain and inflammation treatment. *Molecules* 2018;23:2478.

54. Finnerup NB, Attal N, Haroutounian S, et al. Pharmacotherapy for neuropathic pain in adults: a systematic review and meta-analysis. *Lancet Neurol* 2015;14:162–173.

15 Cannabis Nutrition

Betty Wedman-St Louis
Clinical Nutritionist

CONTENTS

Many people believe in hemp and cannabis, whether for food, medicine, textiles, or as a dietary supplement. While both hemp and marijuana are cannabis sativa L., the difference is the level of psychoactive cannabinoids associated with the use of "marijuana." By definition, hemp contains less than 0.3% THC, whereas "marijuana" can contain 5%–35% THC.

Due to its nutritional content, hemp can be used as food for both humans and livestock. Hemp seed and its oil are popular ingredients in recipes because of its high omega-3 fatty acids, but the legal status of its use in the United States has limited its availability and use prior to the February 6, 2004 Ninth Circuit Court of Appeals ruling. Circuit Judge Betty B. Fletcher wrote that the DEA "cannot regulate naturally-occurring THC not contained within or derived from marijuana—i.e. non-psychoactive hemp products—because non-psychoactive hemp is not included in Schedule 1. The DEA has no authority to regulate drugs that are not scheduled, and it has not followed procedures required to schedule a substance" [1].

This legal action excluded hemp stalks, fiber, oil, and cake made from hemp seed and sterilized hemp seed from Schedule 1 status. The benefits of hemp oil products, CBD, and other cannabinoids like cannabinol (CBN) and cannabigerol (CBG) could be used to augment the body's naturally occurring endocannabinoids. The phyto-cannabinoids from hemp are supplements to the body's own endocannabinoids for functioning in the nervous system and immune system.

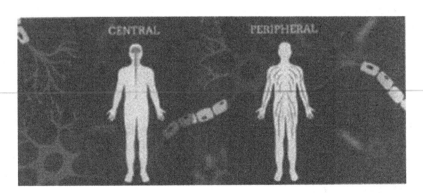

These phytocannabinoid supplements serve as therapeutic agents in one of human-ity's most valued ancient crops [2]. As a nutrition or dietary supplement, cannabis meets the FDA criteria of approval for over-the-counter use [3]:

- Benefits outweigh the risks.
- Potential for abuse and misuse is low.
- Consumer can tell when medication is needed.
- Can be adequately labeled.
- Health professionals are not necessary for its safe and effective use.

HEMP & 2018 FARM BILL

But as Jane Wilson of the American Herbal Products Association (AHPA) stated following the passage of the 2018 Farm Bill, "the good news is that the Drug Enforcement Agency (DEA) is not out of the picture for any governance role for hemp and the USDA will take the helm as the primary regulatory authority for domestic production of hemp" [4]. She went on to state that hemp—any constituent, concentrate or extract—is eligible to be used in dietary supplements according to the FD&C Act "as long as the level of THC present does not exceed 0.3%."

Unfortunately, the 2018 Farm Bill does not clarify the FDA regulatory status of CBD containing dietary supplements. FDA has pointed to DSHEA (Dietary Supplement Health and Education Act) in support of its position that CBD cannot be used in dietary supplements until it is approved as a new drug. Drug claims made about products not approved by FDA that state CBD and/or other cannabis-derived compounds offer therapeutic benefits could be declared unapproved and unsubstantiated and is in violation of the law. Scott Gottlieb, M.D., FDA Commissioner, declared that CBD "regardless of whether the substances are hemp-derived are not approved for use in food or dietary supplements and FDA will take action against companies illegally selling cannabis and cannabis-derived products, or those making unsubstantiated health claims" [4].

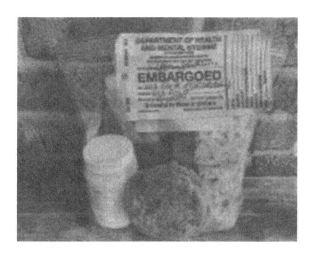

Adding to the confusion, on December 20, 2018, FDA granted GRAS (generally recognized as safe) status for hemp seed-derived food ingredients submitted by Fresh Hemp Foods, Ltd. and which can apply to other companies. These ingredients can be used in juices, smoothies, protein drinks, plant-based alternatives to dairy products, soups, dips, spreads, sauces, dressings, plant-based alternatives to meat products, desserts, baked goods, cereals, snacks, and nutrition bars [5].

SAFETY OF CANNABIDIOL (CBD)

Cannabidiol (CBD) is a component of cannabis sativa and constitutes up to 40% of the extraction from the plant [6]. But hemp/CBD concentrations are highly variable and depend on the growing conditions, phenotype, and part of the plant used for extraction. As Bergamaschi et al. reported, CBD is well tolerated and safe in humans at high doses with chronic use in numerous studies principally using animal or human cell lines [7].

Iffland and Grotenhermen [8] confirmed the safety of CBD use in humans reported by Bergamaschi et al. and reported that CBD has a better side effect profile than other drugs which could improve patient compliance and adherence to treatment. But toxicological parameters like CBD effect on hormones were still lacking.

CBD has been proposed as a potential treatment for opioid addiction, so safety and pharmacokinetics were reviewed by Manini et al. [9]. High doses—up to 800 mg or 10–15 mg/kg—were well tolerated, and further studies on CBD as an inhibitor of opioid-seeking behaviors and endogenous opioid-mediated reward pathways were recommended.

The phytocannabinoid components in cannabis are no different than phytochemicals derived from other plants eaten for health benefits. They can interact in an additive and synergistic way to modulate physiological function [10]. Martin elaborates on how a large number of dietary food compounds can exert effects on the human genome to modulate gene expression and target apoptosis with dietary bioactive agents [11]. The health benefits of food botanicals are further reviewed by Lui for additive and synergistic combinations in *The American Journal of Clinical Nutrition* [12]. A misplaced fear about herb-drug interactions has led physicians to not recommend botanicals like cannabis and may be an issue related to the use of hemp/CBD products.

DRUG-INDUCED NUTRIENT DEPLETION

A challenge facing many healthcare professionals today is the problem of polypharmacy prescribing and the resulting drug-induced metabolic imbalances. According to the CDC (Centers for Disease and Control) data, over 50% of Americans take prescription medications for management of diabetes, cardiovascular disease, stroke, hypertension, pain, mood, and sleep disorders [13].

The following is a brief look at common medications and potential nutrient depletions along with metabolic effects of the nutrient depletion. No studies exist on pharmaceutical imbalances to the endocannabinoid system, but full spectrum cannabis products have been indicated to reduce many of the complications caused by polypharmacy.

Drug	Nutrient Loss	Health Consequence
Metformin [14–17]	Coenzyme Q10	↑ blood pressure, CHF, pain, memory loss, fatigue
Beta-blockers [18–20]	Coenzyme Q10	HTN, CHF, pain, fatigue, joint aches, arrhythmia, ↓ cognitive function, insulin resistance
	Zinc	↓ immunity & wound healing, smell & taste issues, pain, insulin resistance, depression
	Melatonin	Sleep disturbances, impaired glucose, ↑ oxidative stress
Thiazide diuretics [21–25]	Magnesium	Muscle cramps, fatigue, restless legs, irritability, anxiety, insomnia
	Coenzyme Q10	(see above)
ACE inhibitors [26,27]	Zinc	(see above)
Angiotensin II receptor Antagonists [28,29]	Zinc	(see above)
HMG CoA	Zinc	(see above)
Reductase	Coenzyme Q10	(see above)

(Continued)

Drug	Nutrient Loss	Health Consequence
Inhibitors [30–33]	Vitamin E	Dermatitis, muscle weakness, ↓ antioxidant capacity, ↓ immunity
	Vitamin D	Osteoporosis, hearing issues, depression, muscle weakness, MS, schizophrenia, ↓ immunity
	Carnitine	↑ blood lipids, abnormal liver function, fatigue, blood glucose imbalance
	Omega-3 fatty acids	Neurochemical imbalance, skin disorders, chronic inflammation, cognitive impairment, insulin resistance, joint pain
	Selenium	↓ antioxidant protection, fatigue, muscle aches, RBC fragility, decreased conversion T4 to T3
	Copper	Hair color loss, anemia, fatigue, nervous system disorders
Non-steroidal anti-inflammatory drugs (NSAIDs) [34,35]	Tryptophan	Neurochemical imbalance, anxiety, depression, psychiatric disorders, insomnia
	Melatonin	(see above)
	Zinc	(see above)
Acetaminophen (Tylenol) [36,37]	Glutathione	↓ antioxidant capacity, liver damage, fatigue, ↓ immunity hair loss

CLINICAL ENDOCANNABINOID DEFICIENCY

As Ethan Russo, M.D., presented in 2004 [38], the theory of clinical endocannabinoid deficiency (CED) can be manifested by careful review of the polypharmacy nutrient deficiency data. Many neurotransmitter disorders, mood, pain, and digestive issues could result from an underlying endocannabinoid deficiency due to low levels of anandamide (AEA) and 2-arachidonoylglcerol (2-AG). When naive endocannabinoid levels are decreased, a lower threshold for pain and derangements of digestion, mood, and sleep result [39]. Various strategies to treat CED can be considered. A full spectrum CBD extract with terpenes and flavonoids is encouraged [40]. Lifestyle interventions should also be considered such as the importance of regular exercise to induce endocannabinoid signaling [41].

WESTERN MEDICINE VS. EASTERN MEDICINE

In July 1999, UCSF pharmacologist Lester Bornheim presented a paper at the International Cannabinoid Research Society about cannabidiol metabolism and described the political environment about cannabis as "the fact that cannabinoids affect so many systems makes them more difficult to study and to develop therapeutic drugs. The FDA doesn't approve of polypharmacy in general. To get a drug combination through the FDA is very difficult. And here you're talking about something with hundreds of different compounds and you have to prove that every one of them is really safe."

"It gets down to the basic difference between Western medicine and Eastern medicine. Eastern medicine uses herbal extracts with hundreds of different compounds and they believe that the combination has value. Western medicine says, if it works, there's probably one component that's doing the job and everything else is complicating the issue. Let's find that ingredient. Let's make it 100 times more active with chemical substitutes, and then bombard the body and knock out the problem" [42]. Cannabis clearly falls into the category of a holistic herbal medicine.

CANNABIS AS HERBAL HEALTH PRODUCT

Cannabis has been used for millennia in cultures throughout the world as a medicinal plant. It is only recently that Western medicine has evolved to include herbal treatments like acupuncture, homeopathy, and herbal extracts. Extractions from the whole cannabis plant can provide the full effect of cannabis benefits as anti-inflammatory and antioxidant.

Using the whole plant and the nutrients in each component starts by looking at the raw acid form of cannabinoids. The leaves (discarding the stems) can be made into a slurry for an afternoon "pick-me-up" by cancer patients, athletes, and tired homemakers. The raw leaves have anti-inflammatory benefits beyond what decarboxylated leaves can provide. The THCA (tetrahydrocannabinolic acid) in the raw leaves does not convert to THC (the psychoactive cannabinoid) until it is heated to 220°C for an hour. THCA can stimulate appetite, reduce nausea, and offer neuroprotective benefits along with the CBDA (cannabidiolic acid) adding antidepressant and anticancer potential. Raw cannabis leaves also have a wide array of terpenes like myrcene, limonene, and pinene. Raw leaves have carotenoids—beta carotene, alpha carotene, lutein, zeaxanthin, and lycopene—which can benefit eye health and immune function [43]. Lutein is a noted nutritional carotenoid because of its role in cognition and macular pigment [44].

Raw leaves can also be used in salads and anywhere leaf lettuce would be needed, i.e., a sandwich. Ten to 12 leaves per day is a usual amount for juicing. One or two raw buds may be added to increase the cannabinoid content. Sipping the juice or smoothie three to four times throughout the day can provide improved absorption of the nutrients instead of consuming it at one sitting. Stems are not consumed because they contain calcium carbonate in the hairs along the stalk and these can make the beverage an irritant to the gastrointestinal tract.

The chloroplasts in the raw leaves contain chlorophyll which does not have the most pleasant taste for humans, but it is critical in the plant's nutrition. Some botanists compare the role of chlorophyll in cannabis to hemoglobin in the human red blood cell. Chlorophyll is popular in many "green drinks" sold by nutraceutical companies. It is a beneficial compound in raw cannabis leaves because of its detoxification potential and anti-inflammatory properties.

HEMP SEED OIL

Cold-pressed hemp seed oil will contain more terpenes than a decarboxylated hemp seed oil but either can be used as an olive oil substitute for salad dressing. To enhance cannabinoid and terpene absorption from raw cannabis, a modest amount of hemp seed oil can be used since terpenes and cannabinoids are both highly lipophilic and not water soluble. The hemp oil purchased in a health food store is different than the hemp/CBD extracts. Standard hemp oil is usually produced by cold pressing the seeds, whereas CBD extract is usually made by a super critical CO_2 extraction of the hemp plant itself and not the seeds. Hemp seed oil is a nutritional food, but it does not have the naturally occurring terpenes, cannabinoids, and flavonoids found in full spectrum CBD extracts.

CANNABIS ROOTS

The roots of the cannabis plant have a long history of medical use, but their therapeutic potential has been overlooked [45]. The first mention of beneficial properties in cannabis roots dates back to 77 AD in Natural Histories by Latin naturalist Pliny the Elder [46]. Herbalists around the world have treated many conditions from fever and infections to gout, arthritis, and sexually transmitted diseases with hemp root preparations either as a decoction or crushed extract of the raw root [47].

Topical use features the fresh ground up root and juice mixed with fat (oil or butter) applied directly after pounding and crushing the root into a salve. The French physician Francois Rabelais wrote about boiling the root in water to soothe muscles or stiff joints, gout pains, and rheumatism [48]. In general, the historic record indicates that cannabis root was usually extracted with boiling water and applied topically to treat gout and arthritis [49].

A composite of medical use of cannabis roots extrapolated from Ryz et al. [45] is given as follows:

Gout, arthritis, pain	Boiled roots decoction
Fever	Boiled roots
Inflammation	Boiled roots
Skin burns	Raw root juice or decoction mixed with butter
Tumors	Boiled roots
Childbirth (hemorrhage)	Juice + decoction
Gastrointestinal tonic	Pulverized root + wine
Infection	Boiled root or pulverized + wine

Cannabis roots contain many different active compounds including triterpenoids, friedelin, and epifriedelanol [50,51]. Friedelin is found in cannabis and other plants like algae and lichens, and used in Ayurvedic medicine as an aphrodisiac [52]. Friedelin extracted from the bark of Mesu daphnifolia, a ubiquitous tree in Malaysia, was shown to have cytotoxic activity against various female malignancies—breast cancer, cervical carcinoma, and ovarian cancer cell lines [53]. Epifriedelanol is also abundant in nature, but no research is available about the specific activity of these compounds in cannabis roots. Choline has also been reported as a compound in cannabis roots [54].

Lignans are another compound found in cannabis roots which have important antioxidant activity through antiviral, antidiabetic, antitumor, and anti-obesity function. The Chinese pharmacopeia has references to the therapeutic use of hemp roots for pregnancy and obstetric issues such as "the juice of the root is thought to have a beneficial action in retained placenta and postpartum hemorrhage" [55].

HEMP SEEDS

The most nutrient dense part of the cannabis plant is its seeds which not only provide protein, magnesium, iron, and zinc but are an excellent source of plant-based omega-3 fatty acids. One ounce of hemp seeds contains about 6,000 mg alpha linolenic acid and offers as much protein as soybeans with high amounts of the amino acid arginine, the metabolic precursor for the production of nitric oxide (NO). Nitric oxide is the signaling messenger in the cardiovascular system and is responsible for regulating muscle cells and blood pressure [56].

The nutrient profile of hemp seed provided by Rodriguez-Leyva and Pierce per 100 grams is given as

Energy	567 kcal (2,200 Kj)
Protein	24.8 g
Fat	35.5 g
Carbohydrates	27.6 g
Calcium	145 mg
Iron	14 mg
Magnesium	183 mg
Vitamin A	3,800 IU
Vitamin D	2,277.5 uI
Vitamin E	90 mg

Totals:

Saturated fat	8.48 g
Monounsaturated fat	14.8 g
Polyunsaturated fat	36.2 g

CANNABIS BUDS

For hundreds of years, the cannabis bud has been considered the most important part of the plant, but the tide is turning on using raw cannabis bud for its health benefits instead of smoking. Raw fresh cannabis bud is more exciting as a super food than broccoli or kale. Fresh bud means harvesting just before full bloom. Once the flower is harvested and drying begins, there are significant changes in the chemical compounds once the trichome resin glands begin to degrade.

The benefits of raw cannabis buds can be used in juices, smoothies, salads, sauces, and salad dressings. The buds need to be stored by wrapping in a clean towel and placing them in the refrigerator like any other salad ingredient or vegetable.

HOME GROWING YOUR CANNABIS

More and more individuals are exploring home production of cannabis to ensure adequate safety and availability for their personal use. This is an area where the differences between state laws predominate and can change annually. Leafly staff provided an updated state roster on January 15, 2019 [57].

Alaska allows an adult over 21 to grow and process no more than six plants with no more than three plants that are mature.

Arizona allows a medical cannabis patient or their qualifying designated caregiver up to 12 plants if they live more than 25 miles from the nearest medical marijuana dispensary.

California allows an adult over 21 no more than 6 plants at a time grown only at their residence where it cannot be seen and locked up.

Colorado allows growth of up to six plants per person with no more than three plants in mature/flowering stage at any time. No more than 12 plants are allowed per residence.

Connecticut—no home cultivation

Delaware—no home cultivation

District of Columbia allows up to six plants and no more than three mature plants.

Florida—not permitted

Hawaii may be grown at qualifying patient or their designated caregiver's residence.

Illinois—not permitted

Maine allows maximum of 6 plants, 12 immature plants and unlimited seedlings per resident for personal use.

Maryland—not permitted

Massachusetts allows up to 6 mature plants per person for personal use with max of 12 per residence.

Michigan allows up to 12 plants for personal use.

Minnesota—not permitted

Montana allows 4 mature plants, 12 seedlings per registered cardholder.

Nevada allows up to 6 plants per residence if more than 25 miles from nearest retail cannabis shop & up to 12 plants per household.

New Hampshire—not permitted

New Jersey—not permitted

New Mexico allows qualified patients to apply for a license to grow their own supply allowing 4 mature plants and 12 seedlings.

New York—not permitted

North Dakota allows up to 8 plants if more than 40 miles from dispensary

Ohio—not permitted

Oklahoma allows no more than 6 mature plants and up to 12 total.

Oregon allows recreational consumer 21 years or older up to 4 plants per residence. A medical marijuana patient may possess up to 6 mature plants.

Pennsylvania—not permitted

Rhode Island allows up to not to 12 mature plants and up to 12 seedlings.

Vermont allows two mature plants and seven immature plants per registered patient.

Washington allows 6 plants for personal medical use and up to 15 plants for medical use if healthcare professional determines need.

West Virginia—not permitted

CANNABIS EDIBLES

Most of humanity's 10,000+ years of using cannabis has focused on its use as edibles. It is a proud culinary tradition that dates back thousands of years across the globe without prohibitions imposed on this plant.

Bhang (circa 1,000 BC) is a cannabis edible preparation associated with springtime in the Hindu festival Holi. Shiva, the Hindu god of transformation, recognized its ability to "release anxiety." Bhang is a recognized Ayurvedic medicine treatment for fever, digestive disorders, and immune building. Bhang is made by grinding cannabis into a paste and mixing it with milk and spices along with almonds or pistachios. Government shops throughout India sell bhang, and each one can vary the recipe to include ginger, fennel, anise, cardamom, or rose water to meet an individual's choice.

On the African continent, Morocco is known as the hash-making culture that has reigned since 1000 AD. Mahjoun or mazhoum is a hashish-powered edible made with figs, dates, and ground nuts. Honey, turmeric, cardamom, ginger, and cinnamon are added for flavoring, but each family closely guards their secret recipe.

The most famous cannabis edible is Alice B. Toklas's hashish fudge made from spices, nuts, fruit, and cannabis. It was a last minute addition from artist Brion Gysin according to David Bienenstock that sparked media scandal when published in a French cookbook in 1954 [58]. The American edition of the book omitted the recipe but later editions in the 1960s included Hashish Fudge, and the recipe was passed around as "pot brownies" while being featured in the 1968 film *I Love You Alice B. Toklas*.

In the 1970s, cannabis edibles took on a new cause. Mary Jane Rathbun began selling her cannabis-infused brownies to make ends meet and became San Francisco's "Brownie Mary" by distributing her treats in the gay community. She soon recognized that her cannabis brownies helped restore their appetites and reduced some of their AIDS/HIV symptoms. By 1996 "Brownie Mary" helped pass California's Prop 215 and was making rounds at local AIDS and cancer centers despite being arrested three times. Due to her volunteering work, Donald Abrams, M.D., at San Francisco General Hospital, studied how cannabis improved patient appetites and did not inhibit immune function.

According to David Bienenstock, the first packaged cannabis edible for mainstream retail shop distribution was produced by Scott Van Rixel, a master chocolatier. He founded Bhang, a company dedicated to cannabis-infused chocolate in a childproof package with labeling to meet FDA standards. It was labeled as 73.5% cacao and listed 60 mg of THC with less than 2 mg each of CBD and CBN. The bar could be broken into four pieces resulting in a 15 mg dose of THC being the first time edibles declared what was in a serving of the product.

CANNABIS-INFUSED EDIBLES TODAY

Cannabis edibles were considered one of the top 10 food trends in 2018 undoubtedly because edibles are convenient, discrete, and a delicious way to deliver CBD and/ or THC. Many individuals prefer edibles to smoking because there is no odor, no second hand smoke, AND longer lasting benefits [59]. But cannabis-infused edibles are not without dangers from intoxication from high doses that cause behavioral impairment, extreme sedation, agitation, or anxiety.

Although "marijuana edibles" are still illegal under Federal and many state statutes, food products containing cannabis sativa L. are currently common in states that either permit or decline to prosecute "medical" or "recreational" products [60]. These products range from beverages, candy, and baked goods to oils and honey. Edibles are becoming commonplace, and advances in technology enable producers to create a wide variety of cannabis goods. More people are learning better practices for proper dosing edibles as the popularity of various edibles varies from state to state. Gummies rule with their many flavors—mango, watermelon, blueberry, apple, grape, orange, pineapple, raspberry, strawberry—with "Game Day Gummies" produced for the Denver Broncos fans.

Legalization of cannabis in a growing number of U.S. states and Canadian provinces continues to raise concerns about food safety issues in edible production. Steven Burton of Icicle Technologies stated that "there are many food safety hazards associated with cannabis production and distribution that could put the public at risk" [61]. Pests and pathogen contamination—salmonella and E. coli— were of particular concern since cannabis edible producers may not be subject to federal regulations that cover food and pharmaceutical operations. Producers of cannabis edibles need to be treated the same as other food product producers and have comprehensive food safety programs—GMPs (good manufacturing principles), HACCP plans, supplier verification, and recall procedures—in place for state and federal regulators.

CANNABIS MEETS FOOD SCIENCE

Cannabis users have long made their own homemade edibles by making it themselves from personally tailoring the extract and controlling who consumed the product. Mass production of cannabis-infused food products with no quality standards or regulations creates a new challenge for food science. Product developers need to understand the cannabinoid ramifications (THC vs. CBD), how to combine nonpolar cannabinoids into non-polar bases like butter or oil, and remove or overpower the aldehydes that give cannabis its grassy flavor and green color. Once formulation challenges are achieved, dosing and blending of the fatty cannabis mixture needs to produce a product that is not too strong or too weak in cannabis effect.

Quality control is critical to ensure food safety in composition and microbiology. Chromatographic techniques using high performance liquid chromatography (HPLC) are used for detecting and quantifying cannabinoids in the edible product. Quality control laboratories need to develop protocols for measuring cannabinoids, pesticide residue, and microbiological contaminants, so they can conform to FDA standards and print an accurate label [62]. Quality assurance professionals need to be sure that their cannabis is coming from legal and reputable sources because supply chain sources may have adulterated or contaminated product.

EDIBLES PACKAGING

Some cannabis edible products for retail sale are packaged to resemble commercially available products that appeal to children—gummy candy, lollipops, cookies—and children may unintentionally consume these products, especially in states that have legalized recreational and medical cannabis use [63]. Child-resistant packaging has been implemented by numerous companies and has become mandatory in some states.

Colorado has implemented new medical and retail packaging which requires the use of a universal symbol on the front to indicate a marijuana product [64]. The new universal symbol is a visual indicator that helps consumers and non-consumers easily identify marijuana products and avoid unintentional ingestion. The symbols can be viewed on the Colorado Marijuana website: www.colorado.gov/pacific/marijuana/news.

DOSING CHALLENGES

There are differences between how THC and CBD are absorbed orally than when inhaled. Smoking or vaping allows the cannabinoids to directly enter the bloodstream through the lungs. When ingesting cannabinoids in edibles, they pass through the liver for metabolism which slows down utilization by the body. Other medications being processed by the liver could change the metabolic effect and need to be considered. Despite the potential promises of edibles for treatment of a variety of ailments, one of the biggest challenges for users and regulators is avoiding intoxication [65]. For a healthy adult user, the duration of intoxication can last hours to several days related to the amount of overconsumption of the edible dose. Pharmacokinetics of orally consumed cannabis is difficult to predict which makes edibles more difficult to dose due to individual responses and whether the edible was consumed on an empty stomach (effects are quicker) or eaten after a meal.

As the cannabis edible enters the gastrointestinal tract, the delta 9-THC is absorbed into the bloodstream and travels via the portal vein to the liver where it undergoes first-pass metabolism. In the liver, the cytochrome P450 enzyme system hydroxylates delta 9-THC to 11-hydroxytetrahdrocannabinol (11-OH-THC) which is a potent psychoactive metabolite that readily crosses the blood-brain barrier [66].

A standard dose of a cannabis-infused edible is considered as 10 mg THC [67], but each user needs to be conscientious of their tolerance and consider the time of the day when consuming it. If an edible product contains THC and CBD, the CBD can block some of the intoxicating effect. Products with a CBD:THC ratio of 1:1 are therapeutic and produce less impairment than THC-dominant products [68].

As the CBD:THC ratio increases, the likelihood of intoxicating effects decreases and the medicinal effects for pain and anxiety relief increase. A 4:1 ratio of CBD:THC offers medicinal effects with little or no impairment. [Example: a person feels can feel impaired after a 5 mg THC edible serving but has less or no impairment when using a 20mg CBD + 5 md THC edible.]

A cannabis-infused edible dosing chart provides a general guideline in advising consumption. If no effects from an edible are felt after 1–2 hours, another low dose can be consumed. Allow 8–24 hours before trying another dose to avoid over consumption [69]. Some individuals may not be able to absorb cannabis cannabinoids via oral consumption due to liver detoxification issues and sublingual or vaping may be their only choice for symptom management.

EDIBLE DOSING CHART

THC	CBD	Effect
1–2.5 mg	----	Improved focus, mild pain relief
2.5 mg	2.5 mg	Improved pain relief, improved sleep
10–15 mg	10–15 mg	Stronger symptom relief, better sleep, more pain relief
15–20 mg	-----	Euphoria, deep sleep
15–20 mg	50–100 mg	Improved pain relief, anti-inflammatory

Finding the right dose is challenging in the cannabis-infused edible market since body type (amount of fat), gender, and age along with awareness of cannabis tolerance due to smoking or vaping all need to be considered. Individuals should be advised not to mix edibles with alcohol (beer, wine, liquor) because of the increased risk of intoxication.

LABELING CANNABIS EDIBLES

Focus groups with 94 consumers and non-consumers of edibles in Denver and Seattle were conducted to collect information on labeling usefulness, attractiveness, ease of comprehension, and acceptability [70]. Some participants had concerns that too much information was on the label which would result in consumers not reading the label. Others indicated the consumption advice was not clear, and web—and video-based education would be useful to alert consumers about the possible risks of edibles.

Discrepancies between federal and state cannabis laws have resulted in inadequate regulation and oversight, leading to inaccurate labeling of some products according to Vandrey et al. [71]. In 2017, Bonn-Miller et al. [72] examined the label accuracy of CBD products sold online and found that 26% contained less CBD than labeled which could negate any potential clinical response in patient symptom management. The THC content in some medical cannabis products could be sufficient to produce intoxication or impairment, especially among children [73].

Here is a warning statement found inside a cannabis-infused edible purchased in Las Vegas, Nevada.

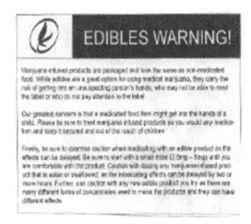

INDEPENDENT CANNABIS EDIBLE STUDY

Patients continue to bring the author their cannabis-infused edible products for "approval" including their stories about how they reacted to consumption of an edible. Inaccuracies and inconsistencies in product labels were commonplace, so numerous cannabis edible samples were purchased for analysis by a Florida laboratory with competence and calibration certification. A summary of four cannabis edible products follows. Certificates of Analysis for the samples are attached (see the Section "Certificates of Analysis for Cannabis Edibles").

Kush Cakes sold on Amazon as "premier Relaxation Brownie." Label states "formulated by a pharmacist" and indicates no more than one brownie per 24 hours.

Cost $5 each (56 g)	
Result	CBD 0.00 mg/g
	THC 0.00 mg/g

Cannabis Chocolate "To Whom It May" (California company) with "high CBD" marked on bottom of box

Cost of 4 truffles = $50		
Results	Zak truffle	CBD 0.52 mg/g
		THC 0.00 mg/g
	Ralph truffle	CBD 0.40 mg/g
		THC 0.01 mg/g

CBD Milk Chocolate Bar label states "20 mg 100% active CBD oil"

Cost $10.50 (20 g bar)	
Result	CBD 0.42 mg/g or 8.4 mg per bar
	THC 0.00 mg/g

Hemp Gummies by Serenity label states 10 mg CBD per gummie

Cost $2 per gummie		
Result	5 gummies = 20 g	CBD 2.93 mg/g
		THC 0.00 mg/g
	1 gummie	CBD 0.586 mg/g

Dosing accuracy cannot be achieved if labeling is so incorrect. Cannabis-infused edibles are expensive, and the fastest way for medical benefits to be disregarded is from mislabeling due to poor analysis by the provider.

Continued monitoring is needed to access labeling accuracy for dosing potential. Steep Hill Labs explained the difficulty in getting an accurate analysis at the Pittsburgh Cannabis Conference in 2017.

- First, the cannabis flowers have to be tested for use in the edible.
- After the cannabis oil and terpenes are extracted, another testing determines what extraction level is used in making the product.
- Testing SHOULD be done on the finished product to insure accuracy of cannabinoid and terpene content on the edible label

When cannabis users made their own edibles, consumption was among friends. Mass production for the general public requires adequate testing and accurate labeling, so dosing guidelines can be evaluated for symptom relief. Testing for solvents and microorganisms is critical and needs to be on the label and/or Certificate of Analysis especially for people with immune disorders like Crohn's disease, multiple sclerosis, and lupus erythematosus.

NEW CANNABIS CONSUMERS-A CANNASSEUR

Frozen meals from companies like Earth's Edibles are identified as "cannabis-infused gourmet foods" featuring curries, pastas, pizzas, sauces, and soups along with "gourmet treats" like granola, gummies, and chocolates [73]. Meals are labeled low THC, medium THC, and high THC.

CBD-based cocktails like CBD Mint Julep (bourbon) or CBD Margaritas (Grand Marnier and lime juice) or a CBD Pisco Sour (brandy) are made with CBD-infused simple syrup for a health-focused treat.

Other cannasseurs are using canna-flour from leaves and buds as a natural fiber boost and nutrient dense additive for baked goods like zucchini bread, chocolate chip cookies, and bran muffins.

Today's consumers are more socially conscious and interested in food, so cannabis is a natural new food for them to add to their diet. They are ready to skip the canned cranberry sauce Aunt Mildred always has at Thanksgiving and bring their own homemade Cranberry Orange Canna Relish. The same goes for classic green bean casserole being replaced by Green Bean Canna Casserole at holiday events.

Pumpkin Canna Treats made with cannabis-infused honey replace the boring pumpkin pie and make for an exciting change. Other recipes for those wanting to add cannabinoids into their diet can be found in the Appendix.

CERTIFICATES OF ANALYSIS FOR CANNABIS EDIBLES

CERTIFICATE OF ANALYSIS
4131 SW 47th Ave, Suite 1408
Davie, FL 33314

Product Information:

Sample ID:	D804021-01	Type:	Kush Cakes
Lot Number:	-	Storage conditions:	4 °C
Customer:	Dr. Betty Wedman	Sample size:	56g
	17920 Gulf Blvd., Suite 606 St. Petersburg, FL 33708	Sampled by:	Customer
License Number:	-	Date Sampled:	-
Date Accepted:	04/12/2018	Sampling Location:	-

CBD 0.00 mg/g
THC 0.00 mg/g

1. Cannabinoid profile:
Analysis Method: SOP.T.30.050
SOP.T.40.020

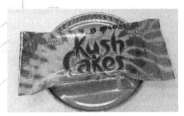

QA Testing	%	mg/g
CBDV	0.000	0.000
CBDA	0.000	0.000
CBGA	0.000	0.000
CBG	0.000	0.000
CBD	0.000	0.000
THCV	0.000	0.000
CBN	0.000	0.000
Total THC	0.000	0.000
-THC	0.000	0.000
-THCa	0.000	0.000
CBC	0.000	0.000

Statement:
This product met stringent quality standards at time of batch/lot release. Any test results reported on this certificate were obtained at time of release.

CERTIFICATE OF ANALYSIS

4131 SW 47th Ave, Suite 1408
Davie, FL 33314

Product Information:

Sample ID:	D804021-04	Type:	CBD 20mg Choc. Bar
Lot Number:	-	Storage conditions:	4 °C
Customer:	Dr. Betty Wedman	Sample size:	20g
	17920 Gulf Blvd., Suite 606 St. Petersburg, FL 33708	Sampled by:	Customer
License Number:	-	Date Sampled:	-
Date Accepted:	04/12/2018	Sampling Location:	-

CBD 0.42 mg/g
THC 0.00 mg/g

1. Cannabinoid profile:

Analysis Method: SOP.T.30.050
SOP.T.40.020

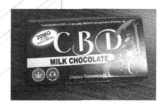

QA Testing	%	mg/g
CBDV	0.000	0.000
CBDA	0.000	0.000
CBGA	0.000	0.000
CBG	0.000	0.000
CBD	0.042	0.420
THCV	0.000	0.000
CBN	0.000	0.000
Total THC	0.000	0.000
-THC	0.000	0.000
-THCa	0.000	0.000
CBC	0.000	0.000

Statement:

This product met stringent quality standards at time of batch/lot release. Any test results reported on this certificate were obtained at time of release.

www.eviolabsfl.com   **Page | 1**

CERTIFICATE OF ANALYSIS
4131 SW 47th Ave, Suite 1408
Davie, FL 33314

Product Information:

Sample ID:	D804021-02	Type:	Ralph Truffle
Lot Number:	-	Storage conditions:	4 °C
Customer:	Dr. Betty Wedman	Sample size:	3g
	17920 Gulf Blvd., Suite 606 St. Petersburg, FL 33708	Sampled by:	Customer
License Number:	-	Date Sampled:	-
Date Accepted:	04/12/2018	Sampling Location:	-

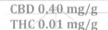

CBD 0.40 mg/g
THC 0.01 mg/g

1. Cannabinoid profile:
Analysis Method: SOP.T.30.050
SOP.T.40.020

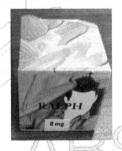

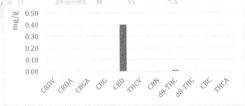

QA Testing	%	mg/g
CBDV	0.000	0.000
CBDA	0.000	0.000
CBGA	0.000	0.000
CBG	0.000	0.000
CBD	0.040	0.400
THCV	0.000	0.000
CBN	0.000	0.000
Total THC	0.001	0.010
-THC	0.001	0.010
-THCa	0.000	0.000
CBC	0.000	0.000

Statement:
This product met stringent quality standards at time of batch/lot release. Any test results reported on this certificate were obtained at time of release.

www.eviolabsfl.com   **Page | 1**

CERTIFICATE OF ANALYSIS

4131 SW 47th Ave, Suite 1408
Davie, FL 33314

Product Information:

Sample ID:	D804021-05	Type:	Hemp Gummy 300mg
Lot Number:	Serenity-30	Storage conditions:	4 °C
Customer:	Dr. Betty Wedman	Sample size:	20g
	17920 Gulf Blvd., Suite 606 St. Petersburg, FL 33708	Sampled by:	Customer
License Number:	-	Date Sampled:	-
Date Accepted:	04/12/2018	Sampling Location:	-

CBD 2.93 mg/g
THC 0.00 mg/g

1. Cannabinoid profile:

Analysis Method: SOP.T.30.050
SOP.T.40.020

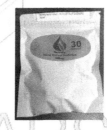

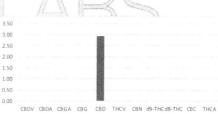

QA Testing	%	mg/g
CBDV	0.000	0.000
CBDA	0.000	0.000
CBGA	0.000	0.000
CBG	0.000	0.000
CBD	0.293	2.93
THCV	0.000	0.000
CBN	0.000	0.000
Total THC	0.000	0.000
-THC	0.000	0.000
-THCa	0.000	0.000
CBC	0.000	0.000

Statement:

This product met stringent quality standards at time of batch/lot release. Any test results reported on this certificate were obtained at time of release.

www.eviolabsfl.com **Page | 1**

REFERENCES

1. Hemp Industries Association USA. LLC v. Drug Enforcement Administration 03-71366, 03-71693 decided February 2, 2004. www.caselaw.findlaw.com.
2. Gray DJ, Baker H, Clancy K, et al. Current and future needs and applications for cannabis. *Crit Rev Plant Sci* 2016;35(5–6):425–6.
3. Regulations of Over-the-Counter (OTC) Drug Products-FDA. www.fda/gov/downloads/aboutfda/centersoffices/cder/ucm148055.pdf.
4. Olivo L. 2018. Farm bill bring victory for hemp, uncertainty for CBD. Nutraceuticals World 1.14.19. www.nutraceuticalsworld.com/contents/view_online-exclu...=MjQwMzg5NzkzNTYS1.
5. FDA responds to three GRAS notices for hemp seed-derived ingredients for use in human food. Dec 20, 2018. fda.gov.
6. Grlie L. A comparative study on some chemical and biological characteristics of various samples of cannabis resin. *Bull Narcot* 1976;14:37–46.
7. Bergamaschi MM, Queiroz RHC, Crippa JAS, et al. Safety and side effects of cannabidiol, a Cannabis sativa constituent. *Curr Drug Safety* 2011;6:000.
8. Iffland K, Grotenherman F. An update on safety and side effects of cannabidiol: a review of clinical data and relevant animal studies. *Cannabis Cannabinoid Res* 2017;2(1):139–54.
9. Manini AF, Yiannoulos G, Bergamaschi MM, et al. Safety pharmacokinetics of oral cannabidiol when administered concomitantly with intravenous fentanyl in humans. *J Addict Med* 2015;9(3):204–10.
10. McCarthy MF. Proposal for a dietary "phytochemical index." *Med Hypothesis* 2004;63:813–7.
11. Martin KR. Targeting apoptosis with dietary bioactive agents. *Exp Biol Med* 2006;231:117–29.
12. Liu RH. Health benefits of fruits and vegetables are from addictive and synergistic combinations of phytochemicals. *Am J Clin Nutr* 2003;78:517S–20S.
13. Centers for Disease Control (CDC). www.cdc.gov.
14. Adams JK, et al. Malabsorption of B12 and intrinsic factor during biguanide therapy. *Diabetologia* 1983;24(1):16–18.
15. Kishi T, Kishi H, Wataanabe T, et al. Bioenergetics in clinical medicine. XI. Studies on coenzyme Q and diabetes mellitus. *J Med* 1976;7(3–4):307–21.
16. Ting RZ, Szeto CC, Chan MH, et al. Risk factors of vitamin B12 deficiency in patients receiving metformin. *Arch Int Med* 2006;166(18):1975–9.
17. DeJager J, Kooy A, Lehert P, et al. Long term treatment with metformin in patients with type 2 diabetes and risk of vitamin B12 deficiency: randomized placebo controlled trial. *BMJ* 2010;340:c2181.
18. Kishi T, Watanabe T, Folkers K. Bioenergetics in clinical medicine XV. Inhibition of coenzyme Q 10-enzymes by clinically used adrenergic blockers beta-receptors. *Res Commun Chem Pathol Pharmacol* 1977; 17(1);157–64.
19. Scheer FA, Morris CJ, Garcia JL, et al. Repeated melatonin supplementation,improves sleep in hypertensive patients treat with beta-blockers: a randomized controlled study. *Sleep* 2012;35(10):1395–402.
20. Fares A. Night-time exogenous melatonin administration may be a beneficial treatment for sleeping disorders in beta blocker patients. *J Cardiovasc Dis Res* 2011;2(3):153–55.
21. Kishi H, et al. Bioenergetics in clinical medicine III. Inhibition of coenzyme Q-enzymes bu clinically used anti-hypertensive drugs. *Res Commun Chem Pathol Pharmacol* 1975;12(3):533–40.
22. Clayton JA, Rogers S, Blakey J. Thiazide diuretic prescription and electrolyte abnormalities in primary care. *Br J Clin Pharmacol* 2006;61:87–95.

23. Pak CY. Correction of thiazide-induced hypomagnesemia by potassium-magnesium citrate from review of prior trials. *Clin Nephrol* 2000;54:271–5.
24. Wester PO. Urinary zinc excretion during treatment with different diuretics. *Acta Med Scand* 1980;208(3):209–12.
25. Odvina CV, Mason RP, Pak CY. Prevention of thiazide-induced hypokalemia without magnesium depletion by potassium-magnesium-citrate. *Am J Ther* 2006;13(2):101–8.
26. Golik A, Modai D, Averbukh Z, et al. Zinc metabolism in patients treated with captopril versus enalapril. *Metabolism* 1990;39(7):665–7.
27. Chakithandy S, Evans R, Vyakarnam P. Acute severe hyponatremia and seizures associated with postoperative enalapril administration. *Anaesth Intensive Care* 2009;37(4):673–4.
28. Braun LA, Rosenfeldt F. Pharmaco-nutrient interactions - a systemic review of zinc and anti-hypertensive therapy. *Int J Clin Pract* 2013;67(8):717–25.
29. Park MH, Kim HN, Lim JS, et al. Angiotensin II potentiates zinc-induced cortical neuronal death by acting on angiotensin II type 2 receptor. *Mol Brain* 2013;6(1):50.
30. Colquhoun DM, Jackson R, Walters M, et al. Effects of simvastatin on blood lipids, vitamin E, coenzyme Q 10 levels and left ventricular function in humans. *Eur J Clin Invest* 2005;35(4):251–8.
31. Harris JI, Hibbeln JR, Mackey RH, et al. Statin treatment alters serum n-3 and n-6 fatty acids in hypercholesterolemic patients. *Prostaglandins Leukot Essent Fatty Acids* 2004;71(4):263–9.
32. Folkers K, et al. Lovastatin decreases coenzyme Q levels in humans. *Proc Natl Acad Sci USA* 1990;87(22);8931–4.
33. Ghayour-Mobarhan M, Lamb DJ, Taylor A, et al. Effect of statin therapy on serum trace element status in dyslipidemic subjects. *J Trace Elem Med Biol* 2005;19(1):61–7.
34. Wharam PC, Speedy DB, Noakes TD, et al. NSAID use increases the risk of developing hyponatremia during an Ironman triathlon. *Med Sci Sports Exerc* 2006;38(4):618–22.
35. Baggott JE, et al. Inhibition of folate-dependent enzymes by non-steroidal anti-inflammatory drugs. *Biochem J* 1992;282(Pt 1):197–202.
36. McGill MR, Yan HM, Ramachandran A, et al. HepaRG cells; a human model to study mechanisms of acetaminophen hepatotoxicity. *Hepatology* 2011;53(3):974–82.
37. Anoush M, Eghbal MA, Fathiazad F, et al. The protective effects of garlic extract against acetaminophen-induced oxidative stress and glutathione depletion. *Pak J Biol Sci* 2009;12(10):765–71.
38. Russo EB. Clinical endocannabinoid deficiency (CECD): can this concept explain therapeutic benefits of cannabis in migraine, fibromyalgia, irritable bowel syndrome and other treatment-resistant conditions? *Neuroendocrinol Lett* 2004;25:31–9.
39. Pacher P, Kunos G. Modulating the endocannabinoid system in human health and disease - successes and failures. *FEBS J* 2013;280:1918–43.
40. Russo, EB. Taming THC:potential cannabis synergy and phytocannabinoid-terpene entourage effects. *Br J Pharmacol* 2001;163;1344–64.
41. Raichen DA, Foster AD, Gerdeman GL, et al. Wired to run: exercise-induced endocannabinoid signaling in humans and cursorial mammals with implications for the 'runner high'. *J Exp Biol* 2012;215:1331–6.
42. Gardner F. Introducing the International Cannabinoid Research Society- and CBD. www.beyondthc.com/lester-bornheim-work-at-ucsf-plus-icrs-99.
43. Johnson EJ. The role of carotenoids in human health. *Nutr Clin Care* 2002;5(2):56–65.
44. Heiting G. Lutein and zeaxanthin:eye and vision benefits. www.allaboutvision.com/nutrition/lutein.htm.
45. Ryz NR, Remillard DJ, Russo EB. Cannabis roots: a traditional therapy with future potential for treating inflammation and pain. *Cannabis and Cannbinoid Res* 2017;2(1):210–16.

46. Pliny (the Elder). The natural history of Pliny. vol. 4. *Bohn's Classical Library*, Henry Thomas Riley. HG Bohm: London, 1856;XX;298.

47. Brand E, Wiseman N. *Concise Chinese Materia Medica*. Paradigm Publications: Taos, NM, 2008.

48. Rabelais F, *Gargantua and Pantagruel*, 1st ed. Norton: New York, 1990;xi:623.

49. Salmon W. *Botanologia. The English herbal: A History of Plants*. I Dawkes: London, 1710.

50. Slatkin DJ, Doorenbos NJ, Harris LS, et al. Clinical constituents of Cannabis sativa L. root. *J Pharm Ci.* 1971;60:1891–2.

51. Sethi VK, Jain MP, Thakur RS. Chemical investigation of wild Cannabis sativa L. roots. *PLants Med* 1997;32:378–9.

52. Aswar UM, Bhaskaran S, Mohan V, et al. Estrogenic activity of friedelin fraction (IND-HE) separated from Cissus quadrangularis and its effect on female sexual function. *Pharmacognosy* 2010;2:138–45.

53. Ee GC, Lim CK, Rahmat A, et al. Cytotoxic activities of chemical constituents from Mesua daphnifolia. *Trop Biomed* 2005;22:99–102.

54. Mole ML, Jr, Turner CE. Phytochemical screening of Cannabis sativa L.II. Choline and neurine in the roots of Mexican variant. *Acta Pharm Jugosl* 1973;23:203–5.

55. Smith FP, Stuart GA. *Chinese Materia Medica: Vegetable Kingdom*. American Presbyterian Mission Press: Shanghai, 1911.

56. Rodriguez-Leyva D, Pierce GN. The cardiac and haemostatic effects of dietary hempseed. *Nutr Metab* (Lond) 2010;7:32.

57. Home cannabis cultivation laws: a state-by-state guide. www.leafly.com/cannabis/home-cannabis-cultivation-laws.

58. Bienenstock D. 7 Cannabis edibles that changed the game. Feb 22, 2018. www.leafly.com/news/strains-products.

59. Giombi KC, Kosa KM, Rains C, et al. Consumer's perceptions of edible marijuana products for recreational use: likes, dislikes, and reasons for use. *Subst Use Misuse* 2018;53(4):541–7.

60. Klein RFX. Analysis of "marijuana edibles" - Food products containing marijuana extracts - an overview, review, and literature survey. *Microgram J* 2017;14(1–4):9–32.

61. Food Safety News. Feb 15, 2018. www.foodsafetynews.com.

62. Cannabis-Infused: Dixie Elixirs & Edibles. Quality Assurance & Food Safety 2014. www.qualityassurancemag.com/article/qa1014-marijuana-edibles-industry-challenges.

63. Cao D, Srisuma S, Bronstein AC, et al. Characterization of edible marijuana product exposures reported to United States poison centers. *Clinical Toxicol* 2016;54(9):840–46.

64. New Colorado rules make marijuana packaging safer for adults, less appealing to children. www.colorado.gov/pacific/marijuana/news.

65. Barrus DG, Capogrossi KL, Cates SC, et al. Tasty THC: Promises and challenges of cannabis edibles. Methods Rep RTI Press 2016 PMCID:5260817.

66. Mura P, Kintz P, Dumestre V, et al. THC can be detected in brain while absent in blood. *J Anal Toxicol* 2005;29(8):842–3.

67. Orens A, Light M, Rowberry J, et al. Marijuana equivalency in portion and dosage. Colorado Dept of Revenue, Denver CO 2015.

68. Grotenhermen F. Pharmacokinetics and pharmacodynamics of cannabinoids. *Clin Pharmacokinet* 2003;42(4):327–60.

69. Grotenhermen F. Harm reduction associated with inhalation and oral administration of cannabis and THC. *J Cannabis Therapeutics* 2001;1(3–4):133–52.

70. Kosa KM, Giombi K, Rains CB, et al. Consumer use and understanding of labeling information on edible marijuana products sold for recreational use in the states of Colorado and Washington. *Int J Drug Policy* 2017;43:57–66.

71. Vandrey R, Rabe JC, Raber ME, et al. Cannabinoid dose and label accuracy in edible medical cannabis products sold online. *JAMA* 2015;313(24):2491–3.
72. Bonn-Miller MO. Loflin MJE, Thomas BF, et al. Labeling accuracy of cannabidiol extracts sold online. *JAMA* 2017;318(17):1708–9.
73. Crippa, JA, Crippa AC, Hallak JE, et al. Δ 9-THC intoxication by cannabidiol-enriched extract in two children with refractory epilepsy. *Front Pharmacol* 2016;7:359.

16 Cannabis, a Bio-Spiritual Remedy for Addiction

Joseph J. Morgan and Kenneth Blum
Substance Abuse Disorders Institute

CONTENTS

Addiction is complex, illogical, cunning, and baffling. It is best to be open minded and think of multifactorial causes and treatments.

- Biological (family history, genetic addiction risk assessment)
- Spiritual (assess current beliefs and during and after working 12-step programs)
- Toxicological/acute environmental change considerations (detox/rehab)
- Emotional components (i.e., comorbid PTSD, anxiety, depression, ADHD, learning disabilities, adjustment disorders, self-esteem, etc.)
- Lifestyle and nutritional choices.

Cannabis may help some people with each of these components. It is a therapeutic intervention warranted to be reviewed with the patient.

Each physical and/or emotional trauma increases the risk for addiction and/or relapse. It is rare in the United States to reach age 24 without having had some emotional trauma; however, genetics, emotional constitution, family history, and social support play a role in susceptibility to substance use, abuse, and developing dependency.

Addiction commonly results from self-medication or prescribed medication for pain, stress, and/or trauma (PTSD). Relapse and cross-addiction or serial addiction, as well as polysubstance addiction, are not uncommon. Both the trauma/PTSD and all aspects of addiction(s) require effective treatment. This typically has included abstinence from all similarly addictive substances. Spiritual transformation involves reframing of sensitivity to others vs. isolation, resentments (bearing grudges), and all other forms of negativity and self-centeredness. Cannabis and nutrition, including healthy diet and neuronutrients to correct deficiencies in the brain reward centers related to dopamine and other neurotransmitter deficits, emerge as safer alternatives.

CASE REPORTS

These two case summaries illustrate how and where cannabis was therapeutic along with cannabis-related adverse reactions.

Case 1 (a first-person format from a doctoral thesis in progress): My addiction started out innocently. Having suffered from back pain years before marriage, I experienced the benefits of oxycodone in easing an undiagnosed anxiety disorder as well as quelling physical pain. But it wasn't until later, after having three girls a year apart and suffering from recurring back pain, post-partum depression that worsened after each birth, and exhaustion, that I began reaching for our well stocked breakfront filled with a large supply of Manichewitz. With that energizing and relaxing wine, coupled with the wine coolers I saw other moms in our well to do cul de sac drinking with impunity, I began to notice dependency and signs of progressive addiction.

I had a supportive loving family who quickly got me help. Rehab treatment helped, but after some success, I relapsed due to increasing anxiety, depression, and cravings. Subsequently, as a direct result of my drug use, I experienced a traumatic physical assault from an intoxicated dealer resulting in physical mutilation and requiring life-saving surgery and subsequent plastic surgical repairs. These events all led to severe untreated PTSD. Cannabis was not offered by the medical and mental health professions. I succumbed to using drugs and alcohol again to treat my physical and emotional pain and PTSD. Another brief yet horrendous set of consequences predictably occurred as a direct result of active addiction and landed me back in rehab.

For 20 years in recovery, I've been working as a therapist in the field of addiction. If only medical cannabis had been available to me to treat anxiety, depression, and to satisfy addictive drug and alcohol cravings, I may have been spared that last relapse that led to the assault and subsequent PTSD. I am sensitive to THC. It makes me anxious. I don't like the psychoactive effect, unless in a microdose which also relieves nausea and my headaches. However, I find hemp CBD, especially as formulated and recommended to me by Dr. Hyla Cass, reduces anxiety, nausea, and cravings for cigarettes. CBD also helps me sleep well. I haven't had drug or alcohol cravings for 20 years which I attribute to my Higher Power and actively working two 12-step programs.

There is limited published information indicating the effectiveness of medical cannabis use to prevent relapse in the post-acute withdrawal period lasting up to 18 months. Cannabis seems quite effective in sustaining sobriety during this especially rough period when individuals are going to 12-step programs and trying to get a handle on the mental, emotional, and spiritual changes necessary to maintain a sound and sober life. There is much evidence in the recovery community attesting to the imperative aid cannabis offers for achieving and maintaining a critical power over a previously powerless situation. It is my hope that the people I work with will be institutionally given a much needed assist of the nonaddictive alternative medical cannabis offers. It is my contention that once made available, much more anecdotal and scientific support for the use of medical cannabis will flood forth.

Case 2: An only child, a currently middle-aged optometrist's parents were traumatized immigrant war refugees who had experienced starvation. They quarreled often, separated several times, and divorced before he was 9 years old. He liked being away from the small apartment he shared with his mental health-challenged mother. She had refractory agitated depression and severe fibromyalgia (not recognized decades ago) and diagnosed as paranoia. She was a prescribed sedative heavy user. Heavily sedated at times; unpredictably enraged at others. Before age 13, he was mugged twice in his urban neighborhood where his friend's families were relocating due to increasing crime and demographic change. Ice cream, milkshakes, pizza, lamb chops, and being away from home in perceived safe places brought him solace. As a chubby adolescent, music and marijuana were shared with friends. However, he often felt like a lonely outsider in his neighborhood and at school.

To escape, he went to his ancestral homeland for the last 2 years of high school. There he was traumatized by war, including the fear of being killed. Seeing horrifically injured people, watching distant bombings, and observing bomb laden jets return empty and military convoys return from the front with newly destroyed armored vehicles were further trauma. He experienced teacher and consumer goods shortages. In college, after temporarily dropping out from a lack of direction and fueled by too much alcohol and pesticide-laced marijuana, he refocused on academics. He no longer used marijuana and felt it interfered with retention while studying. He reduced his alcohol use and went to optometry school.

Anxious and fearing poverty and abandonment if he failed, anxiety and insomnia worsened. In optometry school, he was a rare user of marijuana and a moderate user of alcohol, prescribed benzodiazepines, and various classes of sleeping pills. Weight gain accelerated. He graduated, began in a low-pressure, patient-centered professional group practice, married a teetotaler, had children, and has had a successful career. But he felt lonely, uncertain, angry, fearful, and anxious. A psychiatrist diagnosed General Anxiety Disorder and Adjustment Disorder of Adult Life. He was prescribed psychiatric medications that did not help and caused social withdrawal, loss of libido, and apathy. Food, especially bread, pizza, pretzels, and ice cream, was his feel good drugs. He ate a lot of processed foods. Fearing a career-ending arrest or positive urine drug screen, he abstained from marijuana for over 30 years.

By his mid-30s, he had metabolic syndrome with prominent central obesity. He was prescribed lipid-lowering drugs and oral antidiabetic drugs. By age 50, despite lifelong regular exercise, his BMI was 38 and he had completely lost control of ability to regulate caloric intake. With type 2 diabetes and a rising HbA1C, he could barely walk more than 200 yards without resting from obesity-related foot pain. He blamed poorly made shoes. He was using CPAP for obstructive sleep apnea. Consultations with diabetes educators resulted in a 3 lb. weight loss.

He made peace with dying from a complication of uncontrollable overeating and worsening obesity. However, he moved to join an old friend's smaller practice. His senior partner was an enthusiastic medical marijuana patient for chronic pain. Thus, he too became a western-state legal medical marijuana patient. A recommended a pesticide-free CBD tincture (AC/DC or Charlotte's web that assayed at 1:17 ration of THC: CBD) by a knowledgeable cannabis physician reduced his carb craving and overall appetite within the first 2 days. This began a slow journey to a 70 lb. weight loss and vitality. Assayed, pesticide-free THC-dominant *indica* (body relaxing) medical cannabis helped with lifelong anxiety and insomnia more than FDA-approved anxiolytics, antidepressants, and all other types of neuropsychiatric medications prescribed over decades (including SSRI, SNRI, benzodiazepines, lithium, typical and atypical antipsychotics).

He was introduced by a new acquaintance, who had lost over 150 lbs., to a 12-step program for food addicts. That program viewed flour and sugar as addictive and deadly white powders to be *completely* abstained from. He was told that unlike drug, alcohol, and gambling addictions, for which complete abstinence is required in recovery, food addicts have to deal with the beast coming out of the cage at least three times a day. Desperate and immediately compliant with food restrictions, including weighing and measuring most foods, eating simple non-processed foods like eggs, yogurt, oatmeal, shredded wheat, berries, beans, lots of salad with raw and cooked vegetables, his weight loss accelerated. He spoke with his 12-step program sponsor for 15–30 minutes at least five times a week, read program literature and that of Alcoholics Anonymous, went to meetings, and spoke daily with other food addicts in his program about experiences. He used the tools of the program. Despite several stress-related food/binge relapses that resulted in a maximum 20 lb. weight gain over a 5-year period, he has managed to keep off at least 60 of the 70 lbs. lost for over 2 years.

Feeling his food addiction was reasonably controlled and becoming increasingly upset over the unpredictable and sometimes crazy behavior of a newly alcoholic family member, he found Al Anon and began seriously working its 12-step program. As a state legal medical cannabis patient, he currently uses a hybrid medical cannabis vape for occasional PTSD flares and a body-relaxing *indica* tincture or oil at least 3× a week for insomnia. Nocturnal THC-dominant cannabis almost always causes food binges ("munchies") not suppressed with CBD. He finds nocturnal CBD to be too stimulating/arousing; it exacerbates his chronic insomnia. Nocturnal sex is an effective therapy for insomnia. He feels cannabis (THC) before nocturnal sex is most effective/relaxing for insomnia but that THC-dominant cannabis has kept him from losing those last 10 lbs. Moreover, he knows if he uses THC cannabis by day, he won't be able to control food cravings.

Genetic Addiction Risk Score (GARS) testing via cheek swab revealed a Reward Deficiency Syndrome (RDS) with six gene variants associated with addiction. Having had GARS and undergoing genetic counseling for RDS allowed him to understand the biological basis of his addiction. He learned some people are born with addictive craving behavior, and most other addicts have stress-induced craving behavior. Substances can chronically deplete dopamine in the brain reward center which can cause withdrawal or toxicity-induced craving. As tolerance develops, larger doses are needed for a high. Thus genes, environment, stress, and the drugs of choice are all important factors for addiction and relapse risk. Having four or more (out of 21) gene variants in GARS is RWD associated with increased addiction and relapse risk. Seven or more gene variants qualify RWD associated with increased risk of alcoholism. His HIPPA-protected written report noted, "Certain genes potentially impact how well an individual can control or moderate his desire for alcohol, drugs, and even food." About half of your overall addiction risk is genetic. People continually lacking dopamine don't feel satisfaction in their lives, have difficulty coping with stress, and carry an elevated risk for behaviors that are known to increase dopamine in the pleasure centers of the brain.

His risk variant genes included COMT and OPRM1 (coding for the mu opioid receptor), both associated with reduced sensitivity to opioids. Four of his six risk variants were associated with increased risk of addiction to glucose, opioids, and cannabis. He felt his results explained his previously puzzling lack of expected pain relief from opioids prescribed for pain from fractures and dental procedures, and his addictive craving reactions for starchy food. He is grateful he never had an opioid abuse problem and is aware of this potential risk. The genetic counselor explained Reward Deficiency Syndrome related to food, music, and cannabis all boosting dopamine in his brain reward center.

He has completed all 12 steps in Al Anon and enthusiastically attends at least two meetings a week. He feels working the 12-step program with a sponsor has fundamentally transformed his life for better and he is able to replace self-centeredness, defiance, loneliness, anger, resentment, critical judgment of others, and frustration with caring about others. He avoids judgment of others and practices framing all that life deals him into gratitude and acceptance. He finds peace in yoga, exercise, listening to the music of his adolescence and college-era concerts along with daily formal and informal prayer, and meditation.

He reports using a tincture or oil extraction of THC-based *indica*, body-relaxing cannabis increases the quality of his sleep and thus next day functioning. He rarely takes FDA-approved medications for insomnia, unless traveling out of state without legal access to cannabis at his destination. He uses CBD with breakfast and sometimes before going out to self-serve buffets.

DEFINING ADDICTION

Recovery from any addiction, an attraction to a false god, requires rejecting of a lie (about a substance or behavior or lifestyle) and finding a replacement transcendental meaning. If cannabis could possibly replace more harmful mind-altering substances like alcohol and opioids and reduce inpatient detox and drug rehab, it would provide a valuable therapy.

The American Society of Addiction Medicine (ASAM) defines addiction as "A primary, chronic disease of brain reward, motivation, memory, and related circuitry. Dysfunction in these circuits leads to characteristic biological, psychological, social and spiritual manifestations. This is reflected in an individual pathologically pursuing reward and/or relief by substance use and other behaviors. Addiction is characterized by an inability to consistently abstain, impairment in behavioral control, craving, diminished recognition of significant problems with one's behaviors and interpersonal relationships, and a dysfunctional emotional response. Like other chronic diseases, addiction often involves cycles of relapse and remission. Without treatment or engagement in recovery activities, addiction is progressive and can result in disability or premature death." [1]

Neuroscientist Kenneth Blum has for decades pioneered and refined a concept of addiction as "Reward Deficiency Syndrome" with a genetic basis and proffers specific neuronutrients as a therapy to reduce cravings and relapse [2]. The basic premises are biological rewards which underlie substance addiction and all addictive behaviors. A dopamine deficiency in the brain reward center results from genetics, stressors, and adverse effects from prolonged substance use or behavioral habits. To feel ordinary pleasure, interactions of neurotransmitters regulate the dopamine and other neurotransmitter activity in the mesolimbic system reward center, particularly in the nucleus accumbens. Those who lack pleasure are predisposed to use any means, substance, or behavior to activate dopamine release to relieve stress, and feel healthy, whole, or experience pleasure.

The Genetic Addiction Risk Score (GARS) results impact on initial addiction, and subsequent relapse risks may be lessened with Precision Addiction Management (PAM) tablets over a longer period based on genetic risk profile. Talk therapies and steps that promote natural dopamine and endorphin release, including healthy diet, yoga, exercise, mediation, orgasmic sex, and music as well as other support systems promote a "pro-dopamine" lifestyle. PAM and the above measures help with successful recovery, reducing cravings and relapse, via induction of dopamine homeostasis. Reward Deficiency may be summarized as vulnerability to addiction, and relapse may be the result of the cumulative effects of dopaminergic and other neurotransmitter genetic variants and elevated stress levels. Dopamine homeostasis may be a preferred goal to combat relapse [2,3].

CANNABIS USE DISORDER (CUD)

An individual diagnosed with cannabis use disorder (F 12:10 or F 12:20) in the current Diagnostic and Statistical Manual, 5th edition, (DSM-V) must meet all of the following [4]:

- A problematic pattern of cannabis use with clinically significant impairment or distress, as manifested by at least 2 of the following, occurring within a 1 year period:
  Cannabis is often taken over a longer period or larger amounts than intended.
  Persistent desire or unsuccessful efforts to reduce or control cannabis use.
  A great deal of time spent in activities to obtain cannabis, use it, or recover from its effects.
  Craving, or a strong desire or urge to use.
  Recurrent use resulting in not meeting major expectations at school, work, or home.
  Continued cannabis use despite having persistent or recurrent social or interpersonal problems caused or exacerbated by the cannabis.
  Important social, occupational, or recreational activities are forsaken or reduced because of cannabis use.
  Recurrent cannabis use in contexts in which it is physically hazardous.
  Cannabis use is continued despite knowledge of having a persistent or recurrent physical or psychological problem that is likely to have been caused or exacerbated by cannabis.
- Tolerance, as defined by either of the following:
  A need for markedly increased amounts of cannabis to achieve intoxication or desired effect.

A markedly diminished effect with continued use of the same amount of cannabis.

• Withdrawal, as characterized by either of the following:

Withdrawal syndrome for cannabis:

Stopping cannabis use that has been heavy and prolonged (i.e., usually daily or almost daily use over a period of a least a few months).

Three (or more) of the following signs and symptoms develop within approximately 7 days after stopping heavy cannabis use:

Irritability, anger, or aggression.

Nervousness or anxiety.

Sleeping-related difficulty (e.g., insomnia, bad dreams).

Diminished appetite or weight loss.

Restlessness.

Depressed mood.

Epidemiologists from the National Institute of Health in 2012–2013 published results of face-to-face interviews with 36,309 respondents ≥18 years old participating in the National Epidemiologic Survey on Alcohol and Related Conditions-III [5]. Prevalence of 12-month CUD was greater among men (3.5%) than women (1.7%). Women experienced shorter duration from onset of cannabis use (mean 4.7 years) to onset of CUD than men (mean = 5.8 years). In both men and women, prevalences of CUD were greater among young adults, Blacks, and those with lower income and greater among Native American women relative to White women. CUD was highly comorbid with other substance use disorders, PTSD, antisocial personality disorder (PD), and borderline and schizotypal PDs. Quality of life for individuals with CUD was low regardless of gender [5]. They concluded, DSM-5 CUD among men and women is highly prevalent, comorbid, and characterized by low quality of life.

Historically, CUD excluded medical cannabis patients. This study suggests alternatively CUD, in the absence of personality disorder (PD) and other substance abuse, is rare in medical cannabis patients, especially Caucasians and there are demographic risk factors. However, cannabis is a potentially mild addictive substance, like a caffeine habit, but potentially far more intoxicating in a dose-dependent manner. Given how widespread medical and recreational use are, this data supports cannabis safety for well-adjusted non-PD patients in a supervised medical setting.

The cannabis withdrawal syndromes resemble that of caffeine—next day headaches, insomnia, and irritability. CUD criteria do not distinguish toxic properties of contaminants from those of cannabinoids. If THC is the intoxicant in cannabis, why is there not a dronabinol use disorder of equal severity? Why does dronabinol even at a dose of 20 mg three times a day not treat CUD or reduce marijuana use? [6]. In contrast an alcoholic will, for example, substitute beer or whiskey for vodka. Alcohol is alcohol. An opioid addict can effectively substitute, for example, buprenorphine or oxycodone for heroin or vice versa to prevent withdrawal.

As more states and other jurisdictions legalize cannabis, users will have access to cannabis products and spend less time looking for and thinking about how to obtain and where to use cannabis. Moreover, the CUD diagnostic criteria of involving "a great deal of time is spent in activities necessary to obtain, use cannabis, or recover from its effects" at least partly will be resolved by decriminalization and/or legal cannabis access. No more fear of arrest, incarceration, and job loss is time saving.

The "La Guardia Study" of 1944, conducted by the New York Academy of Medicine, refuted the "gateway to hard drug" hypothesis proffered by the Federal Bureau of Narcotics, then led by Harry Anslinger [7]. This detailed study of drug use in New York City took years and reached 12 conclusions for understanding of what is currently deemed CUD by the American Psychiatric Association and why Schedule 1 status for cannabis, unlike heroin in Schedule 1, makes no scientific sense:

1. The introduction of marijuana into this area is recent as compared to other localities.
2. The cost of marijuana is low and therefore within the purchasing power of most persons.
3. The distribution and use of marijuana is centered in Harlem.
4. The majority of marijuana smokers are Blacks and Latin-Americans.
5. The consensus among marijuana smokers is that the use of the drug creates a definite feeling of adequacy.
6. The practice of smoking marijuana does not lead to addiction in the medical sense of the word.
7. The sale and distribution of marijuana is not under the control of any single organized group.
8. The use of marijuana does not lead to morphine or heroin or cocaine addiction, and no effort is made to create a market for these narcotics by stimulating the practice of marijuana smoking.
9. Marijuana is not the determining factor in the commission of major crimes.
10. Marijuana smoking is not widespread among school children.
11. Juvenile delinquency is not associated with smoking marijuana.
12. Publicity over the catastrophic effects of marijuana smoking in New York City is unfounded.

EVIDENCE FOR THERAPEUTIC INTERVENTION WITH CANNABIS

Older medical literature on this topic is fascinating. Birch described, in the first volume of The Lancet, his experience in India with a 24-year-old serial alcoholic and oral opium addict, who once had a responsible position and who resembled "an exhumed corpse." He was treated with increasing doses of a cannabis tincture with "the happiest result" including return of appetite, normal sleep, resolution of delusions, and regaining his ability to walk. He returned to work after 6 weeks. Birch also treated addicts to chloral hydrate with cannabis and commented, "The chief point... was the immediate action of the drug in appeasing the appetite for chloral or opium and in restoring ability to appreciate food. It seems to supply the place of the poison... I think it will be found there need be no fear of peremptorily withdrawing the deleterious drug if hemp be employed..." [8] Dr. Birch withdrew opium and chloral hydrate, an addictive sedative of that era abruptly, substituted with cannabis for a reduction of harm and gradually tapered off the cannabis.

A larger patient series, with similar results, was reported by JB Mattison in 1891 [9]. He describes more than 10 years of experience with cannabis with habitués, active and former users of opium, chloral, and/or cocaine. "In these, often, it has proved an efficient substitute for the poppy. Its power in this regard has sometimes surprised me." He described a surgeon who had been injecting morphine twice daily for 10 years who recovered with less than a dozen doses of cannabis tincture. He points out that very high doses of cannabis should be used for detox and in addicts to other substances, approximately three to six times what one would use to treat a nonaddict. He concludes by saying doctors should "steer clear of narcotic shoals on which many a patient has gone awreck… at times hemp will fail, so do other drugs. But the many cases in which it acts well entitle it to a large and lasting confidence."

In a Canadian medical cannabis patient study, published in 2016 by Lucas et al., $N = 473$, 80% reported substitution of cannabis for prescribed drugs, 52% reported substituting cannabis for alcohol, and 33% used their medical cannabis to substitute for illicit substances [10]. Those substituting cannabis for prescribed drugs were more likely to report difficulty affording sufficient quantities of cannabis. Patients less than 40 years old are more likely to substitute cannabis for all three classes of substances—alcohol, benzodiazepines, and opioids.

A study by Kral et al. surveyed 653 urban California heroin injectors or nonmedical opioid users about hard drug and cannabis use [11]. About half reported cannabis use in the past 30 days. The mean and median number of times opioids were used in past 30 days was significantly lower for people who used cannabis than those who did not use cannabis (mean: 58.3 vs. 76.4 times; median: 30 vs. 60 times, respectively; $p < 0.003$). In multivariable analysis, people who used cannabis used opioids less often than those who did not use cannabis (Beta: -0.346; 95% confidence interval: -0.575, -0.116; $p < 0.003$). Cannabis access or use once again clearly showed an impressive public health benefit of substitution and reduction in opioid use.

The use of cannabidiol (CBD) to inhibit reward-facilitating effects of morphine in rats by Katsidoni et al. indicates cannabidiol attenuates cue-induced reinstatement of heroin seeking [12]. They investigated the effects of cannabidiol on brain reward function and on the reward-facilitating effect of morphine and cocaine using the intracranial self-stimulation (ICSS) paradigm. CBD inhibited the reward-facilitating effect of morphine, but not cocaine suggesting that CBD interferes with brain reward mechanisms responsible for the expression of the acute reinforcing properties of opioids, thus indicating that CBD may be clinically useful in attenuating the rewarding effects of opioids.

REFERENCES

1. American Society of Addiction Medicine. Short and Long Definition of Addiction. www.asam.org/quality-practice/definition-of-addiction.
2. Blum K et al. 2018. Introducing precision addiction management of reward deficiency syndrome, the construct that underpins all addictive behavior. *Frontiers in Psychiatry.* 27 November 2018. doi:10.3389/fpsyt.2018.00548.
3. Blum K et al. 2017. Substance use disorder a biodirectional subset of reward deficiency syndrome. *Frontiers in Bioscience* (Landmark Education) 22:1534–48.

4. American Psychiatric Association. Diagnostic and Statistical Manual of Mental Disorders (DSM–5) 2013, Washington DC: American Psychiatric Publishing. ISBN-10: 0890425558.

5. Kerridge BT et al. 2018. DSM-5 cannabis use disorder in the National Epidemiologic Survey on Alcohol and Related Conditions-III: Gender-specific profiles. *Addictive Behaviors* 76:52–60. doi:10.1016/j.addbeh.2017.07.012. Epub 2017 Jul 14.

6. Levin, FR et al. 2016 Feb 1. Dronabinol and lofexidine for cannabis use disorder: A randomized, double-blind, placebo-controlled trial. *Drug Alcohol Depend* 159:53–60. doi:10.1016/j.drugalcdep.2015.11.025. Epub 2015 Nov 27.

7. Mayor's Committee on Marihuana. The Marihuana problem in the city of New York: Sociological. Medical, Legal, and Pharmacological Studies 1944. Available at www.druglibrary.net/schaffer/Library/studies/lag/lagmenu.html.

8. Birch, E.A. 1889. The use of Indian hemp in the treatment of chronic chloral and chronic opium poisoning. *Lancet* 1:625. Reprinted in Marijuana: Medical Papers 1839–1972 by Tod E Mikuriya, 2007, Nevada City, CA: Symposium Publishing.

9. Mattison J.B. 1891. Cannabis indica as an anodyne and hypnotic. *St luius Medical and Surgical Journal* 56:265–271. Reprinted in Reprinted in Marijuana: Medical Papers 1839–1972 by Tod E Mikuriya, 2007, Nevada City, CA: Symposium Publishing.

10. Lucas, P et al. 2016. Substituting cannabis for prescription drugs, alcohol, and other drugs among medical cannabis patients: The impact of contextual factors. *Drug and Alcohol Review* 35:326–33. doi:10.1111/dar.12323. Epub 2015 Sept 14.

11. Kral AH, et al. 2015. Is cannabis use associated with less opioid use among people who inject drugs? *Drug Alcohol Depend* 153:236–41. Published online 2015 May 22. doi:10.1016/j.drugalcdep.2015.05.014.

12. Katsidoni V. 2013. Cannabidiol inhibits the reward-facilitating effect of morphine: Involvement of 5-HT1A receptors in the dorsal raphe nucleus. *Addiction Biology* 18:286–96. doi:10.1111/j.1369–1600.2012.00483.x. Epub 2012 Aug 2.

17 Cannabis Use in Chinese Medicine, Ayurvedic Medicine, & Different Religions

Betty Wedman-St Louis
Clinical Nutritionist

CONTENTS

Different religions regard cannabis use based on historic perspective and healthcare professionals need to access the religious attitude of their patients before recommending cannabis as medicine. Currently, many religious sects are opposed to the use of intoxicants—Islam, Bahai, Latter-Day Saints (Mormons)—by their members. Some Christian faiths (Catholicism, Protestantism), Buddhism, and Judaism have supported the use of medicinal cannabis. Hinduism, Taoism, and ancient Scythia & Assyria have used cannabis in religious ceremonies for centuries. Here is a brief overview in how these cultures have used hemp.

Cannabis has been documented in Chinese medical texts over 2,000 years for pain and mental illness with the achenes (seeds) of cannabis used for more than 1,800 years. Currently, China is one of the world's major hemp cultivators with a 600 AD agricultural text describing the cultivation of hemp, Qi Min Yao Shu (translated as "Essential Techniques for the Welfare of the People").

ANCIENT SCYTHIA & ASSYRIA

Ancient cultures used cannabis incense for religious ceremonies with hemp plants burned on wooden tripods according to Herodotus, a Greek historian from the fifth-century BCE. Assyrians used cannabis incense during funeral rituals and to ward off evil spirits.

Scythians were a nomadic population that traveled throughout Europe, Central Asia, and Russia. As expert horsemen, they used cannabis in religious ceremonies by creating a teepee or tent supported by three wooden sticks and covered them with woolen felt. Inside the tent, they placed hot stones on the ground and threw hemp seeds onto the stones to [produce a vapor they inhaled.

BUDDHISM

India and Tibet share a border and a tradition of using cannabis in religious activities. Tibet is a predominately Buddhist nation whereby cannabis is used for meditation and awareness during religious ceremonies. Being a Buddhist means living in a way that is honorable and respecting the sanctity of life. The five basic precepts for Buddhists are: abstain from harming living beings, one cannot steal, or lie, avoid sexual misconduct, and no intoxication. The use of drugs for medical purposes is allowed, so the Dalai Lama has declared that medical cannabis use is permitted.

HINDUISM

The Vedas, the oldest and most sacred Hindu text dating back to 1500 BCE, indicate cannabis is one of the five sacred plants. Ancient Hindus believe that the gods sent hemp out of compassion for humans so they could attain happiness. Some Hindu stories state that cannabis came from a drop of nectar that descended from heaven.

Since ancient times, people have consumed "bhang," a cannabis drink made with milk and almonds during Hindu festivals. Another legend says that Shiva, a Hindu god, created cannabis from his own body as the elixir of life so it holds a sacred place in the Hindu faith.

In the 1890s, the British colonization of India had medical authorities worried about the use of cannabis in Hindu culture, but they soon declared that cannabis use was so embedded in the culture and harmless in moderation.

JUDAISM

In *Cannabis: A History* by Martin Booth, Sara Benetowa (later known as Sula Benet), an etymologist from the Institute of Anthropological Sciences in Warsaw, Poland, wrote a treatise in 1936 entitled, "Tracing One Word Through Different Languages." This was a study on the word "cannabis" used in Hebrew texts. She demonstrated that the ancient Hebrew word for cannabis was Kaneh-Bosem and that over the course of time, the two words were fused into one, kanabos or kannabus. The Webster's New World Hebrew Dictionary (page 607) identifies hemp as kanabos. Kaneh-bosem is mentioned five times in the Old Testament with the first being Exodus 30:23 when Moses was directed by God to anoint the meeting tent and all its furnishings with a specially prepared oil containing Kaneh-bosem.

TAOISM

Taoism is based on the philosophy of Lao Tzu and became the official religion of China in the Tang Dynasty (618–907 CE). Taoism is an ancient Chinese belief system related to doing what is natural and maintaining balance in the universe.

Cannabis was used in ritual incense—burners to produce "hallucinogenic smokes" according to the Taoist encyclopedia Wushang Biyao. It was also used to eliminate selfish desires, induce feelings of well-being, and achieve a state of naturalness when used by Taoist priests and shamans, but not shared with common people.

CHINESE MEDICINE

Traditional Chinese Medicine (TCM) has a long history of using cannabis. It is considered one of the 50 fundamental herbs of TCM and named for the Chinese goddess Ma Gu ("hemp maiden") which is associated with the elixir of life. The Chinese term for anesthesia is composed with the Chinese character that means hemp. Hua Tuo, A Han Dynasty physician in 200 AD, is said to be the first person to use cannabis as an anesthetic during an acupuncture procedure. Mixing ma fei san (dried, powdered plant and wine) allowed pain control during the procedure.

Chinese medicine is designed to consider all influences to the body, mind, and spirit in order to determine a diagnosis and treatment. Chinese herbal medicine is based on polypharmacy to combine substances that provide synergistic properties to potentize the force of the medicine. Using cannabis alone would be considered unhealthy and may cause imbalances in the body by overtaxing the liver. Therefore, acupuncture can be combined with cannabis to increase endocannabinoid functioning.

In the mid-1800s, the British colonized China and made them legalize opium for taxation revenue. The Opium Wars opened China to world trade issues and pushed cannabis use to an illegal status. The achenes ("seeds") are the only part of the plant that remains used in modern TCM practice.

AYURVEDIC MEDICINE

An Interview with Dr. Muhammed Majeed, Founder, Sami-Sabinsa Group

Question: **What role cannabis has played in Ayurvedic medicine? Since Ayurveda is the world's oldest medical system, could you give me insight into its use?**

Reply: Ayurveda is the oldest system of medicine that has flourished for thousands of years because of its methodical evaluation of a patient and systematic methods of healing. The concept of Shodhana or internal purification plays a very important role in Ayurveda's palliative and treatment aspects (which includes Panchakarma). The Shamana or Mitigative therapy is conducted with the help of internal medication and diet, which is followed after Shodhana. Thus, Ayurvedic treatment, while correcting the disease, also helps to rejuvenate the body, which is important for longer, healthy life. Acharya Charaka while quoting the uses of Ayurveda says

"Protection of the health and the treatment of a diseased are the uses of Ayurveda."

Question: **Life-force energy puts so much emphasis on nature and plants that it must play a role in Ayurveda. What is that role?**

Reply: Nature and plants are the main sources for Ayurveda for the treatment of diseases. Ayurveda puts forth the belief that nature and man are identical. A man is composed of the same components (Pancha Mahabhuta) as nature. Thus the constitution of a person (Prakriti) depends on nature. A human body can adapt to these natural medicines easily and get healed in a natural way. This approach towards healing can sustain health for a longer duration of life. Thus nature is a comparative parameter to assess one's health and plants are the keys to correct the disturbances in the nature of a person in a natural way.

Question: **Since Ayurveda defines health as a harmony among the body, mind, and spirit, how does cannabis play a part in that balance?**

Reply: Cannabis possesses the properties Laghu (light for digestion), Teekshna (sharp acting), and Vyavaayi (spreads swiftly). It mitigates Vaata and Kapha doshas. The fast acting property of cannabis makes it an intoxicating plant and thus is used after Shodhana or Purification in Ayurvedic medicines. Even after Shodhana, its dosage is 2–4 Ratti, which is equal to 250–500 mg. It is used in the management of mental disorders like depression and schizophrenia, brain related conditions such as epilepsy and seizures, and also reducing pain.

By this short introduction to cannabis and its properties mentioned in Ayurveda, we can say that Bhanga or cannabis helps to manage Vaata dosha which is vitiated in mental disorders. Vitiated Vaata dosha can bring disturbances in functions of mind (Chitta vrittis) and can cause excitement and aggression. This affects the body too, as the body functions according to the mind. Intensified Vaata can cause increased sensitivity and excruciating pain in the nerves and spinal system. Cannabis can manage both the conditions as it mitigates Vaata. Because of its Kapha mitigating property, cannabis can impart activeness in mind and treat Tamas (Chaotic phase of mind). Thus, it can bring out a balance in mind, body, and spirit. Small doses of cannabis with milk and ghee always help to activate the mind and help in proper functioning too. Natural medicines promoting the health of mind and the body can always potentiate the spirit towards positivity.

REFERENCES

Abel EL. *The First Twelve Thousand Years.* 1980. McGraw Hill, New York.
Brand EJ, Zhao Z. Cannabis in Chinese Medicine: Are Some Traditional Indications Referenced in Ancient Literature Related to Cannabinoids. *Front Pharmacol* 2017;8:108.
Chopa IC, Chopra RN. The Use of Cannabis Drugs in India. *Bull Narc.* 1957 Jan 4–29.
Durant W. *The Story of Civilization - Our Oriental Heritage.* 1935. MJF Books, New York.
Iverson LL. *The Science of Marijuana.* 2008. Oxford Press, New York.
Rosenberg Z. Development of pharmacology in Chinese medicine and biomedicine. In: R Scalzo, ed. *Protoc J Bot Med.* 1997. Harvard MA.

18 Legal Landscape

Robert T. Hoban
Hoban Law Group

Medicinal forms of cannabis are more accessible than ever before. Within over a majority of the United States in 2019, it is as simple for patients as walking into a dispensary and buying a variety of widely available marijuana products—the historical stigmas associated with cannabis become less and less prevalent each day, and instead, cannabis use no longer seems strange to many. And, this societal shift is not confined to simply the United States, but also in a growing number of countries around the world—for example, Canada federally legalized marijuana in 2018, much to the chagrin of many other countries. Not very long ago, however, such widespread acceptance of cannabis—whether marijuana[1] or hemp, both derived from the genus cannabis—would have been unthinkable.

Over the past several decades, but particularly accelerating since the 2000s, the legal landscape of cannabis as medicine continues to evolve and transform on an ongoing basis. During that time, we can see the emergence of the early stages of a forward-looking model of cannabis regulation takes shape. Specifically, three independent lanes—"swim lanes," if you will—appear primed to carry cannabis regulation onward: (1) over-the-counter cannabis available via marijuana dispensaries; (2) pharmaceutical drugs approved by the U.S. Food and Drug Administration ("FDA"); and (3) hemp-derived supplements, cosmetics, and other similar products.

However, despite all of the progress already achieved concerning cannabis policy reform in general, marijuana remains federally illegal within the United States, though hemp is federally lawful. Effectively, marijuana remains scheduled—ever since 1970—as a Schedule I controlled substance as within the Controlled Substances Act (the "CSA"), alongside the likes of heroin, LSD, and ecstasy. Juxtaposed against Schedule I, Schedules II–V of the CSA gradually relax the regulation of substances within such schedules, allowing for various, though still restricted, medical, and research uses. As part of inclusion within Schedule I of the CSA, the highest level of government restriction, marijuana continues to be considered to possess a high potential for abuse and addiction, without an accepted medical use or acceptable safe use. This characterization under U.S. federal law operates in stark contrast to the rapid development of the marijuana industry among the majority of state laws from coast to coast within the United States.

Some might wonder, if marijuana is widely lawful among many states' laws, and the federal government is exercising discretion in enforcing federal law against state-lawful marijuana operations, is there any real harm in allowing marijuana to remain

---

[1] The federal Controlled Substances Act schedules "marihuana;" for purposes herein, we use the commonly used spelling, "marijuana."

within Schedule I of the CSA? There are clear ramifications, in the medical context particularly, to marijuana remaining within Schedule I of the CSA. For example, although a majority of American states legalized various forms of marijuana, whether medicinal and/or adult-use, the ability to appropriately and adequately research marijuana remains severely stunted and is a major setback to the continued advancement of cannabis policy reform.

As a Schedule I substance, only facilities duly registered with the U.S. Drug Enforcement Administration ("DEA") may cultivate marijuana, and researchers may only obtain marijuana for research studies from certain DEA-authorized sources. To date, despite the submission of additional applications from third parties which have not been acted upon by DEA, the University of Mississippi remains the sole institution permitted by DEA to cultivate marijuana domestically for purposes of research. However, the quantity and quality of such marijuana provided through the University of Mississippi remains in question—critics suggest the marijuana available is inferior to that available in state-lawful marketplaces around the United States, thus limiting the research able to be conducted. Moreover, if the research is specifically for the creation of a new drug, the researcher must then submit an investigational new drug (IND) application to the FDA. Collectively, these threshold requirements unavoidably require present obstacles—including significant amounts of resources in time, effort, and money—to the furtherance of cannabis research.

In the event Congress re-scheduled marijuana to another schedule within the CSA, or even removed marijuana entirely from the CSA, these impediments to research would likewise be relaxed, if not entirely withdrawn. So far, however, efforts to re-schedule or de-schedule have been unfruitful. In 2016, DEA and its sister agencies considered an administrative petition to re-schedule marijuana. As part of the petition's evaluation, the Department of Health and Human Services re-iterated the U.S. federal government's prior conclusions concerning marijuana: there exists a high potential for abuse, no accepted medical use, and no acceptable level of safety for use, even under medical supervision. These conclusions give little weight to, and seem to fly in the face of, mounting evidence—some anecdotal, others clinical in nature—which seem to suggest treatment under Schedule I is inappropriate for marijuana. Yet, the status quo continues. To that end, Capitol Hill remains similarly short on solutions. In fact, no Congressional effort to re-schedule marijuana has survived the initial committee-level review.

With cannabis policy reform seemingly gaining momentum, to truly understand those proposed policy reforms, it is important to consider the historical context and evolution of legislation and regulation related to cannabis in order to reconcile the policy reforms considered now.

However, prior to the Marihuana Tax Act of 1937 (the "Tax Act"), and even as early as the 1600s, there existed a rich history of cannabis cultivation and use within the United States. Americans cultivated cannabis, including hemp for industrial and other purposes. Cannabis even appeared in the *United States Pharmacopeia* beginning around 1850. Perhaps surprisingly, in the Jamestown Colony of Virginia, it was unlawful for farmers to *not* grow hemp; even this country's forefathers grew hemp, including George Washington on his farm in Virginia. Even into the 1900s, cannabis continued to be widely produced, with various cannabis products—including medicinal products forms—sold over-the-counter.

The perspective concerning started to evolve in the early 1900s. Eventually, in the 1930s, a variety of political lobbying campaigns—rumored to include actors such as then-Federal Bureau of Narcotics Commissioner Harry Anslinger and even traditional paper companies fearful of competing products derived from hemp—lobbied hard to further regulation cannabis—both marijuana and hemp. Those efforts ultimately culminated in the passage of the Tax Act.

The Tax Act represented a first step towards the harshly restrictive federal marijuana prohibition now in place within the United States. Although the Tax Act did not make cannabis—either marijuana or hemp—illegal *per se*, the Tax Act imposed restrictions, taxes, and conditions upon marijuana cultivation that effectively ended cannabis cultivation and use in America over the course of the coming decades. And, importantly, the Tax Act reflects where Congress first defined marijuana, a definition which has been carried forward to date in the CSA's definition of marijuana. At the same time, this definition of marijuana also presented the first instance of Congress distinguishing marijuana from hemp—at that time, Congress only recognized certain portions of the cannabis plant as hemp, though such understanding has evolved to the present definition of hemp.

Building upon the elimination of cannabis production and usage caused by the Tax Act, by the 1970s, President Nixon declared a "war on drugs." Correspondingly, Congress enacted the CSA—and its inclusion of marijuana as a Schedule I substance—cementing the prohibition on marijuana. Between the 1970s and the 1990s, hundreds of thousands of Americans were incarcerated for marijuana-related crimes. For patients who might benefit from cannabis usage, marijuana's inclusion in Schedule I of the CSA not only possessed the threat of incarceration, but also stymied research and development of useful medical applications of cannabis.

However, beginning in the 1990s, states slowly started to recognize their independence in creating state-level cannabis policy reform, increasingly taken cannabis policy reform into their own hands either through voter initiatives or legislative action. In 1996, California became the first state to authorize medical marijuana and end marijuana prohibition under state law, through Proposition 215, also known as the Compassionate Use Act of 1996. Under Proposition 215, California authorized the use of medical marijuana by Californians for therapeutic purposes of treating cancer, anorexia, AIDS, chronic pain along with a number of other illnesses. Continually since then, a majority of U.S. states established medical marijuana regulatory regimes—and, even more recently, beginning with Colorado and Washington in the 2013, also creating adult-use marijuana regulatory schemes.

This widescale transformation of cannabis policy is attributable to many different, though interlinked, causes. For example, there exists undisputed momentum in public support for marijuana legalization, particularly among younger generations, who were not as deeply exposed to the stigmatized messaging concerning marijuana which dominated conversations and marketing campaigns through the early years of the war on drugs. Moreover, there continues to be calls for cannabis policy reform based upon, and to rectify, the disproportionate impact of cannabis illegalization on minority populations. And, for those still leery of the societal impact of cannabis, as numerous states establish regulatory programs, many realize a number of the fears commonly associated with marijuana legalization are largely unfounded and grow increasingly more comfortable with the idea of cannabis policy reform. Outside of the United States, there continues to be an international shift in cannabis reform as well, even by the U.S. neighbors, Canada and Mexico. Accordingly, the calls for cannabis policy reform are even now reaching the halls of Congress, due to the factors referenced above and perhaps others as well, stimulating growing support among lawmakers at the Capitol for permanent cannabis reform.

To illustrate the dramatic shift in public support surrounding cannabis, consider several polling resources over the past several years. According to a 2017 Quinnipiac University poll, 93% of participants supported the legalization of marijuana for medical purposes. Separately, a *New York Times* poll in 2018 resulted in 71% agreeing that the government should not enforce federal laws against marijuana users in states that have legalized medical or adult-use marijuana use. October 2018 surveys from the national analytical group Gallup showed that 66% of the population support the legalization of marijuana, as compared to 12% in 1969. In demonstrating the generational gap in terms of perspective concerning marijuana, a 2018 Pew Research Center Poll also found that 74% of millennials strongly supported federal marijuana legalization, whereas support for marijuana legalization among baby boomers exposed to the war on drugs remains low.

In addition to the shifts in cannabis policy within the United States, significant international movement surrounding cannabis reform continues to occur and seems to be accelerating. Several countries—such as Canada and Colombia—federally legalized marijuana and established regulatory programs which even allow for the import and export of cannabis around the world. Moreover, in the past decade, tens of additional countries have either decriminalized cannabis, legalized its medical use, or legalized its personal use in small amounts. Countries considering or engaging in cannabis policy reform in some form or fashion include, without limitation, Spain, Netherlands, Uruguay, Peru, Jamaica, Portugal, Switzerland, Denmark, Argentina, Cambodia, Costa Rica, Czech Republic, Chile, Colombia, Croatia, Macedonia, Malta, Finland, Belize, Ukraine, Belgium, Philippines, Ecuador, Italy, Luxembourg, Thailand, Russia, Mexico, Israel, Romania, Norway, Australia, Turkey, Zimbabwe, and Germany, among others.

Additionally, the World Health Organization's ("WHO") Expert Committee on Drug Dependence, an independent group of experts in the field of drugs, recently recommended the reclassification of cannabis in the Single Convention of 1961 and the 1971 Convention on Psychotropic Substances. The WHO committee's recommendation will be considered by the United Nations Control Narcotic Board, which will decide whether and how to amend the treatment of cannabis pursuant to these treaties.

Changes in the international landscape could well affect the United States, as well. For example, in continuing to oppose the re-scheduling or de-scheduling or marijuana and limiting its own authority, DEA continues to cite its control obligations under the Single Convention of 1961 as justification to oppose cannabis policy reform. If WHO's recommendation is accepted and the Single Convention of 1961 is correspondingly amended, DEA could no longer cite treaty control obligations, and

DEA and its sister agencies could likely then re-consider a petition similar to the one presented in 2016.

Another contributing factor to the momentum gained in favor of cannabis policy reform are the experiences in states with successfully implemented regulated marijuana regulatory regimes. Many states with established programs experience firsthand that many of the negative perceptions concerning marijuana are not realized, while many others find therapeutic benefit otherwise unavailable through other medications.

Without any federal regulatory oversight (as marijuana remains a federally controlled substance), state regulatory schemes vary across the board. However, states newly establishing medical marijuana programs frequently draw from successfully implemented components of other states' medical marijuana programs. In general, state-level medical marijuana programs often contain similar themes:

- Registration of patients in a state registry;
- Registration of caregivers, where allowed, in a state registry;
- Parameters concerning a physician's recommendation for a patient, generally relating to a bona fide physician-patient relationship and integrating use of medical marijuana with other forms of care and treatment;
- Medical conditions for which medical marijuana may be recommended by a physician such as AIDS, HIV, cancer, and PTSD, among others;
- Licensure for businesses which cultivate, process, distribute, and/or sell medical marijuana, as well as manufacture, distribute, and/or sell medical marijuana products;
- Additional regulations concerning operations of facilities, age restrictions, packaging and labeling of products, and other miscellaneous regulations.

Given the lack of uniformity, there exists great disparity over implementation of medical marijuana regulatory programs, and access by patients thereto. For example, among the states, there are inconsistencies in which type(s) of professionals—or, in some cases, non-professionals—may recommend medical marijuana to a patient and in the regulations which govern those professionals' recommendations. Requirements of medical professionals often include

- A professional medical license (e.g., M.D., D.O.) in good standing;
- Licensure in good standing to practice in a state, respectively;
- Valid, unrestricted DEA certifications;
- Completion of state-specific courses relating to the recommendation of medical marijuana, where required;
- Records concerning the physician's "bona fide" physician-patient relationship, detailing the incorporation of other forms of care and treatment alongside a medical marijuana treatment regimen.

However, despite common logic suggesting it best to rely upon recommendations from medical professionals, the available research on medical marijuana for physicians, and there familiarity with medical marijuana, is even lacking. As a result, without the benefit of definitive research, patients may enter a dispensary and often rely on the advice of "budtenders"—salespeople at dispensaries—in selecting specific strains or product types of medical marijuana in order to treat certain medical and disease conditions. Generally, states prohibit budtenders from providing medical advice to patients as budtenders lack the medical expertise legally required to provide any medical advice; however, such a scenario should not be surprising given the budtenders may possess the greatest familiarity with the available products types.

Separately, states often independently establish which conditions are authorized to be treated with medical marijuana, sometimes seemingly without logic. For example, for years, Colorado did not allow patients to access medical marijuana to treat PTSD despite access being allowed for numerous other conditions, causing patients to lack transparency with their treating physician in order to obtain a recommendation.

Ultimately, these conundrums—professionals' medical recommendations which are lacking as compared with budtenders providing quasi-medical advice, the discrepancy in allowing access to medical marijuana for certain conditions, among other issues—serve to deepen the need for further and more definitive research into medical marijuana. And, while states continue to develop their own independent regulatory marijuana programs, in the event cannabis policy reform came to fruition within the United States, there could be uniformity implemented across state-level programs where authorized—providing a long-term solution for the over-the-counter cannabis lane.

Yet, for now, the status quo concerning federal marijuana regulation within the United States continues, though the appetite to enforce federal law concerning marijuana and interfere with state-regulated cannabis programs wavers from administration to administration.

During the Bush administration in the early 2000s, the federal government staunchly enforced federal law, with thousands of arrests concerning marijuana and seizures of property throughout the country. During this time, a string of Supreme Court cases also disfavored established state-level medical marijuana programs. For example, in the early 2000s, the Supreme Court supported the federal government's right to enforce federal prohibition laws in states with regulated marijuana programs and refused to create an exception to federal marijuana laws for patients with medical conditions.

Comparatively, during the Obama administration thereafter, the federal government afforded state-level marijuana regulatory programs relative freedom. Through memos by then-Deputy Attorney General David Ogden in 2009, and then-Deputy Attorney General James Cole, in 2013, the Department of Justice—under Attorney General Eric Holder—exercised significant enforcement discretion, so long as marijuana businesses operated in compliance with various factors relating to state-level regulatory compliance. These policy memos, though not law, implicitly condoned the emergence of state-level marijuana regulatory schemes without the federal government directly blessing, encouraging, or advancing an end to marijuana prohibition, signaling an important this was a significant change in course.

Upon the beginning of the Trump administration in 2016, however, uncertainty returned as to whether the federal government would shift its position once more.

In early 2018, then-Attorney General Jeff Sessions rescinded the Obama-era memorandums, replacing those policies with ones of "discretion." Though a negative rhetorical shift, little has changed in practice in terms of the Department of Justice—through its U.S. Attorneys in each respective jurisdiction—interfering with state-compliant marijuana businesses. For the foreseeable future, U.S. federal and state laws concerning marijuana are likely to continue to clash without consequence, while patients enjoy generally uninterrupted access to medicinal forms of marijuana. However, broad cannabis policy reform remains much needed in order to resolve the ongoing conflict between federal and state laws.

Concurrent with the emergence of state-level marijuana programs, several pharmaceutical companies engaged in research and development of pharmaceutical products centered around cannabis or cannabis derivatives. For example, dronabinol—marketed as Marinol or Syndros—is a synthetic form of tetrahydrocannabinol ("THC"), the psychoactive compound in cannabis, approved by the FDA for treatment of certain indications. More recently, in the early 2000s, pharmaceutical companies explored products, such as Sativex, which contained isolated forms of THC and cannabidiol ("CBD"), the cannabinoid often associated with cannabis' therapeutic properties; Sativex was not approved. However, in 2018, FDA approved Epidiolex, an isolated form of CBD for treatment of certain child-onset indications. Continued development by pharmaceutical companies relating to CBD, THC, and many of the other cannabinoids naturally occurring in cannabis is widely expected, thus framing the FDA-approved drug lane going forward.

Lastly, the historically lesser known variety of cannabis, hemp, experienced a recent resurgence under U.S. federal law. In 2014, for the first time since the twentieth century, Congress authorized the domestic cultivation of hemp. More recently, in late 2018 through the Agriculture Improvement Act of 2018 (the "2018 Farm Bill"), Congress further clarified and affirmed its authorization of hemp and ensuring hemp is returned to its status as an agricultural commodity within the U.S. agronomy.

To this end, the 2018 Farm Bill affirmatively and definitively removed hemp from the definition of marijuana under the CSA, instead specifying that the United States Department of Agriculture ("USDA"), and not DEA, shall regulate the production of hemp. Importantly, the 2018 Farm Bill provides that hemp—including cannabinoids, derivatives, and extracts therefrom—is not to be treated as a drug akin to marijuana. This shift in policy is important, as such cannabinoids and extracts derived from hemp are widely used today in various forms of products—supplements, cosmetics, and more—to supplement consumers' well-being, similar to vitamin C, calcium, and other such products. These derivatives of hemp thus serve to establish the hemp-derived product lane.

Yet, even with hemp-derived products there remain conundrums for regulators and the industry alike to resolve—primarily, in sensibly distinguishing as between FDA-approved pharmaceutical drugs, which are able to make claims of treatment of certain indications as approved by FDA, as compared with over-the-counter supplements, cosmetics, and other products unable to make such claims. For its part, FDA appears prepared to begin constructively resolving those uncertainties and creating distinct, bright lines as between those channels. FDA's forthcoming regulations of hemp-derived products, as distinguished from FDA-approved drugs, will of course impact those who may benefit from advances in medicinal applications of cannabis as well as those from derivatives of hemp.

Overall, in the coming years, cannabis policy reform seems to be coming full circle from its production and use as recently as the early 1900s under U.S. federal law. However, in the meantime, there exists a maze of confusing and, at times, conflicting legislation and regulation between federal and state law and among the various states. While there is still quite a ways to go in resolving these and other uncertainties, including whether the federal government enacts cannabis policy reform and uniform regulation of medical marijuana, the future of cannabis is emerging and taking shape as three separate and independent lanes, with medicinal forms of cannabis to surely be embedded therein. Despite these evolutions of policy over the past several decades, globally speaking, we are just scratching the surface in terms of establishing formal and long-term cannabis policy reform—it is merely the beginning, and the future of cannabis policy, including cannabis as medicine, awaits.

19 Medical Certification for Healthcare Practitioners*

Chris D. Meletis
Naturopathic Physician

CONTENTS

Cannabinoid-rich hemp oil has emerged as a promising botanical therapeutic with both clinical experience and published studies to support its use. The Stanley brothers are largely credited for first awakening the public to its benefits. The six Colorado siblings developed a hemp extract low in Δ9-tetrahydrocannabinol (THC), the psychoactive component in marijuana, and high in cannabidiol (CBD), a phytocannabinoid that is not associated with the intoxicating effects of the plant. That hemp extract came to be known as Charlotte's Web after the parents of a little girl named Charlotte Figi convinced the brothers to provide their daughter with CBD-rich hemp oil.[1] Charlotte suffered from a severe type of medication-resistant epilepsy known as Dravet syndrome. She was having 300 seizures per week and her heart frequently stopped. After consuming three to four milligrams of the hemp oil per pound of body weight, Charlotte's seizures disappeared. The case received a lot of publicity in major media outlets such as CNN.[1]

* Author Note: Reprinted from *Townsend Letter*, May 2018, http://www.townsendletter.com/). Permission to reuse granted by *Townsend Letter, The Examiner of Alternative Medicine*.

Since then the demand for hemp as a medicinal has skyrocketed and so too has the number of companies producing it and doctors prescribing it. Its benefits have been demonstrated both clinically and in the scientific literature. Based on that scientific research and clinical observations, I employ hemp oil in clinical practice to support the health of patients with epilepsy, anxiety, depression, post-traumatic stress disorder, schizophrenia, inflammation, and pain among other applications.

WHY MANUFACTURERS AND PRACTITIONERS NEED A CERTIFICATION PROGRAM

When new segments of most fields of commercial enterprise enter the marketplace, there are the initial well-intentioned pioneers. This is also true in the hemp oil marketplace. However, like the dietary supplement industry in its early years, the hemp oil marketplace is a Wild West. Up until now, no entity was ensuring the consumer that optimal quantities of the beneficial cannabinoids found in hemp oil were actually contained in the purchased product. As a manufacturer, in order to maintain a respectable reputation and avoid legal complications, it's important to ensure that the hemp oil you're producing lives up to its label specifications. A 2017 article in *JAMA* tested 84 CBD/hemp oil extracts purchased online and found that although CBD oil labeling had the highest degree of accuracy compared to other products tested, 55% of the CBD oil products tested were either under labeled (more CBD was detected in the product than claimed on the label) or over labeled (CBD content that was negligible or less than 1% of the amount on the label).[2] In this study, the over labeled CBD products contained insufficient levels similar to concentrations that resulted in Food and Drug Administration (FDA) warning letters sent to 14 businesses in 2015–2016. Some of the products also contained more THC than noted on the label. In the United States, only cannabinoid-rich hemp oil brands that contain less than 0.3% of the psychoactive cannabinoid THC are legal. Therefore, certainty surrounding the THC content of a particular brand is essential.

The International Center for Cannabis Therapy (ICCT) found similar inaccuracies when its scientists tested hemp oil products sold mainly in online shops in Europe. Not one of the products tested was legally compliant as European legislation requires zero THC in hemp oil. Furthermore, the vast majority of products contained very little CBD and/or high concentrations of heavy metals and pesticides.

Another challenge that has arisen with the availability of hemp oil is that up until now, healthcare practitioners could not tap into a centralized knowledge base where they could have their cannabis questions answered. Because of hemp oil's relative newness in the dietary supplement arena, there are many healthcare practitioners who are unclear of the proper dosage. Some of them have employed hemp products in their practice with little success not realizing that the product may have contained insufficient CBD. I have also encountered uncertainty among practitioners about the best way to incorporate hemp oil into already-prescribed supplement regimens, whether there are any contraindications to its use, and how its effects differ from marijuana. In interacting with attendees of lectures I have conducted on the endo-cannabinoid system, it became clear to me that a number of healthcare practitioners have many questions and concerns about the prescribing of hemp oil as well as the endocannabinoid system on which it acts.

"It is essential that health professionals know what the cannabinoid content of a product is because depending on the illness being treated, too much or too little CBD can affect the outcome," said Petr Kastanek, PhD the director of the ICCT. "A Dravet syndrome patient for example will get strong relief from seizures using CBD, but too much CBD can actually trigger a seizure."

This echoes my clinical experience that as functional medicine providers we must always remember that all receptors throughout the body have an optimal tolerance—not only receptors for CBD—and there is such a thing as too much. This is particularly the case when there is an endogenous pathway which is being augmented, such as the endocannabinoid system. After all, achieving and sustaining homeostasis is the goal.

The ICCT's certification program will instruct practitioners (based on proven protocols) on the ideal amount of hemp oil. "Due to its non-toxic nature, a healthy patient won't suffer side effects, but flooding the CB_1 and CB_2 receptors with cannabinoids is not necessary or advised," said Petr Kastanek. "Micro dosing cannabinoids to activate the receptors creates a potent medical benefit in ICCT's experience."

Clearly, standards are needed both for all cannabis products *and* for practitioners prescribing them.

THE INTERNATIONAL CENTER FOR CANNABIS THERAPY (ICCT)

The ICCT recognized the need for standards in the cannabis industry and consequently introduced three new certification programs: product certification, manufacturing facility certification, and medical certification for practitioners prescribing CBD and other active constituents of hemp. The ICCT is a Czech-based partnership of qualified doctors and scientists who specialize in the medical application of all forms of cannabis. ICCT scientists have spent decades conducting extensive research on the health benefits of medical cannabis as well as product development and medical treatment with an emphasis on enhancing the patients' quality of life.

The organization's certification programs are based on a decade of research conducted by more than 70 ICCT scientists from the Czech Republic and Israel. I recently became aware of the impressive ICCT's mission, clinical work and the high-caliber of people associated with it. In addition to maintaining my naturopathic practice in Oregon, I accepted the role of Chief Medical Officer–USA of the ICCT.

ICCT CERTIFICATION FOR HEMP OIL MANUFACTURERS

The ICCT certification will standardize CBD-rich products and raw materials for human consumption. It uses metabolomic fingerprinting technology to construct a metabolic profile of the cannabinoid product through the pairing of data-rich analytic techniques with multivariate data analysis. The product will be analyzed for cannabinoid profile, pesticides, and contaminants. Manufacturers also have the option to obtain certification for their manufacturing facility similar to cGMP or

NSF certification. The ICCT certification ensures that the manufacturer is compliant with local and state regulations. It also tests the quality and consistency of raw
materials and provides staff training, product formulation, and compliant labeling.
Annual randomized facility inspection is also a component of the manufacturing
facility certification.

American Nutritional Products was the first hemp oil manufacturer to become
certified by ICCT. "It is because of my 28 years in the supplement industry that I
first realized what challenges were going to lie ahead for cannabis and hemp," said
Maria Watson, president and CEO of American Nutritional Products, Inc. and former co-owner of Vitamin Research Products (VRP). "The supplement world started
out with no known certification body and little control on quality. When we owned
VRP, as an industry leader, we drove the movement to clean up our industry—that
now needs to happen in the cannabis space."

THE ICCT MEDICAL CERTIFICATION

Medical certification from ICCT for healthcare practitioners involves eight online
webinar modules, plus one bonus lecture on marketing your certification to the
community and to prospective patients. Conducted by myself and other experts,
the webinar modules are based on ICCT research by a team of 70 scientists, the
evidence-based peer-review literature, my experience in clinical practice, and proven
protocols based on clinical studies. Practitioners enrolled in the certification course
will also learn vital information that ensures patients do not overdose on CBD.
Additionally, the modules will address other topics crucial to the proper prescribing
of hemp oil including:

THE ENTOURAGE EFFECT OF HEMP OIL

The entourage effect is a concept originally proposed by Doctors Mechoulam and
Ben-Shabat two decades ago. It originally referred to the ability of certain endocannabinoid system components to enhance the beneficial effects of the two most
important actors in this system: anandamide and 2-arachidonoylglycerol.[3,4] Since
then the definition of the entourage effect evolved. It now can refer to the fact that
components of cannabis or hemp oil other than THC and CBD—such as phytocannabinoids and terpenes—can actually act synergistically to THC, CBD, or each
other. The ICCT certification online course will explain why the entourage effect is
important in clinical practice.

CBD RECEPTORS AND PAIN PERCEPTION

Hemp oil may be the answer to today's opioid and pain crisis. Opioid overdose is
associated with more than 115 deaths per day in the United States.[5] Finding an alternative to their use is therefore critical.

The endocannabinoid system is closely associated with pain management. The
receptors in this system including CB_1 and CB_2 are activated by endogenous endocannabinoids. However, CBD as a phytocannabinoid and other phytocannabinoids

in hemp oil also affect receptors in this system as does THC, the psychoactive component of cannabis.[6,7]

The certification course will include an in-depth discussion of endocannabinoid receptors and their role in pain management.

HEMP OIL AND NEURODEGENERATIVE CONDITIONS AND MOOD DISORDERS

An abundance of evidence indicates hemp oil impacts the pathophysiology, progression, cause, and ecology of neurodegenerative conditions, mood disorders, and epilepsy. The certification program will help the busy healthcare provider digest this research and discover how it can be applied in clinical practice.

THE GUT-BRAIN AXIS AND CANNABINOIDS

An increasing amount of evidence points to an interplay between intestinal and neurological systems and that this connection is modulated by the gut microbiota, the population of microorganisms found in the intestinal tract. This link between neurological and intestinal systems has become known as the gut-brain axis. Intriguing evidence has emerged that the endocannabinoid system is involved in this interaction.[8,9] The certification program will delve deeply into the role of the endocannabinoid system in the gut-brain axis and how this knowledge can be used to reduce inflammation and support the health of patients with anxiety and depression.

LEGAL CONSIDERATIONS OF PRESCRIBING HEMP OIL

Based on the expertise of a leading attorney in this field of practice, practitioners who receive their cannabinoid certification will move forward with confidence and reassurance on the clinical application of hemp thanks to information presented in a comfortable and simple manner. A number of questions about the legality of hemp oil often arise. These include: (1) What is the difference between federal and state law and the issues of intrastate commerce? (2) Is it true that hemp oil is legal in all 50 states? (3) Is it likely for a person who tests positive to THC, that it could be from hemp oil use alone? (4) Do I need to have special charting or record keeping if I sell hemp oil to patients? (5) If a product that I sell as hemp contains THC beyond the "Legal Limit" to be considered hemp, what is my risk? Hoban Law Group, the leading cannabis business law firm which has presented on behalf of the industry in front of the 9th circuit court, will answer these questions and discuss legal considerations of implementation of hemp oil therapy in practice.

"If you are carrying a hemp product or selling a product with more than 0.3 percent THC then you are dispensing marijuana," said Jason Searns counsel to Hoban Law Group. "It is legally essential to know without question what you are dispensing. With the legal system and U.S. government delineating the role of hemp oil, it is important for clinicians to adhere to a high standard of education as offered by organizations such as the international research and educational organization ICCT."

The Endocannabinoid System and Immunity, Cancer, Senescence, and Healthy Aging

The endocannabinoid system has been found to play an important role in diverse aspects of health. Hemp oil, through its modulation of this system, is a likely option for many health challenges faced by our patients. For example, endocannabinoids are synthesized by most immune cells and upregulate or downregulate a number of immune functions.[10] The CB_2 receptor is also involved in reducing oxidative stress associated with cellular senescence, indicating the endocannabinoid system is involved in healthy aging.[11] The certification program will help practitioners understand the myriad ways in which the endocannabinoid system is involved in health and how modulating that system through hemp oil can achieve beneficial results.

Essential Facts Practitioners Must Know About Employing Hemp Oil in Clinical Practice

The different delivery mechanisms of cannabis can influence how it affects the body. The certification program will allow healthcare providers to become proficient in understanding these delivery systems. For example, there is a next generation of CBD products moving into the American market. These products have efficient, transdermal properties so they bring the active substances deep into the tissue. It is also important when using hemp oil not to unduly disturb the endocannabinoid system and overwhelm natural production of the endocannabinoids or alter receptor activity. The certification program will help practitioners understand how to achieve the benefits of hemp oil without causing this undesirable effect. Processing and extraction processes commonly used in pharmacokinetics, and pharmacodynamics will also be discussed.

Anti-Inflammatory Properties

CBD and other phytocannabinoids and constituents of hemp oil modulate inflammatory pathways. CBD reduces the inflammatory mediators interleukin-6 (IL-6) and TNF-α in rodent models.[12–14] The certification program will discuss in detail the role of hemp oil in influencing inflammatory pathways in various disease states.

Other Benefits of Certification

The International Center for Cannabis Therapy (ICCT) is a Czech Republic-based partnership of qualified doctors and scientists who specialize in the medical application of cannabis. As Chief Medical Officer–USA, my ultimate mission is to offer a certification program that includes a marketing module conducted by Marketing Unlimited, a firm with 28 years' experience in the natural products industry.

RAISING THE BAR ON HEMP OIL
MANUFACTURING AND PRESCRIBING

ICCT's ultimate goal in offering its certification program is to bring European regulatory standards into the U.S. cannabis market. The only type of products carrying ICCT certification will be those that incorporate the efficient use of cannabinoids in well-constructed products to maximize the medical benefit for patients. The ICCT anticipates that consumers will actually seek out doctors who have obtained its certification in cannabinoid therapy and products that have obtained ICCT's blessing as an assurance of quality and safety.

For more information about the ICCT certification programs, visit www. icctcertification.com and join the ICCT mission of education and empowerment.

REFERENCES

1. Young S. Marijuana Stops Child's Severe Seizures. *CNN.* August 7, 2013. www.cnn. com/2013/08/07/health/charlotte-child-medical-marijuana/index.html. Accessed February 3, 2018.
2. Bonn-Miller MO, Loflin MJE, Thomas BF, et al. Labeling accuracy of cannabidiol extracts sold online. *JAMA.* 2017 Nov 7;318(17):1708–9.
3. Piomelli D, Russo EB. The *Cannabis sativa* versus *Cannabis indica* debate: an interview with Ethan Russo, MD. *Cannabis Cannabinoid Res.* 2016;1(1):44–6.
4. Ben-Shabat S, et al. An entourage effect: inactive endogenous fatty acid glycerol esters enhance 2-arachidonoyl-glycerol cannabinoid activity. *Eur J Pharmacol.* 1998 Jul 17;353(1):23–31.
5. National Institute on Drug Abuse. Opioid Overdose Crisis. February 2018. www.drugabuse.gov/drugs-abuse/opioids/opioid-overdose-crisis. Accessed February 3, 2018.
6. Miller RJ, Miller RE. Is cannabis an effective treatment for joint pain? *Clin Exp Rheumatol.* 2017 Sep–Oct;35(Suppl 107(5)):59–67.
7. Morales P, Hurst DP, Reggio PH. Molecular targets of the phytocannabinoids: a complex picture. *Prog Chem Org Nat Prod.* 2017;103:103–31.
8. DiPatrizio N. Endocannabinoids in the Gut. *Cannabis Cannabinoid Res.* 2016 Feb;1(1):67–77.
9. Storr MA, Sharkey KA. The endocannabinoid system and gut-brain signalling. *Curr Opin Pharmacol.* 2007 Dec;7(6):575–82.
10. Chiurchiù V. Endocannabinoids and immunity. *Cannabis Cannabinoid Res.* 2016 Feb 1;1(1):59–66.
11. Hu Y, Zhou KY, Wang ZJ, et al. N-stearoyl-l-Tyrosine inhibits the cell senescence and apoptosis induced by H_2O_2 in HEK293/Tau cells via the CB2 receptor. *Chem Biol Interact.* 2017 Jun 25;272:135–44.
12. Durst R, Danenberg H, Gallily R, et al. Cannabidiol, a nonpsychoactive Cannabis constituent, protects against myocardial ischemic reperfusion injury. *Am J Physiol Heart Circ Physiol.* 2007 Dec;293(6):H3602–7.
13. Barichello T, Ceretta RA, Generoso JS, et al. Cannabidiol reduces host immune response and prevents cognitive impairments in Wistar rats submitted to pneumococcal meningitis. *Eur J Pharmacol.* 2012 Dec 15;697(1–3):158–64.
14. Li K, Feng JY, Li YY, et al. Anti-inflammatory role of cannabidiol and O-1602 in cerulein-induced acute pancreatitis in mice. *Pancreas.* 2013 Jan;42(1):123–9.

20 Cannabis Training Opportunities for Healthcare Professionals

*Alexander Fossi, Judith Spahr,
and Charles Pollack, Jr.*
Thomas Jefferson University

CONTENTS

INTRODUCTION

The state of education and training regarding cannabis as therapy for healthcare professionals in the United States varies widely by specialty and by state. Within the medical community, education often lags behind policy. Public demand has led to legislators approving the medicinal (and in some cases, recreational) use of cannabis, but medical professionals have had little time to prepare themselves for these changes. Those who are involved in the production and distribution of cannabis in these states have similar blind spots. While the process of cultivating specific cannabis strains and converting cannabis plants into a variety of products is well established, many growers and dispensary staff members rely on anecdotal data or personal experience when it comes to recommending products to medical patients or recreational consumers.

In order for healthcare professionals to develop a process for recommending the appropriate products in the correct doses, there will need to be significant additional education made available to these individuals. In addition, if the cannabis industry is expected to be capable of delivering reliable products in safe and potentially effective doses to patients, professionals in this field will need a great deal of training. It has been said that cannabis researchers are being called on to complete 50 years of medical research in 5 years of real time. Virtually every aspect of the field of cannabis as medicine faces this same obstacle. Patients want effective treatments now, but there has been little time for researchers to evaluate those potential treatments, for doctors to gain the knowledge they need to properly recommend them, or for industry members to consistently produce them and market them in a way that consumers or patients understand and can trust.

These problems are compounded by the prevalence of faulty or unsubstantiated information that is widely available to patients interested in cannabis as medicine. Manufacturers of cannabis medications and pro-cannabis sources often make claims that are not backed by current research, and patients who look for information online or rely on media coverage of cannabis medicine can easily be misinformed as to the risks and benefits. Industry staff in growers and dispensaries may be quite familiar with cannabis products but lack medical knowledge, meaning that patients who have medical questions may not be able to speak to someone who can give accurate and research-supported answers to those questions.

Even when working directly with healthcare professionals, it can be difficult for patients to find a physician or other healthcare professional who is well educated when it comes to cannabis as medicine. Current clinical education curricula rarely include discussions of cannabis beyond as a drug of abuse. When patients ask their providers about cannabis as a treatment option, those clinicians may be unable to answer, unwilling to carry on the conversation owing to a lack of knowledge, and unaware of healthcare professionals to whom they could refer the patient. As a result, many patients are still trying to independently find information, often online.

CLINICIANS

CURRENT STATE OF CLINICIAN KNOWLEDGE

There are a number of studies that examine clinicians' knowledge and confidence among healthcare professionals as well as current medical students (Chan et al., 2017). In most cases, the broad conclusions are similar: clinicians are in support of legal reform to allow medicinal cannabis, interested in increased research, and (appropriately) concerned about risks and side effects (Brooks et al., 2017). However, they are hesitant to recommend cannabis, even when such a recommendation would be warranted given the severity of a patient's condition, the current state of research, and state law. In addition, physicians are not comfortable even discussing cannabis in many cases, and a lack of training contributes to their discomfort and lack of confidence (Hwang et al., 2016; Carlini et al., 2017).

It is not particularly difficult to identify the needs that healthcare professionals have when it comes to their understanding of cannabis as medicine. Indeed, professionals themselves have provided a clear picture of what they lack in a number of studies. They are seeking more education in professional settings, such as at conferences and through peer-reviewed research. They want to know how to conduct conversations with their patients about the benefits and risks of cannabis, to which resources they can refer patients when their own knowledge is limited, and how to gain a clear understanding of the legal environment in the states where they practice.

In ongoing studies, the same results have been found. A recent survey of clinicians who work with families of children with autism found that despite a general support for the use of cannabis where medically indicated and a high degree of interest in the possibility of medicinal cannabis among the families of their patients, these clinicians were not having conversations about cannabis as medicine with their patients (Ross, 2018). Clinicians were not confident that they could field questions and did not know where to get more information. Clearly, there is a level of interest in the topic, but more education is needed so that clinicians do not see their own lack of knowledge as a barrier to having conversations about cannabis as medicine with patients. Each new study finds that regardless of state of practice, discipline, and educational background, the vast majority of clinicians are not well prepared to discuss cannabis as medicine (Worster, 2018).

When it comes to developing specific plans for individual patients, clinicians have a number of areas in which they need to be better informed. Dosage guidelines are very much a work in progress even in conditions where cannabis is commonly recommended, but clinicians need to be more aware of what is known about dosing, as well as the best practices for developing a dosage plan for patients who are new to medical cannabis. Healthcare professionals have also expressed a need for more information on precautions that patients can take as they begin to use cannabis (Ziemianski et al., 2015). Being able to inform patients of the risks, how to limit those risks, and how to find an appropriate dose that works to treat symptoms while avoiding adverse events is crucial for clinicians.

Luckily, there is some understanding of how these knowledge gaps can be fixed. One study considered the results of an educational intervention delivered to healthcare professionals in a hospice setting (Mendoza & McPherson, 2018). In this case, the most surprising result was that providers felt that they had sufficient knowledge prior to the intervention, despite having no previous training in cannabis as medicine. However, providers' knowledge and confidence in their own ability to discuss and recommend cannabis improved significantly following the educational intervention. While providers in most fields are generally in favor of patients having access to medical cannabis, it is necessary to ensure that healthcare professionals have the knowledge to discuss and recommend it where appropriate (Uritsky et al., 2011). Patients who have legal and geographical access to medicinal cannabis can still face barriers to access if there are not a sufficient number of healthcare professionals who are able to help them access it (and understand whether they should be using it, what products they should be seeking out, and what risks the use of cannabis may carry for them).

EDUCATIONAL OPPORTUNITIES TO ADDRESS CLINICIAN NEEDS

Clinicians are generally interested in bolstering their knowledge of medicinal cannabis, but it can be difficult to translate that interest into results. Healthcare professionals are not known for having a surplus of time available for training in a new topic. However, there are a number of existing opportunities to improve their understanding.

The most obvious is through accredited, unbiased continuing education courses. Healthcare professionals are typically expected to complete some amount of annual continuing education, so such courses are a way to provide education without an additional time commitment from participants. These courses also are a good fit for what clinicians say they want: short, easily accessible educational modules that can be completed online.

Of course, it is impossible to cover all of the information on cannabis as medicine in just a short course. In addition, it may be impossible to create a course that applies to clinicians in multiple states, as the varying legal status of cannabis requires individualized information. Nonetheless, such a course is an effective first step, as it represents an easy way for healthcare professionals to fit cannabis education into their existing schedules and at least give themselves a baseline understanding of the most important topics in cannabis.

A more thorough effort to improve the knowledge of healthcare professionals would be to add medicinal cannabis education to medical, nursing, and pharmacy education curricula. Most of the current cannabis information that medical students receive about marijuana relates to it as a drug of abuse. The advantage of adding cannabis as medicine to the curriculum would be that every healthcare professional would be better informed about the topic, meaning that patients are not leaving it to chance whether the healthcare professional they are working with happens to be one that has taken an appropriate continuing education course. If the only clinicians with medical cannabis information are those who actively seek it out, there is a possibility that disparities could be created and some populations would lack access to well-informed clinicians.

Cannabis as medicine is not relevant to some medical specialties. However, ensuring that healthcare professionals have at least some understanding of the topic is still worthwhile, as it seems inevitable that the use of medical cannabis will continue to expand in the United States. Perhaps the most significant difficulty in including cannabis topics in medical education is that the research is evolving so quickly at present. Students who want to maintain a current understanding of cannabis as medicine will have to find ongoing educational opportunities, and cannot assume that the information obtained will continue to be accurate for any significant period of time. This effort would need to be supplemented with continuing education opportunities such as those discussed above.

Education for clinicians can also be offered at professional events or conferences. While it will not be possible to include a full education module in a short presentation, offering brief introductions to the topic and highlighting and distributing vetted literature can still provide clinicians who might otherwise have no knowledge with an understanding of the topic. It may also allow those who might be interested in a more formal certification or continuing education course with information on how to access those resources. Many clinicians lack even basic information about medicinal cannabis research, cannabis laws in their state, or where to refer patients who have questions that they cannot answer. Introducing these topics at a conference or similar event is a way to reach a broad group of healthcare professionals and give them at least a surface understanding of cannabis as medicine.

Finally, it is important that healthcare professionals who are particularly interested in the field of cannabis as medicine can access in-depth educational offerings such as certificate courses or graduate-level degree programs. While time and cost will mean that there are a limited number of clinicians who have interest in such programs, those who choose to make cannabis research or cannabis as medicine a focus of their practice will require long-term formal education.

RESEARCHERS

CURRENT STATE OF RESEARCHER KNOWLEDGE

The education currently available to clinicians is limited by the lack of definitive knowledge in the clinical research space. There are very few individuals or institutions in the United States with a cannabis research background dating back more than a few years, which means that cannabis research programs are in their infancy. Thanks to diverse laws in different states and patchwork regulation from federal agencies, cannabis researchers require a detailed legal understanding of their topic. In some cases, research methods used in pharmaceutical trials and observational research can be adapted for cannabis research. However, given the complex legal situation that cannabis falls into and the general lack of conclusive clinical trial data, researchers will require specific training in how to manage questions that come up when examining cannabis as medicine.

While U.S. research efforts are all fairly new, there are some countries where governments have historically been more supportive of cannabis research, and the more advanced state of research in these places gives us the opportunity to learn from them.

Israel in particular has supported cannabis research for a number of decades. The Israeli researcher Dr. Raphael Mechoulam is well known for his work on a variety of medical uses of cannabis, a project he has been involved with since the 1960s (Jorisch, 2018). He has published hundreds of papers on the subject and has detailed the uses of cannabis in conditions including brain trauma, diabetes, arthritis, and stress (Mechoulam, 2015). The advanced state of research in Israel can serve as a stepping stone for American researchers, who would be well served to seek collaborations with Israeli counterparts. While there are differences (in legal systems, products available, and level of vertical integration throughout the healthcare system), the groundwork laid by researchers such as Dr. Mechoulam can help American researchers make up for decades of lost time in their own country.

Even with these outside sources of information, there is a need for more research-ers who are trained in cannabis research to answer questions not already covered in countries such as Israel. These researchers will need an awareness of how to navigate the relationships between healthcare professionals and the cannabis industry and a nuanced legal background to ensure that their studies do not put themselves or their participants in any legal jeopardy.

OPPORTUNITIES TO ADDRESS RESEARCHER NEEDS

While certificate or graduate courses focusing on cannabis as medicine only apply to a small portion of clinicians, they are likely much more broadly applicable to researchers. This education can foster connections between researchers in train-ing and those who have already spent time working in the cannabis field. With the speed at which research is evolving, collaboration and mentoring allows researchers to avoid duplicating their efforts and accelerate their research. This is especially important as validated scales and other instruments are developed, as using com-mon measurements across research allows for results to be compared effectively. Encouraging collaboration with foreign institutions allows us to take advantage of the broader research base available in countries such as Israel. At present, there are a number of academic institutions, researchers, and clinicians who are involved with collaborations that help to foster effective research.

An additional consideration in addressing the needs of researchers in the cannabis as medicine field is the need to look for ways to improve institutional knowledge of the topic. Many Institutional Review Boards may have difficulty involving individuals with an appropriate level of expertise on cannabis when fielding research proposals that involve the use of cannabis. As they attempt to evaluate ethical and logistical concerns associated with cannabis research, these boards will need access to resources that better educate them on this evaluation process.

Institutional knowledge can also be a resource that improves our ability to dis-seminate new information to members of those institutions. If there is a way to pro-vide in-depth training to centralized departments at academic institutions, they can then in turn train individuals throughout their institutions.

CANNABIS INDUSTRY (GROWERS & DISPENSARIES)

CURRENT STATE OF INDUSTRY KNOWLEDGE

It is difficult to describe accurately the expertise of cannabis industry members because the requirements to grow, sell, and market cannabis vary widely from state to state. Retailers or dispensaries are sometimes required to employ a pharmacist or other healthcare professional, but growers are less likely to have a medical back-ground. Growers generally have a background in biology, horticulture, or a similar field, however.

Many states still use the "budtender" model, where dispensary staff may have a mix of formal training and personal experience, but are not typically required to have a clinical background. While these individuals may have a fairly in-depth understanding of cannabis products, they do not have the training to work with medical patients to develop an ideal treatment plan. This places a heavy burden on on-site pharmacists and recommending doctors, as these individuals have to ensure that medical patients are receiving accurate information and are able to use that information to purchase products that will be effective at treating their symptoms while avoiding adverse events.

This also creates a greater need for patient and pharmacist education; on-site pharmacists may have received just a few hours of training and are then expected to be the sole source of medical advice available to patients at the dispensary. Patients who expect the dispensary staff to be able to respond to medical questions may be disappointed in states where more extensive training is not required, and recommending doctors cannot necessarily assume that their patients will receive extensive guidance at the point of sale.

EDUCATIONAL OPPORTUNITIES TO ADDRESS INDUSTRY NEEDS

The most straightforward way to ensure that patients are receiving accurate medical information is to focus on state-by-state regulations to ensure that qualified healthcare professionals are always on-site and available for patients. The key word here is "qualified"—in many cases, existing certification programs are short and unlikely to prepare healthcare professionals for the variety of scenarios and questions they may encounter. Current certifications may involve just a few hours of training in cannabis as medicine, which is enough to give an overview but insufficient to ensure that patients have access to well-informed healthcare professionals at the dispensary.

A likely obstacle is that many states already have their regulations in place, and it may be difficult to change these policies (not to mention convince numerous industry employees that they need to undergo additional training to continue working at their current retail locations). It may be possible to find ways around the need for better training on-site: for example, creating a more formal system by which physicians can provide specific product recommendations or making it possible for patients to contact cannabis-educated doctors by phone when on-site industry and healthcare professionals are unable to field their questions, would alleviate the concerns raised by a lack of training among dispensary staff.

An alternative to ensuring that pharmacists on-site have extensive cannabis training is to offer training/certifications aimed at growers, budtenders, and other non-medical staff members, so that every employee has enough medical information and other necessary skills to respond to basic questions. Skills such as customer service may not be directly medical in nature, but they will be relevant to growers and budtenders who are interested in ensuring that they are offering an optimal experience to patients. There are certainly risks to asking non-healthcare professionals to field medical questions from patients, but that scenario is already occurring in many states where budtenders are the first point of contact for medical patients visiting a dispensary. Adding training to the mix could only improve the results. Of course, while this helps ensure that everyone involved has some level of knowledge, it would require an additional level of regulation, a voluntary effort by dispensaries and growers, or some outside financial backing to cover the costs of the additional training.

The good news is that for the most part, the education needed for industry members exists. Continuing education courses for clinicians and pharmacists can also apply to or be adapted for budtenders and other industry professionals, and more involved courses are available for those who are interested. The problem is that there is at present no real incentive for industry staff or industry professionals to take these courses. An alternative approach might be to create educational opportunities at professional events, conferences, and so on such that growers and budtenders can access this information without much additional effort on their part. Unless state-by-state regulation is altered (or federal law changes drastically), there is unlikely to be any requirement for most industry professionals to be familiar with the medical properties of their products. This makes it even more important that patients be as knowledgeable as possible so that they have a chance to accurately evaluate claims made by dispensary staff.

PATIENTS

CURRENT STATE OF PATIENT KNOWLEDGE

Patients have access to a wealth of information on the subject of cannabis. Many states provide information on their medicinal cannabis websites, and patients in states where medical cannabis is legal can typically reach out to medical professionals and dispensary staff to discuss their specific cases. However, the availability of quality information is tempered by the quantity of unreliable information that patients may come across. Sources both in favor of and opposed to cannabis are easily accessible online, and for virtually any condition it is possible to find someone who touts cannabis as a miracle cure. Sources that lobby in favor of cannabis legalization may present misleading information to patients. An additional risk with the current model of cannabis legislation is that physicians who choose to become recommenders are generally those most in favor of cannabis as medicine, and dispensary staff have incentives to inflate the value of their product. As such, patients need access to reliable sources of data that are without a vested interest by the cannabis industry, and they need the tools to evaluate claims they may hear from others or see online.

Organizations such as Health on the Net (HON) and DISCERN attempt to provide a way to be sure that health information is medically accurate and of high quality (Health on the Net, 2018; DISCERN, 2018). These organizations can help patients and clinicians as they attempt to determine whether information they find is accurate, although they tend to be more academically focused—patients who search online for information on cannabis as medicine are unlikely to come across the HON or DISCERN sites. Nonetheless, they provide a framework that organizations can use if they wish to publish accurate medical information on cannabis, and clinicians can certainly reference them in conversations with patients. Additionally, websites can be HON or DISCERN certified; if patients are aware of this, they can look for those certifications as a sign that certain information meets at least a baseline level of trustworthiness. That said, these certifications are not always readily apparent and are not in widespread use among those who offer information as cannabis as medicine.

A secondary question is how useful this type of tool really is—while studies have found both HON and DISCERN to be helpful in evaluating health information, some analyses have found that HON does not necessarily predict good quality health information (Khazaal et al., 2012). Even if there is some doubt as to their validity, quality metrics can help sift through a large quantity of information and discard sources that are especially incorrect. Whether healthcare providers choose to use HON, DISCERN, or some other metric for accurate information, having organizations that attempt to certify useful and accurate sources is necessary so that patients know what resources to trust.

The best way to respond to the quantity of inaccurate information is for reliable sources of information to publish accurate cannabis information for patients; at the moment, many healthcare organizations seem to be hesitant to offer cannabis information, likely in part because the research on the topic remains limited. As cannabis as medicine becomes more of an accepted aspect of the healthcare system, it is to be hoped that healthcare organizations will be able to publicize good information for their patients that will help patients not need to rely on subpar sources.

Educational Opportunities to Address Patient Needs

Addressing patient needs requires a different model than that used to educate clinicians or industry professionals. While it is possible to make general recommendations, it is important to remember that different patient populations will require different information. A universally helpful option would be to ensure that patients have access to reliable sources of cannabis information presented in a way that is appropriate to patients with various levels of health literacy. Patients need to be able to evaluate claims they see online or hear from those that work in the cannabis industry, and accurate, understandable resources are the best way to provide them with tools to do so. Even in areas where our current knowledge is limited, it is important for patients to know that the research is not conclusive.

Another way to address patient needs is to promote standardized labeling of cannabis products that follows best practices in providing strain information, composition of cannabis products, directions as to the route of administration, and to whatever extent possible, a description of the beneficial effects and risks associated with a particular product. Concise information that can be understood by patients with any level of health literacy is necessary to ensure that patients take correct doses, that others who come across cannabis medicine products know what they are, and that adverse effects are avoided to whatever extent possible. The Figure 20.1a,b here provide examples of labels that legislators could use to develop regulation or that growers and dispensaries could use as examples for what to put on their products.

(a)   (b)

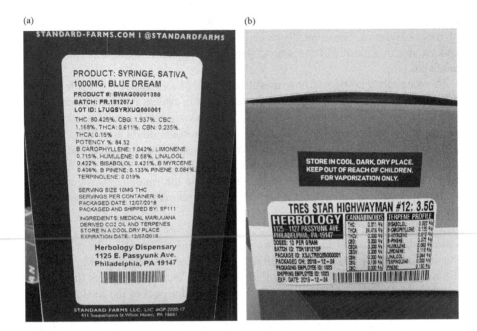

FIGURE 20.1 (a, b) Examples of labels that provide detailed information to patients at the dispensary. Photo courtesy of Herbology Dispensary. Source: Locklund, Sarah. (Photographer). (February 27, 2019). *Sample dispensary product labels.*

Patients knowing where they can go for information, when they should contact their health providers, and how to accurately understand products is paramount; no single educational experience is going to fully equip patients, so they need to know where good sources of information can be found. Ongoing communication with a clinician who is well trained in cannabis as medicine is crucial, and access to print and online documents that can inform patients is important as well. Sites such as Jefferson's Lambert Center offer information on a variety of topics related to cannabis as medicine (Lambert Center, 2019). These documents provide information that helps patients understand products available to them and have constructive conversations with their clinicians and with dispensary staff.

CONCLUSION

One of the essential facts for anyone working in the field of medicinal cannabis to understand is how incomplete our current knowledge is. For researchers, it can be as significant to debunk incorrect claims of the effectiveness of cannabis as a treatment for a given condition as it is to identify cases where cannabis should be used. Healthcare professionals working with incomplete research data need to be able to identify patients who may benefit from medical cannabis while being clear about the limitations and possible adverse affects associated with cannabis treatments. Patients, who have access to information from a variety of sources with differing amounts of reliability, need tools to evaluate claims that they see. They also need to be educated on how to talk to medical professionals about cannabis if they are interested, as well as how to understand the contents of the cannabis products they see at the dispensary.

While there exist opportunities to transmit all of this information, it is important to keep in mind that the speed with which cannabis science is advancing means that education for each of these audiences must be an ongoing process. Collaboration among researchers will help ensure that everyone stays up-to-date on current best practices and available information. Clinicians will need frequent refresher courses and knowledge of who to contact when they come across cases that are not covered by their past education. Growers and dispensary staff need to be trained in how to accurately portray their products and how to create products with the best chance of positive outcomes for patients, which is a process that will require back-and-forth communication between industry, clinicians, and patients. Patients need to know that the information they get today may quickly become outdated, meaning that ongoing communication with healthcare providers is essential to ensuring that they reach the best outcome possible.

REFERENCES

Brooks, E., Gundersen, D., Flynn, E., Brooks-Russell, A., & Bull, S. (2017, Sep). The clinical implications of legalizing marijuana: Are physician and non-physician providers prepared? *Addict Behav, 72*, 1–7.

Carlini, B., Garrett, S., & Carter, G. (2017, Feb). Medicinal cannabis: A survey among health care providers in Washington state. *Am J Hosp Palliat Care, 34*(1), 85–91.

Chan, M., Knoepke, C., Cole, M., McKinnon, J., & Matlock, D. (2017, Apr). Colorado medical students' attitudes and beliefs about marijuana. *J Gen Intern Med, 32*(4), 458–463.

DISCERN. (2018). *DISCERN online*. Retrieved from DISCERN: www.discern.org.uk/index. php, accessed January 2, 2019.

Health on the Net. (2018). *Health on the Net*. Retrieved from Health on the Net: www.hon.ch/en/, accessed January 2, 2019.

Hwang, J., Arneson, T., & Peter, W. S. (2016, Nov). Minnesota pharmacists and medical cannabis: A survey of knowledge, concerns, and interest prior to program launch. *P & T, 41*(11), 716–722.

Jorisch, A. (2018, June 19). A Higher Calling: How Israeli Marijuana Research Changed the World. *Jerusalem Post*.

Khazaal, Y., Chatton, A., Zullino, D., & Khan, R. (2012, Mar). HON label and DISCERN as content quality indicators of health-related websites. *Psychiatr Q, 83*(1), 15–27.

Lambert Center. (2019, February 25). *Resources for Patients*. Retrieved from Lambert Center for the Study of Medicinal Cannabis & Hemp: www.jefferson.edu/university/emerging-health-professions/lambert-center/Resources/Patients.html, accessed February 27, 2019.

Locklund, S. (Photographer), Herbology. (2019, February 27). Sample dispensary product labels.

Mechoulam, R. (2015, Sep). Cannabis – the Israeli perspective. *J Basic Clin Physiol Pharmacol, 27*(3), 181–187.

Mendoza, K., & McPherson, M. (2018, May). Knowledge, skills, and attitudes regarding the use of medical cannabis in the hospice population: An educational intervention. *AM J Hosp Palliative Care, 35*(5), 759–766.

Ross, W. (2018). Autism spectrum disorder: A survey of clinician attitudes and knowledge. Unpublished manuscript.

Uritsky, T., McPherson, M., & Pradel, F. (2011, Dec). Assessment of hospice health professionals' knowledge, views, and experience with medical marijuana. *J Palliat Med, 14*(12), 1291–1295.

Worster, B. (2018). Clinician attitudes towards medical marijuana in Pennsylvania. Unpublished manuscript.

Ziemianski, D., Capler, R., Tekanoff, R., Lacasse, A., Luconi, F., & Ware, M. (2015, Mar 19). Cannabis in medicine: A national educational needs assessment among Canadian physicians. *BMC Med Educ, 15*, 52.

21 Analysis Update—Full Spectrum Cannabis

Robert Clifford, Scott Kuzdzal,
Paul Winkler, and Will Bankert
Shimadzu Scientific Instruments

CONTENTS

INTRODUCTION

Most cannabis testing has been conducted for quality control (QC) purposes in order to verify the cannabinoids, especially the psychoactive delta-9-tetrahydrocannabinol (delta-9-THC) and the non-psychoactive cannabidiol (CBD), are present in high concentrations.[1] QC testing also involves confirming the products are free from contaminants such as pesticides, heavy metals, residual solvents, mycotoxins/aflatoxins, and microorganisms. However, the cannabis plant is much more complex, containing over 500 naturally occurring compounds, such as amino acids, proteins, glycoproteins, enzymes, sugars, hydrocarbons, nutrients, fatty acids, phenols, flavonoids, and terpenes in addition to the cannabinoids. It has been reported[2] that there are more than 100 cannabinoids and over 200 terpenes, volatile unsaturated hydrocarbons found in essential oils, in cannabis.

Dr. Raphael Mechoulam coined the term *entourage effect*[3] while Dr. Ethan Russo popularized it for the synergy between the cannabinoids and terpenoids. Terpenes and terpenoids are terms used interchangeably[4,5]; however, terpenoids are actually terpenes that have been oxidized and contain additional functional groups such as alcohols, esters, and carboxylic acids when a product has been cured and dried. So, one can think of terpenes as being in the hydrated form and terpenoids in the dehydrated form, though there is more going on as the structures differ beyond the loss of water molecules.

Terpenes are extracted from flowers, leaves, stems, bark, roots, and other parts of a plant[6] and have been used to make essential oils. Essential oils may contain a combination of terpenes to generate a fragrance and provide aromatherapy. Smells are processed by the olfactory bulb, which has many sensory nerve fibers and links to the brain's amygdala, which is involved in experiencing emotions, and the brain's hippocampus, also involving emotion as well as memory and the autonomic nervous system. The use of essential oils as a cleansing ritual by the Chinese and Egyptians[7] dates to 3500 BC. The Bible has more than 200 references to essential oils, including the terpenes frankincense and myrrh, which were burned in the temples and represented worship and death and mourning, respectively. Today, essential oil companies such as doTerra[8] have a Medical Advisory Panel stacked with medical personnel, including physicians, orthopedic surgeons, anesthesiologists, ear, nose and throat (ENT) surgeons, holistic integrative medicine physicians, pediatricians, obstetricians, and gynecologists.

While QC laboratories continue to grow in the field of cannabis testing, research and development (R&D) is gaining more popularity at universities and pharmaceutical companies. For example, Northern Michigan University now offers a 4-year degree in Medicinal Plant Chemistry[9] with an entrepreneurial track or a bioanalytical track focusing on biology and chemistry. The University of California, San Diego, recently opened the Center for Medicinal Cannabis Research (CMCR).[10] The UCLA Cannabis Research Initiative (UCLA-CRI)[11] claims to be one of the first academic programs in the world dedicated to the study of cannabis. One of the leading researchers studying the cannabinoid-terpenoid entourage effect within the medical community is Dr. Dedi Meiri[12] of Israel's Technion Institute of Technology in the Laboratory of Cancer Biology and Cannabinoid Research. Dr. Meiri is studying the effect of various species of cannabis on cancer, epilepsy, and glucose metabolism (diabetes). He currently has eight clinical trials underway and operates the *Cannabis Database Project*, which is a medical cannabis patient database.

GW Pharmaceutical[13] is known for Sativex (Nabiximols) treatment for multiple sclerosis (MS) patients, used to alleviate neuropathic pain, spasticity, and overactive bladder. Nabiximols are made with two unknown cannabis cultivars. Different cultivars contain different cannabinoids and terpenes in different concentrations. GW Pharmaceutical also received FDA approval in June 2018 for Epidiolex, a proprietary oral solution of pure plant-derived CBD used to treat seizures associated with Lennox-Gastaut syndrome (LGS) or Dravet syndrome. Stock prices soared the day the product was made available to Americans in November 2018.

Cure Pharmaceutical[14] is taking the opportunity to work in the cannabinoid-terpenoid space that the traditional pharmaceutical industry has avoided. Cure's goal is to remove the pain points of invasiveness by eliminating injections, increasing the drug's bioavailability, increasing palatability for the very young and old, facilitating patient-specific dosing, and delivering faster symptom relief.

Many people are familiar with basic wine and food pairing tips such as red wines are best served with red meats and white wine are paired best with fish or chicken, but it is better to match the wine with the sauce and not the meat. More recently, with the explosion of the craft beer industry, the topic of pairing beer with food has received significant attention. Examples of basic beer pairing include a light beer such as a pilsner for seafood and a heavy beer such as a stout (i.e. Guinness beer) served with beef stew, a common dish in Ireland. The cannabis industry is seeing a similar trend. At related expositions, chefs often present lessons on food/cannabis preparation. Examples[15] include eating mangoes, containing high levels of the terpene myrcene, also found in hops used in beer production, allowing cannabinoids to more easily pass through the brain blood barrier. Broccoli contains the terpene beta-caryophyllene, also found in basil, rosemary, and cinnamon, and has been reported to reduce inflammation, depression, and pain.

TERPENES HEALTH BENEFITS

There are more than 200 terpenes found in the cannabis plant and more than 30,000 found in nature according to some estimates. Terpenes are found on the trichomes, which are the glands where the cannabinoids are found. Terpenes[16,17] are derived from the 5-carbon alkene isoprene with a formula of C_5H_8 or the International Union of Pure and Applied Chemistry's (IUPAC) name of 2-methyl-1,3-butadiene. Terpenes contain multiples of the 5-carbon alkenes, such as monoterpene (10), sesquiterpene (15), and diterpene (20), etc. Thus, the formulas would be $C_{10}H_{16}$, $C_{15}H_{24}$, and $C_{20}H_{32}$, respectively. Plants make terpenes to attract insects by color and aroma for pollination purposes or to repel predators.

Ken Kovash, a cultivator with GI Grow[18], has provided a couple examples of breeding cannabis to produce high levels of THC and high levels of specific terpenes. Shown in Figure 21.1 is the crossbreeding of a male Mendo Express with a female Sour Dog Biofuel BX2. The total THC level was 22%. The total terpene profiles in the flowers are generally in the 1%–2% range. Of the total terpene profile, just under half, or 40%, was pinene and the second most abundant terpene, caryophyllene, was 25%. Shown in Figure 21.2 is the crossbreeding of the same male Mendo Express with a different female called a Bubble Viscious. The THC level was similar to the previous flower at 24%, but the terpene profiles changed significantly with the two most abundant terpenes being myrcene (37%) and limonene (34%).

There are many human benefits to terpenes, including the cannabinoid-terpenoid entourage effect. For example, with its distinct pine odor, pinene[19] functions as a bronchodilator, opening the lungs to improve cannabinoid absorption. Linalool, also found in lavender, has a floral smell. It can act as a sedative and has been reported to have anti-cancer properties. Limonene, also found in citrus fruits, has a citrusy smell and has been reported to have anti-bacterial, anti-cancer, anti-depression, and anti-fungal properties. Table 21.1 lists some examples of common terpenes found in the cannabis plant and that have synergistic effects with the cannabinoids. There is an unlimited number of terpenes and cannabinoids at various ratios and concentrations, so the table only shows the terpene and not the synergistic cannabinoid compounds for each health benefit as this would consume too much space in this chapter. The intention here is to expose the reader and list reference sources for further research.

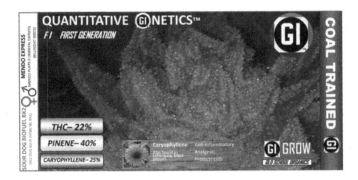

FIGURE 21.1   Crossbreeding a male Mendo Express with a female Sour Dog Biofuel BX2.

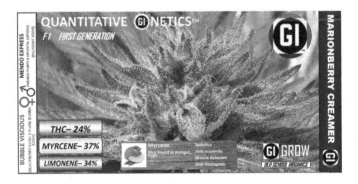

FIGURE 21.2   Crossbreeding a male Mendo Express with a female Bubble Viscious.

TABLE 21.1

Examples of Terpenes, Sources Other Than Cannabis, and Potential Medical Benefits

Terpene	Other Sources	Health Benefits[a]
Alpha-pienene[1,10,52]	Pine needles	Bronchodilator, inflammation, and memory retention
Linalool[1,10,52]	Lavender	Anti-cancer, anti-anxiety, insomnia
Limonene[1,10,52]	Citrus fruits	Anti-bacterial, anti-cancer, anti-depression, anti-fungal
Beta-myrcene[1,10,42]	Hops	Pass cannabinoids through brain blood barrier, anti-septic
Beta-caryophyllene[1,42]	Basil, rosemary, and cinnamon	Inflammation, depression, and pain
Humulene[1,42]	Hops, coriander	Anti-inflammatory, anti-bacterial

[a] The health benefits listed in this chapter are compiled from scientific literature and reported news and may contain anecdotal information. These statements have not been evaluated by the FDA and should not be used to diagnose, treat, cure, or prevent any disease. This chapter is an indication that much research is still needed for this potential powerful plant.

FLAVONOIDS HEALTH BENEFITS

When discussing cannabis cultivars, often referred to as strains, the discussion often involves the cannabinoids and the terpenes. Rarely does the topic include the flavonoids,[20] which provide flavor, color, odor, and pharmacological activity, and assist in pollinating, UV filtering, and preventing pests and fungi, just as the terpenes. Flavonoids are not psychoactive and can be characterized as sweet, sour, bitter, and spicy.[21] Subcategories of sweet include flowery and fruity, with the latter being further subdivided into berries, tropical, and rosaceae, with examples being blueberry, mango, and peach, respectively. Flavonoids are not exclusive to cannabis; they exist in flowers as well as fruits and vegetables. An alternative medicine peer-reviewed journal[22] discusses the potential of flavonoids and terpenoids as containing anti-inflammatory, antitumor, and anti-parasitic properties from Asteraceae, commonly referred as the sunflower family. The flavonoid quercetin is being used in clinical trials for cancer research.[23] Quercetin is also found in red wine, onions, green tea, apples, and berries. Could cannabis with cannabinoids, terpenes, and the flavonoid quercetin have an entourage effect greater than other non-cannabis plants? Of course, more research is needed in this area.

Flavonoids, a secondary metabolite, are also referred to as Bioflavonoids, from the Latin flavus, meaning yellow; but the colors also include reds, blues, and purples with colors dependent on pH and temperature. The other two classes of compounds include isoflavonoids and neoflavonoids, which all have a 15-carbon skeleton, including two phenyl rings and a heterocyclic ring. There are over 6,000 flavonoids found in nature. These are categorized by the subgroups anthoxanthins, flavanones, flavanonols, flavans, and anthocyanidins. Cannaflavins[24] fall under the subgroup flavins and are unique to the cannabis plant. Cannaflavin-A inhibits Prostaglandin E2 (PGE2), responsible for inflammation. Cannaflavin-B and Cannaflavin-C are under research for their potential medical benefits. There are about 20 flavonoids found in cannabis. Other flavonoids found in cannabis[25] include catechins, an antioxidant also found in cocoa, tea, and pome fruits; orientin, an antioxidant and free-radical scavenger powerful enough to reduce radiation damage; silymarin, which helps reduce damage from free radicals and battle cancer; kaempferol, which reduces the risk of various cancers; and apigenin,[26] offering anti-anxiety and anti-inflammatory properties and found in parsley, celery, and chamomile tea. It has been reported that many of these flavonoids are synergistic with cannabinoids such as THC and CBD. In studies, the full plant extract, including cannabinoids, terpenes, and flavonoids, almost always has more medicinal benefits than an extracted isolated compound. Others[27] have stated that isolates are at one end of the spectrum while the full plant is at the other end; in between are tailored cannabinoid formulations, which are far more effective and consistent. Also, CBD is the same molecule whether it comes from hemp or marijuana. The medical benefits are typically determined by the other components, such as flavonoids, amino acids, fatty acids, nutrients, etc., present with the CBD (or THC) as well as the concentration of each cannabinoid and other components.

AMINO ACIDS HEALTH BENEFITS

There are 500 naturally occurring amino acids in nature, but only 20 appear in the genetic code. Of those 20 amino acids, 9 are considered essential amino acids, meaning they cannot be produced by the body and must come from the diet. The nine essential amino acids are histidine, isoleucine, leucine, lysine, methionine, phenylalanine, threonine, tryptophan, and valine. Amino acids contain functional groups consisting of an amine (–NH2) and a carboxyl (–COOH) group as well as a side chain (R group). Peptides form when the amine group of one amino acid combines with the carboxyl group of another amino acid. Amino acids are called peptides when a molecule contains a chain of 2–50 amino acids linked together. To be more specific, chains of 20–50 amino acids are referred to as polypeptides; beyond 50 amino acids, the peptides chains are referred to as proteins. Amino acids have been called the building blocks of life. Lacking enough of an essential amino acid will handicap the synthesis of proteins. In the opposite direction, when one consumes proteins, they are broken down in the body to form beneficial amino acids.

Heart disease is the leading cause of death worldwide but it may be reduced with hemp seeds[28]. Hemp is part of the cannabis sativa family. The hemp seed contains high levels of the non-essential amino acid arginine, which produces the gas molecule nitric oxide, which, in turn, dilates the blood vessels, lowering blood pressure, and reducing heart disease. Some non-essential amino acids, like arginine, are considered conditionally essential amino acids because the body can't produce enough of the amino acid under certain conditions like stress to fight off diseases or cancer.[29]

Juiced or raw cannabis[30] is considered a superfood. In fact, the author considers raw cannabis the new kale. Raw cannabis doesn't contain the psychoactive form of delta-9-THC (called the neutral form) because the plants produce the non-psychoactive form, tetrahydrocannabinolic acid (THCA), referred to as the acid form. Only after heating or other oxidative processes does THCA become THC, a process called decarboxylation. Therefore, eating raw cannabis is for people wanting the health benefits, not the "high." Studies show the consumption or raw cannabis has better medical benefits for fibromyalgia, bowel cancer, and neurodegenerative diseases than any other food. Raw cannabis contains essential amino acids, which can repair damaged cells, transport nutrients, and maintain cell structure. Raw cannabis contains antioxidants and the neuroprotective powers of CBD. Like green leafy food, cannabis contains vitamins such as folate, iron, calcium, vitamin C, and vitamin K, similar to terpenes. It is recommended to add a few raw cannabis leaves to your next salad.

As a side note, amino acids are not only valuable to humans, they also assist with plant growth.[31] The amino acids glutamic acid and glycine amplify photosynthesis and plant tissue growth, arginine enhances flower growth, tryptophan signals hormones for growth regulation, and proline maintains water balance, which makes the plant more resistant to extreme temperature.

FATTY ACIDS HEALTH BENEFIT

In addition to essential amino acids, there are essential fatty acids (EFA),[32] which also must come from diet. These EFAs are known as alpha-linolenic acid (omega-3) and linoleic acid (omega-6). Reports suggest the ratio of these two essential fatty acids may affect the immune system and their optimal range is 1:3 for omega-3 to omega-6. Hemp seeds contain over 30% of these EFAs.[28] Raw cannabis provides the perfect ratio of these EFAs. EFAs help treat skin diease,[28] improve protein synthesis, protect against neurodegenerative diseases, and maintain the balance of the endocannabinoid system.[30] Dr. Ethan Russo coined the term Clinical Endocannabinoid Deficiency (CEDC), leading to the discovery of various diseases such as immune system disorders, chronic pain, and fatigue.[33]

NUTRIENTS HEALTH BENEFITS

Green leafy vegetables are known for their health benefits and nutrients such as calcium, folate, iron, vitamin C, and vitamin K.[30] Cannabis has these same health benefits. One such benefit[30] is the ability to repair DNA. Another benefit is the ability to move oxygen from the alveoli into the blood in the capillaries using a process called diffusion. Oxygen moves from high concentration to low concentration through this process. Calcium helps to build strong bones, while vitamin K assists with blood clotting. Also, these nutrients build up the immune system.

CHEMICAL ANALYSIS OF CANNABIS

The chemical compounds discussed above, except for elements like calcium and iron, are analyzed by a technique called chromatography. The primary chromatographic techniques used are liquid chromatography (LC) and gas chromatography (GC).

High Performance Liquid Chromatography (HPLC) is a mature and powerful technique for separating and quantifying constituents in liquid samples. In practice, a sample is dissolved in a suitable solvent, filtered, and then injected into a high-pressure solvent stream flowing through a chromatographic column packed with tiny particles (stationary phase) that have an active surface chemistry. The chemical interactions between the sample constituents, the mobile solvent stream, and the chemical surface of the particles causes the sample constituents to separate from one another as they migrate through the column bed, a process known as differential migration. At the outlet of the column, a detector responds to the separated molecules as they emerge to produce a series of peaks whose areas indicate the concentration of each component. The result is known as a chromatogram. The time the peaks are detected is called the retention time (RT). Ideally, each of the peaks will have different retention times.

GC has some similarities for separating compounds like HPLC, except the mobile phase is a gas instead of a liquid. GC can have tiny particles used to separate the compounds, an older technique called packed column GC. Newer technology has chemical coating on the walls of the tube. This is referred to as capillary column GC, which is the preferred method for cannabis analysis.

After the column separates the compounds, they pass through a detector, which does exactly what it states as it detects each compound. GC and LC utilize different types of detectors. For example, a GC can use a flame ionization detector (FID), thermal conductivity detector (TCD), electron capture detector (ECD), flame photometric detector (FPD), and a flame thermionic detector (FTD). If one were using a FID detector the technique would be referred to as GC/FID. A GC/FID system could be utilized for terpene analysis with the addition of a headspace autosampler. The headspace autosampler has two functions. The autosampler is an automated robot bringing the next sample in line to be analyzed. The headspace heats up the cannabis sample between 70°C and 275°C, so the volatile terpenes can be separated from most of the cannabis matrix, which contains over 500 compounds, allowing for easier separation in the column.

HPLC also offers different types of detectors, such as UV, photodiode array (PDA), refractive index (RI), electroconductive (EC), and fluorescence (RF), each of which is used for specific applications. For example, HPLC could utilize a fluorescence detector for detection of amino acids, while a UV detector could be used for flavonoids.

GC and HPLC have one thing in common with respect to detection: both instruments can utilize the very powerful mass spectrometer (MS). There are several types of mass spectrometers, but the most common are single quadrupole and triple quadrupole. Examples of single quadrupole mass spectrometers are GCMS and LCMS, while the triple quadrupole mass spectrometers are GC-MS/MS and LC-MS/MS (Figure 21.3). In situations where a single or triple quadrupole mass spectrometer could be used, the acronyms GCMS(/MS) or LCMS(/MS) may be used. A GC-MS/MS could be used in the single quadrupole GCMS mode for the analysis of terpenes. This is important because an analyst using a GC-MS/MS for contaminant testing of pesticides could also operate in the GCMS mode for terpene analysis. An LCMS(/MS) can be used to analyze amino acids and flavonoids. In the LC-MS/MS mode, the same instrument and detector could also measure contaminants like pesticides and mycotoxins/aflatoxins. Generally speaking, an MS(/MS) can replace all other detectors.

Another advantage of MS(/MS) systems is they provide more information about compounds, which overcomes the issue of peaks not being completely separated or resolved. Using an LC-MS/MS provides not only the retention time, but also a fingerprint of the molecule based on molecular weight transitions of how the compound fragments within a collision cell. GC-MS/MS utilizes commercially available libraries filled with transitions of many compounds that can automatically search for matching compounds. For example, libraries containing flavor and fragrance compounds are available.

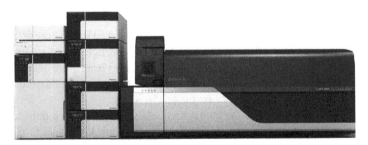

FIGURE 21.3   Shimadzu LCMS-8060 Triple Quadrupole Mass Spectrometer.

For analysis of nutrient elements like calcium and iron, there are several techniques to utilize such as atomic absorption (AA), graphite furnace AA (GFAA), and inductively coupled plasma (ICP) spectroscopy as well as another mass spectrometry technique, inductively coupled plasma mass spectrometry (ICPMS). Each has advantages and disadvantages.

Cannabis samples must be digested in an acid solution, typically done using a microwave oven. Once digested, they are measured by one of these techniques.

AA measures only one element at a time and sensitivity is poorer than other techniques. Sensitivity for most AA elements are in the part-per-million range or milligram/liter (mg/L) for the digested sample. AA has better sensitivity than ICP for Group I and II elements like sodium (Na), potassium (K), calcium (Ca), and magnesium (Mg) and costs less (~$15K–20K). GFAA costs more (~$45–$60K) and still only does one element at time but has sensitivity in the part-per-billion (ppb) or microgram/liter (ug/L) range. Simultaneous ICP can measure multiple elements at the same time with sensitivity in the ppm range, though at a higher cost ($70–$90K). The simultaneous ICPMS, with the highest costs ($120K–150K), is capable of measuring in the ppb range and, in some cases, the part-per-trillion (ppt) range. For the non-chemist, a useful analogy is a ppm is a drop in a kitchen sink, a ppb is a drop in a swimming pool, and a ppt is a drop in a small lake. Another way of putting it is ppt measures 1,000 times lower than ppb, which is a 1,000 times lower then ppm.

CONCLUSION

Cannabis is a very valuable plant with many health benefits when consumed. Cannabis contains beneficial terpenes and flavonoids, some of which are found in fruits, vegetables, and plants while others are unique to cannabis. Cannabis and hemp also contain beneficial amino acids, fatty acids, nutrients, proteins, enzymes, sugars, and phenols that aid the human body. These compounds help prevent disease, cancer, and other medical problems. In the future, universities will be teaching nutritionists the health benefits of cannabis. Taken a step further, these universities will be teaching cannabis to dietitians who will go on to earn a registered dietitian degree. The dietitian recommends food and nutrition plans to promote healthy eating habits for prevention and treatment of illness. They will work in hospitals, clinics, and other healthcare facilities. The food plans will be based on different cannabis cultivars with varying terpene and flavonoid compounds and concentrations depending on the symptoms. It will be a bright day when the federal government in the United States permits the study of cannabis for medical prevention and treatment.

REFERENCES

1. Wedman-St Louis, Betty. *Cannabis – A Clinician's Guide.* Boca Raton: CRC Press/ Taylor & Francis. Chapter 23, pp. 241–246.
2. Jikomes, Nick. Leafy. List of Major Cannabinoids in Cannabis and Their Effects. www. leafly.com/news/cannabis-101/list-major-cannabinoids-cannabis-effects.
3. Russo, Ethan B. 2011. Taming THC: potential cannabis synergy and phytocannabinoid-terpenoid entourage effects. *British Journal Pharmacology.* 2011 Aug; 163(7): 1344–1364. www.ncbi.nlm.nih.gov/pmc/articles/PMC3165946/.

4. Valdez, Enigma. *Terpenes and Testing Magazine*. March 2018. https://terpenesandtesting.com/category/science/terpenes-terpenoids-difference/.

5. Patriot Care. https://patriotcare.org/terpenes-vs-terpenoids/.

6. Ellia. 21 Fun Facts About Essential Oils. February 16, 2017. http://blog.ellia.com/21-fun-facts-about-essential-oils/.

7. Wilson, Savannah. 99 Facts You Never Knew About Essential Oils. https://monq.com/eo/essential-oil/99-facts-essential-oils/.

8. doTerra. Medical Advisory Panel. www.doterra.com/US/en/science-advisory-panel.

9. Paulsen, Mark. Northern Michigan University. Medical Plant Chemistry. www.nmu.edu/chemistry/medicinal-plant-chemistry.

10. UC San Diego. Center for Medicinal Cannabis Research. www.cmcr.ucsd.edu/.

11. UCLA Cannabis Research Initiative (UCLA-CRI). www.uclahealth.org/cannabis/.

12. Meire, Dedi. Technion Institute of Technology. Laboratory of Cancer Biology and Cannabinoid Research. https://dmeiri.net.technion.ac.il/.

13. GW Pharmaceutical. www.gwpharm.com/.

14. Cure Pharmaceutical. www.curepharmaceutical.com/.

15. Horne, Veronica. *Pulse*. Marijuana High Increased with These 6 Foods, February 15, 2017. www.marijuanapackaging.com/blog/marijuana-high-increased-with-these-6-foods/.

16. Kevin. *Softsecrets.com*. Terpenes in Nature. February 17, 2014. www.softsecrets.com/us/news/national/terpenes-in-nature/.

17. Cotton, Simon. The building block for terpenes and rubber, and the molecule that makes the Blue Ridge Mountains of Virginia, blue. July 2008. www.chm.bris.ac.uk/motm/isoprene/isoprenejs.htm.

18. Kovash, Ken. *GI Grow*. Quantitative GineticsTM – Organic Biomedical Seed Bank. http://welloiled.squarespace.com.

19. Kuzdzal, Scott. *The Analytical Scientist*. Unraveling the Cannabinome. September 2015. www.ssi.shimadzu.com/sites/ssi.shimadzu.com/files/Products/literature/Life_science/AnalyticalScientistCannabisTesting.pdf.

20. Bennett, Patrick. *Leafly*. What Are Cannabis Flavonoids and What Do They Do? February 8, 2018. www.leafly.com/news/cannabis-101/what-are-marijuana-flavonoids.

21. Clara. *Harmony*. Beyond Cannabinoids: Facts About The Flavonoids. November 10, 2016. https://meetharmony.com/2016/11/10/beyond-cannabinoids-flavonoids-good-cannabis/.

22. Sulsen, Valeria; Lizarraga, Emilio; Mamadalieva, Nilufar; et al. *Evid Based Complement Alternat Med*. 2017; 2017: 6196198. July 12, 2017. www.ncbi.nlm.nih.gov/pmc/articles/PMC5529648/.

23. ClinicalTrials.gov. A service of the U.S. National Institutes of Health. 2017. https://clinicaltrials.gov/ct2/results?term=quercetin+and+cancer&Search=Search.

24. Wilder, Zoe. *Merry Jane*. Everything You Need to Know About Cannabis Flavonoids. November 7, 2018. https://merryjane.com/health/flavonoids-cannabis.

25. Michelle, C.C., *Compassion Concentrates*. Cannabis Flavonoids 101. July 20, 2018. https://compassionconcentrates.com/cannabis-flavonoids-101/.

26. CBD Professor. *CBD School*. What are Flavonoids in Cannabis? April 14, 2017. www.cbdschool.com/what-are-flavonoids/.

27. Cooper, Jon. *Cannabis Business Times*. Entourage Effect 2.0: The Entourage Effect is Real, but Full-Spectrum Cannabis is Not the Answer. August 9, 2018. www.cannabisbusinesstimes.com/article/ebbu-entourage-effect-cannabis-guest-op-ed/.

28. Bjarnadottir, Adda. *Healthline*. 6 Evidence-Based Health Benefits of Hemp Seeds. September 11, 2018. www.healthline.com/nutrition/6-health-benefits-of-hemp-seeds#section1.

29. Kubala, Jillian. *Healthline*. Essential Amino Acids: Definition, Benefits and Food Sources. June 12, 2018. www.healthline.com/nutrition/essential-amino-acids.

30. Faust, Amber. *Wikileaf.* The Superfood Benefits of Ingesting Raw Cannabis. June 12, 2017. www.wikileaf.com/thestash/benefits-of-raw-cannabis/.
31. Robinson, Randy. *Cannabis Cultivation Today.* Amino Acids: What They Mean to Your Cannabis Grow. July 8, 2016. www.cannabisindustryinstitute.com/news/amino-acids-what-they-mean-to-your-cannabis-grow/.
32. Ward, Elizabeth. *WebMD.* Fat Facts: Good Fats vs. Bad Fats. www.webmd.com/food-recipes/features/good-fats-bad-fats#1.
33. United Patients Group. Top 8 Health Benefits of Consuming Raw Cannabis. February 25, 2017. https://unitedpatientsgroup.com/blog/2017/02/25/top-8-health-benefits-of-consuming-raw-cannabis/.

22 Cannabis for Pets

Betty Wedman-St Louis
Clinical Nutritionist

CONTENTS

As more and more people realize the medicinal benefits of cannabis for their health, a growing number of pet owners want to use it to help their pets. Sarah Silcox DVM, founder and president of the Canadian Association of Veterinary Cannabinoid Medicine, answered questions about medical cannabis for animals at the Toronto Cannabis Conference and Expo in June 2018, but was not available to share her expertise in this book.

The lack of education in veterinary schools and regulatory issues about licensure made it impossible to find a veterinarian to provide recommendations for pet parents despite the growing interest and acceptance for the use of CBD/cannabidiol oils.

Dr. Karen Becker, author of Healthy Pets presented by Mercola.com, featured a "Why Pet Owners Seek Cannabis for Their Pets" in November 2018 [1]. She indicates pet owners across the United States are turning to cannabis to treat their pets when conventional options like pain medication fails to provide comfort for their pet. Cannabis extracts, ointments, and edibles have been reported to provide improvements in pets debilitated by arthritis, seizures, anxiety, and other ailments. According to Dr. Becker, pet owners seek out cannabis products on their own because veterinarians "must walk a fine line when speaking about cannabis for pets."

Like humans, animals have an endocannabinoid system that can use phytocannabinoids for arthritis, cancer, seizures, anxiety, and irritable bowel issues. Using CBD/cannabidiol as a tincture in a small dose can help reduce pain. Increasing the dose gradually based on the weight of the animal is what several companies advise on their websites along with being sure to use full spectrum CBD hemp oils.

Cannabis dosages for animals are not well defined, and it is not uncommon for animals to overdose on high concentrations of CBD and THC found in medical and recreational cannabis products used by humans. Using only a CBD hemp full spectrum product reduces the risk of overdosing. Here is how a CBD product could benefit a pet:

- **GI Tract**—supports digestion and reduces inflammation
- **Immunity**—supports immune system needed for respiratory, digestive, and joint health

- **Neurology**—maintains healthy brain, mood, and nervous system
- **Mobility and joints**—reduces discomfort
- **Mood**—encourages calmness and reduces anxiety
- **Comfort**—assists in "end of life" comfort care

Cannabis CBD is basically used to treat the following conditions according to Susan G. Wynn, DVM, CVCH, AHG of Blue Pearl Georgia Veterinary Specialists' Nutrition and Integrative Medicine Department [2]:

- **Cancer**—to promote cancer cell death
- **Nausea and Vomiting**
- **Pain**—acute and chronic
- **Inflammatory Bowel Disease**—anti-inflammatory and antispasmodic effects of CBD help reduce intestinal permeability
- **Epilepsy or Seizure Disorders**
- **Diabetes mellitus**
- **Glaucoma**

Occasionally, pets may ingest cannabis edibles that contain THC, the psychoactive cannabinoid in cannabis, but human urine drug tests are not an effective way to screen a pet for cannabis toxicity. Intoxication in pets is similar to that in humans and starts 30–60 minutes after ingestion. Unfortunately, it may last longer in a cat or dog than a human—up to 18–36 hours after ingestion. The usual signs of intoxication are depression, dilated pupils, vomiting, and possible agitation or excitement. Death from toxicity is not common but tremors and seizures should be assessed by a veterinarian [3].

LIMITED RESEARCH

While pet parents and the veterinary community wait for research to determine dosing and quality standards for cannabis use in animals, the market is exploding. Hemp products are currently available for cats, dogs, and horses.

Research by Cornell University supports the use of CBD in dogs with osteoarthritis. The study was headed by Joe Wakshlag, DVM, PhD, associate professor and section chief of nutrition at Cornell. Investigators tested CBD oil's pain management properties in a randomized, placebo-controlled, double-blind crossover study. Dogs that received 2 mg/kg CBD oil every 12 hours had reduced pain and increased activity [4].

At Colorado State University Veterinary Teaching Hospital, researchers are evaluating the efficacy of CBD for the treatment of epilepsy in dogs. Each dog will be randomly assigned to receive either CBD or a placebo for 12 weeks and then crossover. The study is still ongoing [5].

Marijuana intoxication in a cat was reported when a 6-year-old Persian cat was brought to a veterinary clinic with strong psychomotor agitation turning into aggression. The cat showed no neurological abnormalities but the behavior changed dramatically. The cat had been exposed to marijuana smoke and was hospitalized until recovery was complete. The cat was returned to its owner and future isolation of the animal from marijuana smoke was advised [6].

A cannabis-based CBD study of 30 healthy Beagle dogs hypothesized that CBD would be tolerated. The dogs were randomly assigned to receive CBD in the form of microencapsulated oil beads (capsule), CBD-infused oil, or CBD-infused transdermal cream at a dose of 10 mg/kg/day or 20 mg/kg/day for 6 weeks. Complete blood panels, urinalysis, and bile acid were performed at 0, 2, 4, and 6 weeks. Elevations in serum ALP occurred in some dogs. All the dogs in the study experienced diarrhea that was not associated with the formulation or dose of CBD. The CBD appeared to be well tolerated but more extensive safety data is necessary to determine if there are any long-term effects of CBD on the liver and an association with diarrhea [7].

COMPLEMENTARY AND ALTERNATIVE VETERINARY MEDICINE

David Ramey, DVM, addresses the controversy in the veterinary profession about the dilemmas for practitioners who may or may not choose to endorse complementary and alternative veterinary treatments [8]. Some states have veterinary practice acts allowing the practice of acupuncture, chiropractic, physical therapy, massage therapy, botanical medicine, and nutraceuticals. Advocates of these practices assert that CAVM (Complementary and Alternative Veterinary Medicine) is holistic and considers the whole patient that standard veterinary practices do not take into consideration.

It took The National Institutes of Health (NIH) a decade to establish NCCAM (National Advisory Council on Complementary and Alternative Medicine). The U.S. Congress passed Public Law 102–170 providing $2 million in funding for fiscal year 1992 to establish an office in NIH to investigate and evaluate promising unconventional medical practices or CAM (Complementary and Alternative Medicine). By 2000, NCCAM was chartered and published its first strategic plan launching CAM or PubMed [9]. Let's see how long it takes the American Veterinary Medical Association to recognize the CAM treatment potential for veterinarians and their patients.

REFERENCES

1. Why Pet Owners Seek Cannabis for Their Pets. http://healthypets.mercola.com/sites/healthypets/archive/2018/11.
2. Leweller H. The lowdown on cannabis in veterinary medicine. DVM 360. May 24, 2016.
3. Meola SD, Tearney CC, Haas SA, et al. Evaluation of trends in marijuana toxicosis in dogs living in a state with legalized medical marijuana: 125 dogs (2005–2010). *J Vet Emerg Crit Care* 2012;22:690–696.
4. Wooten SJ. Cornell takes the lead in cannabidiol research. DVM 360, May 09, 2018.
5. Efficacy of cannabidiol for the treatment of epilepsy in dogs. Colorado State University Clinical Trials. http://csu-cvmbs.colostate.edu.
6. Janeczek A, Zawadzki M, Szpot P, et al. Marijuana intoxication in a cat. *Acta Vet Scand* 2018;60(1):44.

7. McGrath S, Bartner LR, Rao S, et al. A report of adverse effects associated with the administration of cannabinoid in healthy dogs. *AHVMA J* 2018 Fall;52:34–38.
8. Ramey DW. Regulatory aspects of complementary and alternative veterinary medicine. *JAVMA* 2003;222(12):2.
9. The NIH Almanac. www.nih.gov/about-nih/what-we-do/nih-almanac.

23 How To Use Cannabis As Medicine

Betty Wedman-St Louis
Clinical Nutritionist

CONTENTS

For hundreds of years, cannabis has been used as a therapeutic medicine around the world, so when Sir William B. O'Shaughnessy published a summary of his clinical experiences using Indian hemp, pharmaceutical companies took notice. Merck in Germany, Burroughs, Wellcome & Company in the United Kingdom, and Squibb, Parke, Davis & Company, and Eli Lilly & Company in the United States all produced cannabis preparations for joint pain, migraines, stomach aches, muscle cramps, and sleep disorders. Cannabis was an accepted medicine during the second half of the 19th century but its use was declined as single agent pain medications were advocated by physicians who demanded standardization of medicines. It was not until 1964 when the chemical structure of THC (delta 9-tetrahydrocannabinol) was elucidated and its pharmacological effects began to be understood.

Numerous therapeutic effects of cannabis have been reviewed but cannabis-based medicines are still an enigma because of legal issues. Many patients could benefit from cannabinoids, terpenoids, and flavonoids found in cannabis sativa L. These patients suffer from medical conditions including chronic pain, chronic inflammatory diseases (Crohn's disease, IBS), neurological disorders (multiple sclerosis, epilepsy, Tourette's syndrome, Parkinson's), and other debilitating illnesses (depression, glaucoma, PTSD, HIV/AIDS, cancer).

Patients should not be deprived of an opportunity for effective symptom treatment with cannabis despite the lack of randomized controlled clinical trials (RCTs). There is increasing awareness that medicine needs to reconsider its use of cannabis as a botanical medicine with thousands of years of safe and effective use. Many seriously ill and treatment-resistant patients should have the opportunity to use cannabinoids, terpenoids, and flavonoids while government agencies undertake the lengthy and costly RCTs needed to comply with evidence-based medicine.

As Andrew Weil, M.D. wrote in *Self Healing*, July 1999: "It's unbelievable to me that it is still illegal to use marijuana medically in this country. When I published a study in Science on the physiological and psychological effects of marijuana on humans in 1968 while I was still a student at Harvard Medical School, I thought that medical use of the plant would be legalized within five years. I never expected the federal government to take such a harsh stance on what is, after all, an herb for which no fatal dose has ever been established."

HOW CANNABIS WORKS

The chemical compounds (phytocannabinoids) in cannabis bind and interact with the naive endocannabinoids (ECS) in the human body that triggers cannabinoid receptors CB_1 and CB_2 to achieve homeostasis in the body to stop disease. Clinical endocannabinoid deficiency (CECD) has been indicated as the reason for unbalanced cannabinoid levels in the human body according to a 2016 National Institute of Medicine paper (www.ncbi.nlm.nih.gov/pubmed/28861491).

The lack of balanced cannabinoids causes inflammation and leads to chronic pathological conditions when the ECS loses its effectiveness in disease management. A simplistic way of describing this process to patients follows. The immune system responds to an intruder by firing up like a furnace to fry a virus or bacteria and the ECS is responsible for turning down the flame, cooling the fever, and restoring homeostasis.

In 2003, U.S. Patent 6630507 B1 was granted for cannabinoids as antioxidants and neuroprotectants. Every living creature spends their lifetime in a war against free radicals found in the air we breathe, water we drink, and food we eat, so cannabinoid antioxidants can reduce the stress and toxic levels from these external factors. Cells unable to repair the damage caused to endolysosomes will die and trigger inflammation and chronic disease. As the inflammatory process continues and expands for an extended period of time, some receptors are desensitized and start a down-regulation cycle, which can lead to more damage and the difficulty to reduce symptoms.

CANNABIS AS ANTIOXIDANT & NEUROPROTECTANT

Cannabis phytocannabinoids can provide the antioxidant benefits needed to inhibit oxidation. Several lab studies support CBD as an antioxidant and neuroprotectant, but clinical studies are needed to research which cannabinoids, terpenes, and flavonoids are most effective against numerous disorders. The key to successful use of cannabis as a medicine is to select the PROPER DOSE and FREQUENCY along with the cannabis components effective for the condition. The disorders that follow have been selected because cannabis has been used or has been shown to be effective for symptom management. Personalizing the medication to the person is important and recommendations are listed as a guide in clinical management. Over 19,000 PubMed documents can be found on cannabis and this is only a brief overview of a 6-month period along with interviews with physicians who recommend cannabis in their practices.

RESOURCES

Grotenhermen F and Muller-Vahl K. Medicinal Uses of Marijuana and Cannabinoids. Critical Reviews in Plant Sciences. http://dx.doi.org/10.1080/07352689.22016.

Russo EB. Cannabis Therapeutics and the Future of Neurology. Front Integr Neurosci 2018. https://doi.org/10.3389/fnint.2018.00051.

Russo EB. Clinical Endocannabinoid Deficiency: The Latest Evidence. Cann Med 2018. UCLA.

Russo EB. Taming THC: Potential Cannabis Synergy and Phytocannabinoid-Terpenoid Entourage Effects. Br J Pharmacol 2011;163(7):1344–1364.

The Health Effects of Cannabis and Cannabinoids. The National Academies of Sciences, Engineering, Medicine. January 2017.

ALZHEIMER'S DISEASE & DEMENTIA

Alzheimer's disease is the major cause of dementia when the acetylcholine (the memory molecule) in the brain becomes deficient. Research indicates that both THC and CBD can interfere with the buildup of beta-amyloid and neurofibrillary tangles that lead to the disease process in Alzheimer's disease. The phytocannabinoids in cannabis can provide antioxidant and anti-inflammatory activity for neuronal protection.

Concentrations of the body's endocannabinoids—anandamide (AEA) and 2-arachidonoylglycerol (2-AG)—are increased in areas of brain damage and fatty acid amide hydrolase (FAAH) is upregulated in senile plaques causing elevated prostaglandins and other proinflammatory molecules. Neuronal damage increases the production of endocannabinoids, but neuro-inflammation, neurotoxicity, and oxidative stress lead to damage and dysfunction.

Cannabis cannabinoids may slow down the buildup of amyloid plaques and tangles or reduce the inflammatory process leading to their buildup. CBD functions to reduce inflammation and oxidative stress. Its protection stabilizes the mitochondrial membrane needed for cellular energy production. THC has also been shown to inhibit acetylcholinesterase and needs to be considered in the management of Alzheimer's disease.

According to E.B. Russo, M.D. the cannabis components that provide benefits are based on symptom management:

- **Agitation:** THC, CBD, linalool
- **Anxiety:** CBD, low dose THC, linalool
- **Psychosis:** CBD
- **Insomnia/Restlessness:** THC, linalool
- **Anorexia:** THC
- **Aggression:** THC, CBD, linalool
- **Depression:** THC, CBD, limonene
- **Pain:** THC, CBD
- **Memory:** alpha-pinene + THC
- **Neuroprotection:** CBD, THC
- **Reduced Aβ plaque formation:** THC, CBD, THCA

Oral cannabis preparations are good Alzheimer's disease choices since they have extended periods of activity and can easily be incorporated in the daily regime. Sublingual tinctures and oils can easily be provided with a snack and/or at bedtime. Vaping can provide assistance with pain relief or to encourage appetite.

High CBD doses can offer neuroprotective benefits starting with 10–20 mg per day at bedtime and increasing to 100–200 mg daily. THC may be added starting with 2–2.5 mg with the bedtime dose and 1–1.5 mg at daytime doses.

AMYOTROPIC LATERAL SCLEROSIS

Amyotropic lateral sclerosis (ALS) is a neurodegenerative disorder with progressive motor neuron loss, paralysis, and death within 2–5 years of diagnosis. The pathogenesis of ALS is similar to other neurodegenerative diseases like multiple sclerosis due to increased glutamine levels causing excitotoxicity and oxidative damage. As the disorder progresses, neuroinflammation presents as tremors and/or muscle weakness, which develops into full paralysis without affecting cognition. Death usually results from respiratory arrest.

Research studies indicate ALS is a disease characterized by chronic inflammation causing nervous system damage with deleterious effects on surrounding neurons. The endocannabinoid system is believed to be involved in the progression of ALS, so phytocannabinoids could play a role in treatment options. The primary site of the pathology in ALS patients is the spinal cord with lower brain-stem regions in the later state of the disease process.

Weakness begins in the extremities (arms and legs) of the ALS patient, which progresses to dysfunction in chewing, swallowing, and breathing. Slurred speech, difficulty walking, hand and leg cramps, and reduced clearance of saliva (resulting in drooling) progress to the inability to move.

Cannabis offers the antioxidant and anti-inflammatory benefits needed to address symptom management and slow the progression of the disease:

- **Pain**—nonopioid analgesic
- **Spasticity**—muscle relaxant
- **Wasting**—appetite stimulant
- **Dyspnea**—bronchodilator
- **Drooling**—dry mouth
- **Depression**—euphoria
- **Neuronal oxidation**—neuroprotective antioxidant

Oral cannabis preparations of high CBD (100–300 mg/day) with low THC (2–4 mg/day) combine the antioxidant and neuroprotective benefits. Terpenoids like beta-caryophyllene can be added for increased neuroprotection and anti-inflammatory properties.

ARTHRITIS

Arthritis is an inflammatory ailment characterized by joint pain that has been treated with cannabis for thousands of years. The two most common forms of joint inflammation are: rheumatoid arthritis (RA) and osteoarthritis (OA).

- Rheumatoid arthritis is an autoimmune disease, which results in permanent joint damage and disability.
- Osteoarthritis is the loss of cartilage in the hands, hips, knees, and spine.

Pain is one of the primary symptoms of joint disease. The treatment for OA is non-steroidal anti-inflammatory drugs (NSAIDs) but chronic use is problematic due to gastrointestinal and renal side effects. Opiates are usually considered for individuals with severe pain and those who cannot tolerate NSAIDs but abuse potential is problematic.

The Chinese pharmacopeia describes Emperor Shen Nung (2700 BC) as using cannabis for pain and inflammation. Asian cultures from prehistory to present day have continuously used cannabis as a treatment for pain. Europeans and Americans used cannabis for their joint pains until the mid-20th century.

The anti-inflammatory effects of CBD and THC need to be considered in the treatment plans for arthritis. One study in 1973 in the Journal of Pharmacology and Experimental Therapeutics reported that THC had twice as much anti-inflammatory activity as hydrocortisone. A Biological & Pharmaceutical Bulletin study in 2011 revealed that six different cannabinoids inhibited the activity of

COX-2 enzymes, which play a role in arthritis-related inflammation. Other studies suggest cannabinoids may have immunosuppressive properties that could inhibit pro-inflammatory cytokines.

The endocannabinoid system has two receptors that are directly related to pain management. CB_1 receptors are found primarily in the nervous system, and THC is the major stimulant of those receptors. The CB_2 receptors modulate the immune and inflammatory response in the body with CBD as its trigger. Cannabis can be used as a powerful anti-inflammatory to control the pro-inflammatory cytokines associated with arthritis. Beta-caryophyllene, a terpenoid, activates CB_2 receptors and initiates potent anti-inflammatory benefits.

A combination of cannabinoids THC + CBD in a 1:1 ratio is reported to offer pain relief. Begin with a dose of 2.5–5 mg and slowly increase the dose until symptoms are reduced. Adding beta-caryophyllene would also be beneficial. Topical creams can also contribute to pain relief.

ANXIETY DISORDERS—GAD, OCD, PTSD, SAD

Anxiety is second only to pain as the reason many people use cannabis. These disorders can include panic attacks, agoraphobia, obsessive-compulsive behaviors, and even paranoia brought on by acute stress events. Anxiety is a common symptom of those suffering from fear, depression, or excessive worry.

The endocannabinoid system plays a regulatory role in the body's stress response mechanisms because it is intimately connected with the hypothalamus—pituitary-adrenal (HPA) axis. Emotions, stress, depression, anger, and anxiety aren't just psychological but have physical consequences. The stress response begins in the brain when a person confronts danger. The information is sent to the amygdala that sends the distress signal to the hypothalamus for communication with the rest of the body through the nervous system. The sympathetic nervous system triggers a fight-or-flight response providing the body with a burst of energy. If the brain continues to perceive a danger, the hypothalamus releases corticotropin-releasing hormone (CRH), which travels to the pituitary gland triggering the release of adrenocorticotropic hormone (ACTH). This hormone goes to the adrenal glands and prompts them to release cortisol to keep the body on high alert. When the danger passes the parasympathetic nervous system tries to calm the body down after the danger has passed.

In numerous surveys, many people were unable to reduce the stress or danger signals. The chronic low-level stress keeps the HPA axis activated and the effect on the body continues causing health problems associated with chronic stress—increased blood pressure, excess body fat, and weight gain. Elevated cortisol levels increase appetite and the extra calories go unused and get stored as body fat.

Millions of people suffer from anxiety-related disorders, and pharmaceutical companies have developed several drugs—selective serotonin reuptake inhibitors (SSRIs like Prozac and Zoloft) to tranquilizers (benozodiazepines like Valium and Xanax). Alternative treatment with cannabis can be a more favorable option without the negative side effects from the pharmaceuticals. Cannabis has powerful anti-anxiety properties and is safe and well-tolerated.

The five basic types of anxiety disorders can be defined as:

- **Generalized anxiety disorder (GAD)**—chronic worry about events, tense and aching muscles, headaches, trembling, sweating
- **Obsessive-compulsive disorder (OCD)**—odd compulsive behaviors or personal rituals like constant washing hands
- **Panic disorder**—prone to panic attacks, hyperventilation, feeling of doom or death
- **Post-traumatic stress disorder (PTSD)**—witnessing traumatic event, re-experiencing in the mind, "flashbacks"
- **Social anxiety disorder (SAD)**—or social phobias like feeling judged by everyone in the room leading to trembling, sweating when entering room

Both CBD and THC are effective in reducing symptoms of anxiety. Using both in a 2 mg CBD + 1 mg THC or 4 mg CBD + 1 mg THC ratio has been reported with higher levels of CBD ranging up to 50–100 mg CBD for panic and phobia disorders. Terpenoids—limonene and linalool—are important dopamine and serotonin modifiers that can provide calming effects. Sublingual doses taken throughout the day are helpful in mood and symptom management.

ASTHMA

Asthma is a common allergic reaction that causes bronchospasms and airflow obstruction. Cannabis THC can be an effective bronchodilator through activation of CB_1 receptors in the lung tissue. CBD has been shown to be useful because of its effect on the production of pro-inflammatory cytokines—TNFα and IL-6. A Brazil rat study showed CBD to have potent immunosuppressive and anti-inflammatory properties. More research is needed to properly assess the effect of cannabinoids on lung function and how they affect air flow related to obstructive lung inflammation.

Studies have shown that a small amount (200–500 mcg) of inhaled THC is all that is required to dilate the airways especially when terpenoids like pinene are included. The anti-inflammatory effect of CBD at 15–20 mg with 0.5–1 mg THC could produce significant symptom reduction. Sublingual dosing would be more effective than oral consumption during an acute attack. Vaping during a bronchial attack would produce the fastest reaction.

ATTENTION DEFICIT HYPERACTIVITY DISORDER

Attention deficit hyperactivity disorder (ADHD) is characterized by distractibility, hyperactivity, and poor impulse control. Current ADHD treatment is through prescription stimulants but cannabis has been reported to offer an alternative.

Brain scanning studies have shown abnormalities in the gray matter in ADHD and in the connectivity among neuronal circuits within the brain. Other studies have focused on a dopamine neurotransmitter dysfunction as the cause of ADHD. The endocannabinoid receptors, especially CB_1, are very active in the brain, and THC has been shown to improve function.

More research on cannabinoid receptor activity in ADHD is needed but very small doses of THC (2–2.5 mg) or THC + CBD could be tried to improve focus and attention in adults. The effects are not long lasting so a cannabis-infused edible with repeat consumption every 1–2 hours would be needed to maintain a therapeutic dose.

AUTISM SPECTRUM DISORDER

Autism spectrum disorder (ASD) is currently treated with antipsychotic medications, which are not always effective and can have harmful side effects. Fragile X syndrome (FXS) is the most commonly known genetic cause of autism. FXS is associated with the fragile X mental retardation protein (FMRP), which regulates signal transduction in the brain. This FMRP deficiency is believed to increase neuronal excitability leading to hyperactivity, attention disorders, and seizures.

The endocannabinoid system is implicated in behavioral, neurological, and molecular issues related to ASD. Research into cannabinoid receptor function in ASD is ongoing. Both CB_1 and CB_2 are pharmacological targets in animal models. Since CB_2 receptors are considered neuroprotective, CBD extracts have been used in an effect to avoid negative brain development issues in children associated with THC.

A CBD extract dose needs to be calculated based on age, weight, and severity of the child's condition. Begin with a dose of 5–10 mg/kg CBD and titrate up as needed.

BACTERIAL & VIRAL INFECTIONS

Five major cannabinoids—THC, CBD, CBG, CBC, and CBN—have been discovered to be potent against bacterial infections. The specific mechanism of these cannabinoids against bacteria is still unknown and studies are limited. The antibacterial effect of cannabinoids against methicillin-resistant staphylococcus aureus (MRSA) and gonorrhea has a long history. Cannabis was sold as a treatment for gonorrhea in the 19th century because it reduced the inflammation and discharge.

Individuals with weakened immune systems, open wounds, surgical implants, and exposure to bacteria in the workplace and home are likely candidates for a MRSA infection. Many MRSA infections are acquired in hospitals, nursing homes, and prisons.

Viruses are extremely small and always looking for a vulnerable host. A virus enters the body via water, air, or food and attaches to a host cell. Once attached or inside the cell, it takes control of cell function and begins to multiply until the host cell is destroyed and inflammation takes over.

Phytocannabinoids—especially CBD—can be used an immune booster like other antioxidants. Dosing would depend on age and body weight.

BRAIN TRAUMA

Traumatic brain injury (TBI) from accidents, warfare, and contact sports continues to be a significant cause of morbidity and mortality. Concussions can produce headaches, fatigue, nausea, dizziness, and cognitive impairment. Chronic Traumatic Encephalopathy (CTE) associated with football injuries can lead to a degenerative dementia, personality changes, and hallucinations.

The neuroprotective and antioxidant properties of cannabinoids can be used to counteract the glutamate excitotoxicity following a traumatic brain injury. Supplementation with a full spectrum THC, CBD, and acid forms (THCA and CBDA) plus terpenoids like beta-caryophyllene may provide anticonvulsant and neuroprotection needed for treatment of chronic traumatic encephalopathy, brain tumors, and neurofibrillary tangles.

A 1:1 ratio of CBD to THC + terpenoids was reported by EB Russo, M.D. for brain tumors with an 83% 1 year survival rate compared to a 53% rate in the control/untreated group. THCA is noted for decreasing neuronal degeneration even though it is reported not to cross the blood-brain barrier. Juicing raw cannabis leaves is one of the most reliable ways to increase acid forms of cannabinoids and terpenes. Much more research is needed to verify efficacy and dosage for cannabis use in brain trauma but at least it is being considered as a therapy.

CACHEXIA & ANOREXIA

Cachexia is usually associated with the later stages of chronic diseases like HIV/AIDS, cancer, Alzheimer's dementia, chronic obstructive pulmonary disease, and neurodegenerative disorders like ALS. Cannabis has been used as an appetite stimulant in Ayurvedic medicine and the Chinese pharmacopeia for centuries. The endocannabinoid system regulates appetite and the desire to eat via a hunger signaling mechanism. Appetite is a function of homeostatic balance for maintaining body weight. When that balance is altered by physiological and psychological factors, loss of appetite occurs.

Animal studies have shown that CB_1 receptor activation increases food intake, but human cancer patient studies using THC and CBD medications have shown mixed results in reducing weight loss. An Israel study of cancer patients in 2013 indicated reduced weight loss when smoking cannabis as a palliative treatment over 8 weeks. More recent studies including the National Academies of Sciences, Engineering, and Medicine report in 2017 indicates treating cachexia with cannabis is not a very effective method for weight stabilization.

Appetite stimulation dosing can start at 2.5 mg THC sublingually 1 hour before each meal and increase to 5–10 mg THC, if needed. A CBD + THC tincture or extract of 10 mg CBD + 2 mg THC is another possibility. Myrcene and beta-caryophyllene, two terpenoids, could improve the entourage effect.

CANCER

In 1975 the National Cancer Institute published a paper reporting that delta 9-THC, delta 8-THC, and CBD inhibited the growth of Lewis lung adenocarcinoma cells in vitro and in mice. That research was not pursued further at the U.S. National Institute of Health but other countries have continued to build on it. Cannabinoids have been found to exert anti-cancer effects in numerous ways in cell culture and animal models:

- triggering cell death or apoptosis
- stopping cell division
- preventing new blood vessels from growing into tumors
- reducing cancer cell growth throughout the body
- speeding up autophagy

A combination of THC and CBD enhanced the antitumor effects of radiation in a murineglioma model, which indicates cannabinoids can serve as a synergistic treatment with radiation and chemotherapy.

Cannabinoids are useful in managing the symptoms related to cancer treatment neuropathy along with antitumor activity. Human studies are needed to guide in the use of cannabis for treatment of malignancies. Radiation and chemotherapy not only affect cancer cells but damage normal cells as well. Cannabinoids offer the advantage of only killing cancer cells and leaving normal cells unharmed.

A full spectrum cannabis extract would be beneficial as an anticancer agent. Terpenoids have biological properties that offer treatment potential in human breast and prostate cancers. Over 70,000 men and women died of these cancers in 2015. Combination CBD + THC had greater effects for inhibiting cancer cell growth. Cannabinoids offer exciting new dimensions beyond palliative care options for cancer patients.

CBD is a potent inhibitor of cancer cell growth so intravenous administration may offer the best clinical application since oral absorption is slow and unpredictable. Oromucosal treatment has been shown to result in CBD plasma concentration effective to reduce lung cell invasion in vitro.

Sublingual and swallowed tinctures and extracts can be used to manage nausea and vomiting, appetite issues, and pain relief. For best results in nausea and vomiting related to chemotherapy, cannabis needs to be taken 2–3 hours before therapy. Suppositories can be used for pain relief and sleep.

DEPRESSION

An estimated 400 million or more people suffer from depression worldwide according to the World Health Organization. Symptoms can vary from low energy to little interest in life, work, or pleasure. Underlying medical conditions like hypothyroidism, environmental toxins, and nutritional deficiencies may be contributing agents, along with stressful life events. The pathophysiology of depression is believed to be linked to neuroendocrine disturbances in the hypothalamus-pituitary-adrenal (HPA) axis. Anti-depressant drugs are the primary treatment available.

Cannabinoids and terpenes have been shown to offer antidepressant efficacy by increasing serotonergic and noradrenergic signaling. Depressed patients usually have low anandamide and 2-AG blood levels needed for endocannabinoid signaling.

Cannabidiol (CBD) at 5–10 mg can be useful in mood management. Higher doses of CBD 15–20 mg can be gradually considered. Small amounts of THC may be needed if CBD does not adequately improve mood management. A CBD + THC ratio of 5:1 or 10:1 can be used in morning dosing sublingually or as an oromucosal spray. Terpenes linalool (calming and antidepressant) along with limonene (antidepressant) can be added for additional therapeutic benefits.

DIABETES & NEUROPATHY

The number of individuals with diabetes is now at epidemic proportion. Diabetes is a metabolic condition whereby the body does not produce enough insulin (Type 1) or has become resistant to its effect on cellular metabolism (Type 2). Type 2 diabetes or hyperinsulinemia is much more common than Type 1 due in a large part to obesity. The body in Type 2 diabetes becomes resistant to the effects of insulin, which allows glucose to build up in the blood leading to vascular disorders—stroke, blindness, kidney, and nerve damage.

Plant cannabinoids from cannabis can help reduce nerve damage (neuropathy) and reduce inflammation in the retina leading to blindness. Research has shown that CBD and THCV may have a therapeutic benefit but efficacy is lacking.

Oral and vaping CBD in gradually increased doses from 20 mg to 100 mg per day may be considered for neuropathy management. THCV varieties of cannabis are limited but use of it as a therapy needs to be considered when available.

EPILEPSY & SEIZURE DISORDERS

Seizure disorders are potentially life-threatening conditions that invoke brain and nervous system activity. Some people refer to it as "a short circuiting of the body's electrical system." Symptoms range from thrashing movements to loss of consciousness with involuntary spasms throughout the body.

Medieval Arabic medical texts describe epilepsy and the use of cannabis to prevent seizures. Epilepsy is the third most common neurological disease today after migraines and Parkinson's disease. Epilepsy has been treated with cannabis for over 1,000 years but only in recent times have the anticonvulsant compounds in cannabis received scientific investigation. Tetrahydrocannabinol (THC), cannabidivarin (CBDV), tetrahydrocannabivarin (THCV), tetrahydrocannabinolic acid (THCA), and linalool (a terpenoid) have all been considered important in their anticonvulsant activity along with cannabidiol (CBD). Currently, THCA and CBDA—the acid forms of THC and CBD—found in raw cannabis are non-intoxicating compounds like CBD that can be used in high doses for children.

Studies have demonstrated that seizure control is mediated by the endocannabinoid system and THC has produced 100% reduction of seizures. Pharmaceuticals—phenobarbital and diphenylhydantoin—did not have the same threshold for seizure control. Animal studies have shown CB_1 is needed for glutamate excitotoxicity management and anticonvulsant effect was present at lower than sedation levels of THC.

Cannabidiol without THC has been the primary focus of studies leading up to the U.S. Food and Drug Administration approval of Epidiolex for seizures in Dravet and Lennox-Gastaut Syndrome patients. More studies are needed to access the safety and efficacy of all cannabinoids for use in seizure disorders. Dravet syndrome and Lennox-Gastaut syndrome are diagnosed in early childhood and represent some of the most difficult types of epilepsy to treat.

CBD acts as a neutral antagonist of CB_1 and exerts anti-seizure effects due to its antagonistic effect on G-protein-coupled receptor 55 (GPR_{55}) to reduce excitability in nerve cells that are hyperexcited in epilepsy patients. CBD's anti-inflammatory and antioxidant properties also play a role in controlling serotonin receptor 5-HT1A.

THC has been demonstrated to have anti-seizure effects, but its psychoactive potential concerns parents regarding irreversible effects on brain development, which have been found in animal studies.

Initial dosing of CBD at 2–5 mg/kg per day with gradual titration to 25 mg/kg may reduce seizure frequency and provides an adequate safety profile for children. Some pediatric neurologists recommend oral dosing of CBD extract or tinctures + terpene linalool at 10 mg twice a day, with doubling the dose every 3–4 days until seizure control is achieved. Some individuals need as much as 15–20 mg/kg to achieve seizure control. A ketogenic diet is critical for seizure management and needs to be maintained during the use of cannabinoid therapy.

FIBROMYALGIA

Fibromyalgia is characterized by chronic pain throughout the body—in muscles, connective tissues, joint stiffness, and general weakness. Current pharmaceutical treatment includes muscle relaxants, pain medications like opioids and antidepressants. Individuals can develop hyperalgesia related to prolonged stress and physical/emotional trauma. It remains poorly understood but some research is indicating it may be a clinical endocannabinoid deficiency (CECD). Dr. Russo's research has indicated that cannabinoids were more effective than prescription medications in managing symptoms.

A combination CBD + THC may be the best choice to provide symptom management. A starting dose of 4–10 mg CBD + 2–4 mg THC could be used at bedtime with gradual increases in CBD. A 2.5 mg THC + 5 mg CBD dose at bedtime has also been reported as effective in some individuals for sleep and pain reduction.

GASTROINTESTINAL DISORDERS

Cannabis has been used to regulate gastrointestinal issues for thousands of years starting with appetite stimulation to stomach pain, diarrhea, and irritable bowel syndrome to Crohn's disease. The endocannabinoid system regulates all gut function through the millions of neurons that surround the GI tract. Inflammation can occur anywhere along the gastrointestinal tract and can cause many different symptoms: abdominal pain, fatigue, loss of appetite, painful bowel movements, bloody stools, and persistent diarrhea or constipation.

Cannabinoids react with CB_1, CB_2, and $TRPV_1$ receptors to maintain the gut mucosal barrier and regulate GI motility. In the stomach, cannabinoids can inhibit gastric acid production for ulcers and GERD (gastroesophageal reflux disease). Irritable bowel disease (IBD), Crohn's disease, and ulcerative colitis animal studies have shown endocannabinoid changes caused by inflammation.

Cannabis has been reported to relieve abdominal pain, improve appetite, reduce stress, and improve sleep, which all affect the gastrointestinal immune function. Cannabinoids have a profound anti-inflammatory effect through CB_2 by reducing pro-inflammatory cytokines and antagonizing the release of prostaglandins, histamine, and proteases from mast cells. CBD has been shown to be a key modulator in the intestinal inflammatory environment.

Oral cannabis tinctures and oil extracts of CBD improve gut transit and inflammation. A dose of 10–20 mg CBD calms the gut and can be increased as needed. CBG (cannabigerol) would be a helpful addition to the CBD.

GLAUCOMA

Glaucoma is the leading cause of blindness worldwide after cataracts. Studies in the 1970s reported smoking cannabis lowered intraocular pressure. The elevated intraocular pressure (IOP) results from a blockage in the flow of fluid that helps the eye maintain its rigid shape. This fluid usually circulates between the front of the lens and the back of the cornea. Elevated intraocular pressure builds up when the fluid from the anterior chamber of the eye becomes restricted. Increased pressure in the eye causes decreased flow of nutrients to the optic nerve leading to blindness.

Endocannabinoid receptors are found throughout the eye. Both CB_1 and GPR_{18} receptors play a role in intraocular pressure. Several clinical studies have found that cannabinoids reduced IOP. Oral, inhalation, and intravenous cannabinoids all had a positive effect with a single dose of 5 mg THC lasting 3–4 hours. For adequate IOP management, the dose would need to be taken three to four times daily. A 5 mg THC + 5 mg CBD oral extract could also be used. Vaping 2–5 mg THC over short durations of 3–4 hours could be another alternative.

Eye drops would be an efficient route of administration if only they were available. A West Indies product called Canasol was previously available and had the ability to lower intraocular pressure by 50% within 15 minutes.

HIV/AIDS

Human immunodeficiency virus (HIV) attacks the immune system, which provides an opportunity for infections and cancer to proliferate by triggering a lethal wasting syndrome and painful nerve damage. The physical discomforts suffered by HIV patients frequently leads to depression and anxiety. Many of the medications used to keep the virus under control cause nausea and vomiting, which gradually subsides but acutely ill individuals have poor appetites and lose weight.

The destructive process of the virus can progress into AIDS (acquired immune deficiency syndrome) causing cachexia or wasting syndrome. Fatigue and diarrhea are common as the disease progresses. Although combination antiretroviral (ARV) therapy has improved immunity and survival, it does not significantly benefit neuropathic pain. Some nucleoside-analogue HIV reverse transcriptase inhibitors (didanosine and stavudine) can contribute to painful episodes.

Patients with chronic neuropathic pain (burning sensation of the skin) are treated with opioids and NSAIDs. Cannabinoids have been shown to modulate pain perception and offer greater pain relief. In fact, cannabinoids are effective within the entire nervous system, which could affect gastrointestinal function to aid appetite, nausea, and vomiting symptoms.

Oral cannabis for broad spectrum symptom management can be used 30–60 minutes prior to a meal and at bedtime. A combination low THC with medium CBD levels could address appetite and pain. A sublingual dose of 2–3 mg THC + 10–15 mg CBD could be gradually increased to 5 mg THC + 20–25 mg CBD before each meal. For insomnia, 5 mg THC orally 1 hour before bed is usually sufficient. Suppositories are also an effective means of sleeping through the night.

Beta-caryophyllene and Cannaflavin A, a cannabis flavonoid, are both anti-inflammatory molecules with no side effects and could be useful.

HUNTINGTON'S DISEASE

Huntington's disease (HD) or Huntington's chorea is a degenerative genetic neurological disorder similar to multiple sclerosis. It affects the nervous system leading to loss of muscle control and dementia. Once HD symptoms of ataxia and poor coordination begin, dystonia and behavioral issues indicate eventual death. Treatment choices include physical and speech therapy, neuroleptics (tranquilizing psychiatric pharmaceuticals), and gastric tube feedings when eating and drinking become difficult.

A mutation in the Huntington protein (HTT) with unstable repetitions leads to the diagnosis and progression of Huntington's disease. The mutated proteins cause toxic effects on neighboring neurons in the cerebral cortex causing cognitive deficiencies leading to dementia. Widespread neurodegeneration leads to cognitive deficits in attention, memory, and executive function, which usually does not occur until 35–50 years of age.

Cell culture studies have indicated cannabinoids can modulate the toxic effects of the protein aggregation responsible for destroying portions of the brain. Animal studies indicate that CBG (cannabigerol) could modulate some of the HD symptoms.

A cannabinoid combination of CBD and THC would possibly be the best therapeutic regime for CB_1 and CB_2 receptor activation. Dosing 1.5–3 mg THC + 20–50 mg CBD initially once or twice a day, and increasing to 3–5 mg THC + 100–300 mg CBD would provide antioxidant and neurological benefits. Beta-caryophyllene would also be helpful for neuroprotective action.

INSOMNIA

Insomnia is the difficulty to fall asleep or maintain sleep, which can affect mental and physical performance and mood. Common pharmacological treatments include benzodiazepines (Valium), sedative-hypnotic drugs (Ambien), opiates for pain, and antidepressants for symptom management.

Many sleep studies using cannabis in the 1970s and 1980s focused on THC because of its sedative properties. Research showing CBD was effective for reducing anxiety, which may be a factor in sleep disorders, is a more current adaptation. But CBD alone has been shown to be inferior to THC or THC + CBD. CBD can be stimulating for some patients and can disrupt the benefits of cannabis treatment when consumed in the evening.

Cannabis-infused edibles with 5–10 mg THC eaten 1 hour before bed can provide a 5–6 hours duration of sleep without residual effects in the morning. Oral cannabis extracts and tinctures are also effective for sleep quality and duration. They can also be used if a person awakens during the night and cannot fall back to sleep. A dose of 3–5 mg THC sublingually 30–60 minutes before bed can be increased to 5–10 mg THC if needed.

MIGRAINE HEADACHES

Migraines are recurring severe headaches that can last hours to days. Some individuals have auras or flashes of light signaling the start of a migraine. Others report nausea and vomiting occurring with a migraine. Tension headaches affect more than 80% of the population and can be severe in intensity, but migraines are considered an endocannabinoid imbalance.

Cannabis has been a treatment for migraines for more than a thousand years and was the treatment of choice in medical journals—The Lancet, Journal of the American Medical Association, Merck's Archive—until the 1930s.

Ethan Russo, MD has hypothesized that a clinical endocannabinoid deficiency (CECD) may be a cause of migraine pathophysiology. According to Dr. Russo, migraine is a hyperalgesic state similar to fibromyalgia and IBS with elevated AEA membrane transporters and FAAH activity lowering the pain threshold in the individual. A trigger for the headache—hunger, flashing lights, food chemicals, hormonal changes—causes a chemical reaction in the brain that should stimulate endocannabinoids to restore equilibrium but it does not.

Based on research, two approaches can be used for the treatment of migraine headaches. A prophylactic approach is a daily dose of 1–2 mg THC taken upon awakening or the usual time of day when headaches are likely to occur. A symptomatic approach can be used to relieve the pain and nausea at the onset of the migraine. Sublingual or vaping 10 mg THC can be helpful to reduce vomiting and nausea at the onset. A combination of 10–25 mg THC and 10–25 mg CBD dose can help reduce the severity of symptoms. Terpenoids myrcene and limonene can be added for sedation.

MOVEMENT DISORDERS/DYSTONIA

Dystonia is a neurological condition characterized by twisting and turning movements produced by muscle contractions that result in abnormal postures. The overactivity of muscles required for normal movement pushes activation of other muscles and causes pain. Minimum research is available on dystonia but one report of

cannabidiol use has indicated improvement. Five patients with dystonia secondary to Wilson's disease (a disorder of copper metabolism) had improved movement
control with CBD. Others have reported high doses of CBD exacerbated tremor in
Parkinson's patients with levodopa-induced dystonia and oral THC (dronabinol) did
not improve symptoms of cervical dystonia.

Oral doses of CBD 100–600 mg/day may provide improvement in movement
disorders but side effects of high dose CBD include hypotension, dry mouth, light-
headedness, and sedation. Gradual titration of 50–100 mg CBD per day may be a
more tolerable way to achieve symptom management.

MULTIPLE SCLEROSIS

Multiple sclerosis (MS) is a chronic inflammatory disorder of the central nervous
system—brain, spinal cord, and optic nerves—producing spasticity or tremors in
muscles, insomnia, and neuropathic pain. Vitamin D deficiency and smoking have
been recognized as contributing factors in neuronal inflammation.

Research has shown cannabinoids useful in the treatment of MS because of their
neuroprotective properties. Cannabinoids reduce inflammation that occurs from
overstimulated macrophages and microglial cells that cause demyelination and cell
death. Both THC and CBD have shown neuroprotective properties in animal studies
but most research has focused on the use of THC.

THC, whether inhaled or oral, provides nerve pain, muscle pain, anxiety, and
insomnia relief. Symptom management probably requires dosing every 3–4 hours.
A THC and CBD combination of 2–5 mg THC + 15–20 mg CBD has been used for
pain and insomnia. CBD creams and salves have been shown to reduce muscle loss
and inflammatory cytokines in a Tehran University study.

NAUSEA & VOMITING

The emetic reflex that consists of nausea and vomiting is a protective reflex occurring
in many animals. Nausea and pain are warning signs of toxicity to the gastrointestinal tract while vomiting is the means to expel the toxin. Multiple stimuli—visual,
olfactory, and pain sensors are processed through the vomiting response. Irritants can
be food, medications, radiation, and cytotoxic drugs.

Nausea is a complex neurological phenomenon that can be triggered by numerous
illnesses and chemotherapy. Numerous studies have shown the use of cannabinoids
to treat nausea and vomiting with CBD, the non-psychoactive cannabinoid, as effective for chemotherapy-induced nausea and a replacement for anti-nausea drugs like
Zofran and Compazine.

Cannabidiol (CBD) regulates nausea through 5HT1 receptors or serotonin
receptors, which are G-protein coupled channels in the central and peripheral
nervous system. A 5 mg CBD tincture used every 3–4 hours during the day can
reduce nausea symptoms. If a THC and CBD combination is needed for improved
symptom management, a CBD + THC ratio of 10 mg CBD +1 mg THC may be
considered.

OSTEOPOROSIS

Osteoporosis or as the Greek translation calls it "porous bones" occurs when bone cells that normally form new bone do not maintain adequate bone mass to prevent stress fractures. These bone fractures are most common in hip and vertebrae.

Israeli and German studies have shown the endocannabinoid system plays a role in bone recycling to sustain bone density. CB_2 receptors encourage the mineralization and slows the action of osteoclasts to break down bone cells. Beta-caryophyllene, a terpenoid, has also been shown to support bone remodeling.

Topical creams or salves may offer the best promise for improving bone remodeling once the determination of lost bone density has been identified. A high CBD with beta-caryophyllene cream or salve could be applied to hip, leg, and arm areas daily. Supplementing with CBD tinctures and extracts could provide an ongoing enhancement of bone structure but the addition of beta-caryophyllene would not be beneficial since it would be destroyed in the digestive process.

PAIN

Pain is the number one symptom for which people seek medical assistance. Over-the-counter analgesics are the primary source of pain relief but severe symptoms are treated with opiates following surgery or trauma. Chronic pain requires an analgesic without concern for abuse.

The endocannabinoid system is involved in homeostatic and physiological functions of the body, which include pain and inflammation. Pain is unpleasant and a very complex phenomenon to define. Acute pain is a brief event that can easily be resolved. Ongoing nociceptive pain or pathophysiological changes within the nervous system (neuropathic pain) is a burden on the sufferer and affects social interactions, occupation, emotions, finances, and state-of-well-being.

The prevalence of persistent, debilitating pain limits productivity as nociceptors present in the skin, blood vessels, muscle tissue, and body organs signal tissue damage. Chronic pain is associated with higher rates of depression, anxiety, sleep disturbance, and reduced physical activity, which reduce an individual's quality of life.

Cannabis has been used to treat pain for centuries but it was made illegal, and many new synthetic drugs were developed to treat pain, but each has side effects. All people are at risk of chronic pain. Some suffer as joints age (e.g. arthritis), others from genetic predisposition (e.g. migraine), others as a component of another disease (e.g. cancer, heart disease), or as a result of surgery (e.g. severed nerves) or following an injury (e.g. lower back or neck). Pain is a very individual and subjective experience and adequate treatment with cannabinoids can reduce inflammation and stimulate the release of the body's natural opioids.

The benefits of cannabinoids for pain focus on the combination of THC and CBD. Cannabigerol (CBG) is a more potent analgesic than THC because it is a more potent GABA uptake inhibitor, but it is less available in most cannabis strains. THCV is not as psychoactive as THC and has been shown to reduce pain in animal studies. Vaporizing THC (2–7 mg) provides fast onset pain relief compared to oral administration. A THC + CBD ratio of 2 mg THC + 10 mg CBD in an oral tincture can achieve pain relief in 45–60 minutes. Patience is needed to find the right dose and frequency. The best way to describe the pain relief from cannabinoids is to identify that a single dose of cannabis is equivalent to a 60 mg codeine dose, which rates poorly on efficacy compared to non-steroidal anti-inflammatory drugs.

CBD can improve mood through activation of serotonin receptors and is a valuable addition in pain therapy. CBD-rich topicals can be effective as an anti-inflammatory that can treat joint and neuropathy pain. The anti-inflammatory and immunosuppressive actions of CBD are helpful in treating rheumatoid arthritis pain and diabetic neuropathy.

High CBD oral tinctures and extracts 25–100 mg taken throughout the day every 1–2 hours have been shown to aid neuropathic pain. Myrcene, a terpene, has analgesic properties, which can add more therapeutic benefit with CBD. Beta-caryophyllene is also a powerful anti-inflammatory that can be used in topicals.

PARKINSON'S DISEASE

Parkinson's disease (PD) is a form of neural degeneration expressed as bradykinesis, rigidity, postural instability, and tremor. Inflammation from oxidative stress and mitochondrial dysfunction contribute to the onset of symptoms. PD is a difficult degenerative brain condition to treat because of a deficiency in the neurotransmitter, dopamine. Available drugs do not halt the disease progression so tremors, rigidity, and dementia result. Treatment with cannabidiol and cannabinoid acids hold promise but clinical trials are needed. The current use of L-dopa as a replacement therapy for dopamine loss induces an irreversible dyskinetic state with involuntary movement so cannabinoids offer a promising alternative.

Cannabidiol (CBD) offers neural protection against progressive degeneration of nigrostriatal dopaminergic neurons along with causing an up-regulation of copper-zinc superoxide dismutase. As an antioxidant, CBD reduces hyperexcitability and increases mitochondrial protection leading to reduced tremors, less muscle rigidity and less side effects from levodopa (L-dopa) medication.

Oral cannabidiol initiated at 15–20 mg per day can improve sleep and provides modest pain relief. Titration of the dose to 25–50 mg per day may be needed for improved symptom control. Modest amounts of THC are sometimes recommended (2–5 mg) to improve pain, anxiety, and depression symptoms. The terpenoid beta-caryophyllene combined with CBD in a cream or salve can provide additional support for leg, back, and arm pain.

Vaping is also a fast and effective method for symptom management especially when THC is added to the regime.

SKIN DISORDERS—ACNE, DERMATITIS, PSORIASIS

The gastrointestinal tract and skin are both complex immune and neuroendocrine organs with a host of microbes that govern their physiology. Animal tests have identified that anandamide (AEA) and 2-AG, primary endocannabinoids in the body, are produced in the skin at the same concentration as found in the brain. These endo-cannabinoids regulate skin cells—follicles, sebocytes, sweat glands, melanocytes, keratinocytes, and macrophages needed for healing. This system plays a protective role in reducing allergic inflammations of the skin.

High dose CBD in topical creams or salves offer promise for improving sebum production in acne due to its anti-inflammatory properties. Terpenoids—limonene and linalool—would add further anti-inflammatory effects in both teen and adult acne, as well as contact dermatitis. Topical treatments of THC + CBD creams and tinctures have been helpful in psoriasis and eczema. A full spectrum cannabis product would offer the most effective option until further research is available.

TOURETTE'S SYNDROME

Gilles de la Tourette syndrome (commonly called Tourette's syndrome) is a developmental neurological disorder characterized by chronic motor and phonic tics. Tics are an uncontrollable, repetitive movement of muscles that appear as a jerking motion. Tics can be minor in some people and totally debilitating for others. To date, little research has been done on the endocannabinoid role in tics development or symptom management.

Whole plant cannabinoids would be the best advice for patients wanting to explore the use of cannabis to manage their disease. THC tincture and extracts beginning with 2–3 mg THC as needed has been used as a therapy with increased doses titrated up weekly as needed. Vaping is a fast action treatment that could also be considered.

WOMEN'S HEALTH

Women have relied on cannabis for centuries as a therapy for menstrual issues, endometriosis, and menopause. The endocannabinoid system plays a vital role in the uterus and throughout pregnancy, regulating fertility, sexual desire, and post-partum depression. Recent observational studies are indicating women are also using cannabis for hot flashes in menopause.

Today, a woman will experience an average of 450 menstrual cycles or "periods" in her lifetime. For women who suffer from menstrual cramps or dysmenorrhea, these periods represent lots of pain and discomfort. Over 50% of the women in an Association of Reproductive Health Professionals survey reported severe symptoms of dysmenorrhea. Lifestyle modifications of diet and exercise plus OTC medications are the current treatment options. The endocannabinoid link to menstrual cramps has yet to be elucidated but cannabis in a 2:1 or 3:1 ratio of CBD to THC could be considered to reduce pain. CBD alone at doses of 5–20 mg has also been shown to reduce pain.

Women with endometriosis suffer from cells outside of the uterus clustering around the ovaries, gastrointestinal tract, and peritoneum of the abdomen instead of just in the uterus. This abnormal condition causes inflammation and pain associated with the menstrual cycle, pain during sex, and infertility. Limited treatment options are available to treat it but cannabis has been useful in pain reduction.

Dosing THC + CBD at a ratio of 1 mg THC + 3 mg CBD could be considered and care should be taken to avoid high THC products until further research is available.

Polycystic ovary syndrome (PCOS) has been linked to fatty acid imbalance in addition to endocannabinoid deficiency. Fatty acid amide hydrolase (FAAH) breaks down anandamide, which is usually deficient in women with PCOS, so a high omega-3 fatty acid dietary supplement and high CBD extract or tincture would be effective in symptom management.

Use of cannabis in pregnancy is discouraged until more research can attest to its safe use. Some women use cannabis to control nausea and vomiting during the early stages of pregnancy but the science is not available on whether THC crosses the placental barrier and enters the fetal bloodstream where it could alter the developing endocannabinoid system.

Menopause symptoms are common with the decline in estrogen—night sweats, pain during intercourse, and low libido. Fatty acid imbalance can make the symptoms worse because poor fatty acid amide hydrolase (FAAH) results in increased mood changes and emotional responses during menopause. More research is needed on how cannabis regulates FAAH and body temperature but high CBD in tinctures and extracts can be effective in symptom management. Suppositories are also an excellent way of symptom management. A high CBD and low THC: 5 mg CBD + 1 mg THC or 10–15 mg CBD + 2 mg THC could aid sleeping and hot flashes control.

Cannabis Vocabulary— A Glossary

Marijuana, sacred grass, weed, dama are all words used to identify cannabis. When the Marijuana Tax Act in 1937 made cannabis illegal, new terms were contrived by the counterculture which evolved into the "pot culture."

Agricultural hemp: varieties of cannabis sativa L. plant that contain less than 0.3% THC in dry weight material grown for industrial purposes.

Alcohol extraction: a method using alcohol to strip cannabis of its trichomes and essential oils.

Buds: died flowers of cannabis plant.

Budtender: a person who works the counter at a cannabis dispensary who show's the dispensary's products, answers questions, and makes suggestions on product purchases.

Cannabinoid: a chemical constituent of cannabis.

Cannabidiol (CBD): second most common phytocannabinoid in cannabis and referred to as CBD, the non-psychoactive component of cannabis which has been shown to have analgesic, antispasmatic, antiseizure, and other health benefits.

Cannabidiolic Acid: the acid form of cannabidiol which research has shown displays more antimicrobial activity than CBD alone.

Cannabidivarin (CBDV): non-psychoactive cannabinoid used in management of epilepsy.

Cannabigerol (CBG): non-psychoactive cannabinoid with antibacterial benefits.

Cannabinol (CBN): mildly psychoactive cannabinoid produced from the degradation of THC.

Cannabichromene (CBC): cannabinoid with anti-inflammatory and antiviral effects.

Clone: a clipping from a cannabis plant which is rooted and grown as an asexual means of propagation.

CO_2 extraction: high pressure CO_2 that becomes liquid capable of serving as a solvent in stripping away cannabinoids and essential oils from cannabis plant material.

Cure: a process after harvest when the cannabis flower is trimmed and dried and placed in airtight containers for slow drying to maximize flavor.

Dab: a small amount of concentrated cannabis extract about the size of a grain of rice.

Decarboxylation: the process of converting the acid form (THCA) into the active form (THC) which occurs at heat of 240°F or more along with some decarboxylation happening naturally as raw cannabis cures.

Dronabinol: international non-proprietary name for synthetic THC product approved for nausea and vomiting in chemotherapy patients and to treat appetite loss in people with AIDS/HIV.

Dry sieve or dry sift: separation process using a variety of screens and agitation to separate trichomes from plant material which is also known as "kief."

Endocannabinoids: natural cannabinoids produced in human body and other vertebrate animals for regulation of biological systems.

Endocannabinoid System (ECS): has components of receptors, regulators, and cannabinoids in brain, CNS, body tissues, organs, and immune system.

Edibles: cannabis product consumed orally instead of smoking.

Flower: another name for "buds" which are produced when light exposure in the growing process changes to less than 12 hours daily.

Gland: trichome filled with cannabinoids and essential oils found on external surface of plant around the female flowers.

Hash or Hashish: resin glands (trichomes) of cannabis plant that has been sieved into different consistencies for use.

Industrial Hemp: cannabis plant containing no more than 0.3% tetrahydrocannabinol.

Joint: cannabis or "marijuana" rolled in non-tobacco paper.

Juicing: process of reducing cannabis to a liquid in a juicer or blender so nutrients from the plant material can be consumed.

Kief: concentrate composed of trichomes.

Marinol: brand name for dronabinol.

Nabilone: a synthetic cannabinoid similar to THC with 1 mg nabilone = 7–8 mg dronabinol.

Nabiximols: synthetic cannabinoid approved in many countries for muscle spasticity in multiple sclerosis as oromucosal spray containing 2.7 mg THC and 2.5 mg CBD.

Phytocannabinoids: cannabinoids produced in plants.

Rick Simpson Oil (RSO): whole plant cannabis oil administered orally or applied to skin.

Solvent: substance that dissolves another substance and because cannabinoids and terpenes are oils, solvents used to extract them include alcohol, petroleum-based liquids, and liquid CO_2.

Spice: also known as "black mamba," "bliss," "Bombay blue," "fake weed," K2, "moon rocks" is a mix of herbs and manmade chemicals with mind-altering effects.

Sublingual: a method for using tinctures where the liquid is placed and held under the tongue for absorption by porous membranes lining the mouth.

Synthetic cannabinoids: cannabinoids synthesized in a laboratory.

Terpene: volatile aromatic molecules that provide the aroma for cannabis.

Tetrahydrocannabinol (THC): main cannabinoid found in cannabis plants that is responsible for psychoactive properties and other medical benefits.

Tetrahydrocannabivarin (THCV): minor cannabinoid found in some cannabis strains.

Tincture: liquid extraction of cannabis made with alcohol or glycerin for administration sublingually.

Topicals: lotions, creams, and balms used to treat pain and skin conditions.

Vape: vaporizing and inhaling cannabis.

Vaporization: heating the cannabis concentrate to about 360°F (193°C) to turn the THC into a gas that can be inhaled without carcinogens associated with burning the plant.

Cannabis Patient Guide

Cannabis is a herbal medicine used since ancient times. Marijuana is the common name for cannabis sativa, a hemp plant that grows naturally throughout temperate and tropical climates. Cannabis contains over 80 unique compounds that interact in your body. Cannabinoids are the major compounds while terpenes and flavonoids help activate the cannabinoids for

- Appetite
- Energy
- Immune function
- Memory
- Nervous system
- Sleep
- Stress management

CANNABINOIDS

THC is the abbreviation for delta 9-tetrahydrocannabinol, the most well-known cannabinoid because of its euphoric "high" feeling. It also has many health benefits—pain relief, appetite stimulation, nausea, and spasm reduction.

THCA is the raw acid form of THC found in the raw plant leaves and bud. It does not produce the "high" like THC and can improve immune function and reduce inflammation.

CBD or cannabidiol, is the second most common cannabinoid and has proven pain and seizure reduction along with anti-anxiety and anti-inflammatory properties. CBD is non-psychoactive but it can cause drowsiness at high doses.

CBDA is the raw acid form of CBD that has been shown to have strong pain and nausea reduction benefits.

CBN or cannabinol inhibits cancer cell growth and is the most sedative cannabinoid that also has antidepressant effects.

CBC or cannabichrome is anti-inflammatory, anti-viral and used to treat anxiety and stress issues.

CBG or cannabigerol relieves glaucoma symptoms and has antibacterial, anti-tumor benefits.

TERPENES

Terpenes are the essential oils of cannabis and they provide the odor of the plant. There are more than 100 terpenoids in cannabis. Here are five that can help influence which cannabis product will work best for you.

- Limonene (citrus) anti-anxiety, antidepressant, GERD
- Beta caryophyllene (spicy) anti-inflammatory, antifungal, relieves pain
- Linalool (floral/lavender) anti-anxiety, relieves pain, anti-inflammatory
- Alpha-pinene (pine) antifungal, antibacterial, anti-inflammatory
- Myrcene (earthy) relieves pain, sedative, promotes sleep, muscle relaxer

HOW TO USE CANNABIS/MARIJUANA

Cannabis is available in many forms—smoking, vaporizing, drinking it in liquid form, swallowing it as a capsule, eating it in edibles, or rubbing it on the skin. A full spectrum cannabis product offers benefits of cannabinoids, terpenes, and flavonoids but the strength and dose needs to be customized for each person through trial and error.

A log is recommended to allow for more personalization of symptom management. Here is a simple way to get started.

Date	Rate Symptom	Product Used	Results After
	1–10 (1 = less pain, 10 = bad)	Tincture, capsule, edible, patch	1 hour (1–10)
Example	Pain = 8	Tincture under tongue	Pain = 3

COMMON WAYS TO USE MARIJUANA/CANNABIS

- Smoking or vaporizing is the most popular way for fast effect usually within 1–3 minutes, lasting 1–3 hours.
- Tinctures and sprays are liquids that are placed under the tongue. Lollipops are held in the mouth while they dissolve. Onset of symptom relief takes 15–30 minutes and lasts 1–2 hours.
- Edibles are products that are swallowed—chocolate candy, cookies, drinks, capsules. Faster effect comes from consuming on an empty stomach with onset usually 60–90 minutes after consumption and lasting 4–6 hours.
- Patches, lotions, and salves release measured doses of cannabinoids into the bloodstream without going to the liver so effects are noticed in 15–30 minutes and last 3–6 hours. These products are a favorite for those suffering from muscle pain and cancer pain.
- Suppositories are made with cannabis oils for use rectally or vaginally with effect in 30 minutes and lasting 3–6 hours. Rectal suppositories are used for irritable bowel, back pain, and cancer therapy.

DOSING GUIDE

Cannabis is a combination of cannabinoids, terpenes, and other compounds that can effect each person in a different manner. There is not one standard starting dose. A CBD only product can be started at 10–15 mg for an adult and increased slowly until full benefit for symptom management is achieved. A CBD + THC product can include 2–5 mg THC with 10–25 mg CBD to get a combined effect—especially for pain relief.

Use of cannabis products are recommended to start at bedtime to reduce anxiety about uncomfortable reactions. Adjusting the dose with a slow increase over a period of days and weeks is needed until symptom relief is achieved.

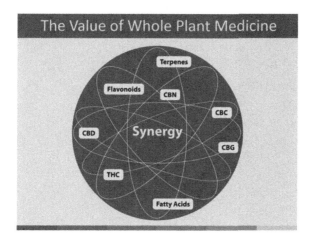

HEALTH EFFECTS OF CANNABIS

Symptom	THC	CBD	CBC	CBG
Pain	*	*	*	*
↓ inflammation		*	*	*
↑ appetite	*	*		
↓ nausea/vomiting	*	*		
↓ seizures		*		
↓ GI contractions		*		
↓ muscle spasms	*	*		
Aids sleep		*		
↑ nervous system		*		
Treats psoriasis		*		
↓ bacteria		*	*	*
↓ cancer cell growth		*	*	*
↑ bone growth		*	*	*

WHAT TO DO FOR AN "OVERDOSE"

If too much THC is consumed through oral consumption or even second hand smoke, recognize the side effects:

Mild = dry mouth, dizziness, rapid heart beat
Moderate = vomiting, walking problems, anxiety
Severe = breathing difficulties, loss of consciousness

Mild and moderate side effects from too much THC can be treated by laying down in a safe place and sleeping off the effects. Severe side effects may require emergency medical attention. Knowing an individual's tolerance level of cannabis is important. Although CBD is non-psychoactive, high doses can cause drowsiness.

Recipes

CHOCOLATE CHIP CANNA COOKIES

1 cup canna butter
3/4 cup brown sugar
1 egg
1 teaspoon vanilla extract
1–1/2 cups all-purpose flour
1/2 cup canna flour
1 teaspoon baking soda
1 1/2 cups chocolate chips

Combine canna butter, brown sugar, egg, and vanilla in mixing bowl. Beat thoroughly. Stir in flours, baking soda, and chips. Mix well. Drop by spoonfuls onto a lightly oiled baking sheet. Bake in 375°F oven 10–15 minutes, or until browned around edges. Makes 20 cookies.

PUMPKIN CANNA TREATS

1 prepared pie crust
1 cup pumpkin puree
2 eggs
1/2 teaspoon pumpkin pie spice
1/2 cup cannabis-infused honey
4 ounces soft cream cheese

Cut pie crust into 6–3 inch rounds with cookie cutter. Lightly oil six muffin pan cups. Place one pie crust round in each muffin cup and press into bottom so edges are flush with top of cup. Beat together pumpkin, eggs, spice, honey, and cream cheese. Fill each crust to top with filling. Bake in 350°F oven about 10–15 minutes, or until crust is golden brown and pumpkin center is firm. Makes six.

CANNA PIZZA

  1 prepared pizza crust
  1–6 ounce can tomato paste
  1/2 cup canna oil
  1/2 teaspoon salt
  2 teaspoons dried basil
  1 clove garlic, minced (optional)
  1 cup shredded Mozzarella cheese
  2 teaspoons dried oregano leaves
  Added toppings, as desired

Place pizza crust on lightly oiled baking pan. Combine tomato sauce, canna oil, salt, basil, and garlic in bowl. Mix well. Spread evenly over crust. Sprinkle on cheese and oregano. Add extra toppings, if desired. Bake in 400°F oven 15–20 minutes until crust is golden brown. Makes four servings.

CANNABIS LEAF PESTO

  1 cup chopped fresh organic cannabis leaves (no stems)
  1 cup fresh basil leaves
  2 cloves fresh peeled garlic
  1 cup freshly grated Parmesan cheese
  1/2 cup toasted pine nuts
  4 teaspoons cannabis-infused olive oil
      (1 tsp = 5 mg THC + 5 mg CBD)
  1/2 cup extra virgin olive oil
  1 teaspoon sea salt

Combine all ingredients in food processor or blender. Blend until smooth. Store in covered container in refrigerator until ready to use as sandwich spread, vegetable dip with yogurt, tossed into pasta, or as topping for baked salmon. Makes two cups.

BANANA CANNA BREAD

  1/2 cup soft canna butter
  3/4 cup sugar
  2 eggs
  1 cup mashed ripe bananas (2 medium)
  1–1/2 cups all- purpose flour
  1/2 cup canna flour
  2 teaspoons baking powder

Cream together canna butter, sugar, and eggs until smooth. Add bananas. Stir in flour, canna flour, and baking powder. Mix well. Pour into greased and floured 9 inches × 5 inches loaf pan. Bake in 375°F oven 45–50 minutes or until browned on top. Makes ten servings.

SWEET POTATO CANNA FRIES

2 large sweet potatoes, peeled
3 tablespoons canna oil
1/2 teaspoon sea salt
1/4 teaspoon garlic powder, optional

Cut potatoes into 1 inch × 3 inches wedges. Place in large bowl with canna oil. Toss. Sprinkle with salt and garlic powder. Arrange potato wedges in single layer on lightly oiled baking sheet. Bake in 425°F oven 15–20 minutes until tender and golden brown. Makes two servings.

GREEN BEAN CANNA CASSEROLE

2–10 ounce cans cut green beans or 3 cups fresh cut steamed green beans
2–10 ounce cans condensed cream of mushroom soup
1/4 cup cannabis-infused butter
2 cups cornflakes
1/2 cup grated Cheddar cheese

Place green beans in lightly oiled casserole dish. Spread soup evenly over green beans. Combine butter and cornflakes. Sprinkle over green beans. Top with grated cheese. Bake in 325°F oven until bubbly and cornflakes are crisp. Makes six servings.

CRANBERRY ORANGE CANNA-RELISH

3 cups raw cranberries
1 navel orange
1 apple
1/4 to 1/2 cup cannabis-infused honey

Chop one cup amounts of cranberries in food processor or blender. Place chopped cranberries in mixing bowl. Peel orange and dice. Add to cranberries. Slice and dice apple. Add to cranberries. Stir in honey and store overnight in refrigerator. Makes four cups.

APPLE SPINACH CANNA SALAD

3 tablespoons canna oil
1–1/2 tablespoons wine vinegar
1 tablespoon Dijon mustard
1 tablespoon cannabis-infused honey
1/2 teaspoon sea salt
1 apple, cored & sliced thin
2 tablespoons chopped onion or scallions
1/2 pound fresh spinach, washed
1/4 cup toasted pecans

Combine canna oil, vinegar, mustard, honey, and salt in bowl. Blend thoroughly. Add apples, onion, and spinach. Toss to coat with dressing. Place pecans on top and serve immediately. Makes 2 servings.

BUTTERNUT SQUASH CANNA SOUP

1 large butternut squash (about 3 pounds)
3 tablespoons olive oil
1/2 cup chopped shallots or scallions
1 teaspoon sea salt
2–4 cloves garlic, minced or pressed
3 tablespoons canna oil
1/4 teaspoon ground nutmeg
4 cups vegetable or chicken broth

Preheat oven to 425°F and line baking sheet with parchment paper. Cut butternut squash in half and remove seeds. Place squash on baking sheet. Drizzle with about one tablespoon olive oil. Sprinkle on salt. Roast squash face down until tender and cooked thoroughly, about 45–50 minutes. Remove from oven. Cool about 10 minutes before scooping out flesh into bowl. Discard skin. Saute one tablespoon olive oil and shallots until shallots are golden. Add garlic and remove from heat. Combine shallot mixture, butternut squash, canna oil, and nutmeg in blender or food processor. Pour in enough broth for blending. Heat mixture with additional broth until ready to serve or let cool and refrigerate for later use. Makes six to eight servings.

Index

A

Absorption, 135
Acetylcholine, 19
Acid forms, of cannabinoids, 186
Acne, 290–291
Acquired immune deficiency syndrome (AIDS), 285–286
Activated microglia, 52
Acute pain, 289
Acute phase, 131–132
Addiction, 215
    cannabis use disorder, 220–222
    case reports, 216–219
    defined as, 219–220
ADHD, *see* Attention deficit hyperactivity disorder (ADHD)
Agonist, 164
    of cannabinoid receptor type 1, 45, 73, 81, 89, 95, 120, 131
    of cannabinoid receptor type 2, 3, 38, 81, 89, 131, 133
    GPR_{55}, 53
Agricultural hemp, 1–4
Agriculture Improvement Act (2018), 1, 235
Akkermansia muciniphila, 75
Alice B, 200
Allosteric modulator, 164
α-humulene, 18
α-pinene, 17
ALS, *see* Amyotropic lateral sclerosis (ALS)
Alzheimer's disease, 275–276
    CB_2 receptors in, 62
American Herbal Products Association (AHPA), 192
American Nutritional Products, Inc., 240
American Society of Addiction Medicine (ASAM), 219
Amino acids, health benefits of, 262
Amygdala, CB_1 receptors in, 120
Amyotropic lateral sclerosis (ALS), 276–277
Anandamide (AEA), 64, 81, 82, 132
Ancient Scythia & Assyria, 225–226
Anorexia, 281
Antagonist, 164
Anthocyanidins, 28
Antibiotics, to treat inflammation, 31
Antidepressant, cannabidiol as, 89–96
Anti-inflammation, 31
Antioxidants, 275

activity, of flavonoids, 31–32
    properties, of cannabidiol, 83
Antipsychotic, cannabidiol as, 96–102
Anti-relapse properties, of CBD, 103
Antiretroviral (ARV) therapy, 285
Anti-stress drug, cannabidiol as, 83–89
Anxiety, 63
Anxiety disorders, 278–279
Anxiolytic drug, cannabidiol as, 83–89
Apigenin, 29
Appetite, 281
2-arachidonoylglycerol (2-AG), 81, 132
Arthritis, 277–278
ASAM, *see* American Society of Addiction Medicine (ASAM)
ASD, *see* Autism spectrum disorder (ASD)
Asthma, 279
Atomic absorption (AA), 265
Attention deficit hyperactivity disorder (ADHD), 279–280
Autism spectrum disorder (ASD), 117–118, 123–124, 186, 280
    CBD cannabis-based treatment approaches for, 119–121
    clinical studies of CBD treatment in, 121–122
    elevated E/I ratio in, 118–119, 123
    treatment, challenges and limitations, 122–123
Autoimmune disorders, 65
Autoimmunity, 65–66
Ayurvedic medicine, 227–228

B

Bacterial infections, 280
Becker, Karen, 269
β-caryophyllene (BCP), 3, 18
β-myrcene, 3, 17
β-pinene, 17
Bhang, 200, 226, 228
Biocompatible polymer PLGA, 149
Bioflavonoids, 261
Bisabolol, 19
Brain-derived neurotrophic (BDNF) levels, 95–96
Brain function, terpenoids, 20
Brain trauma, 280–281
Brief Psychiatric Rating Scale, 63
Buddhism, 226

Printed in the United States
by Baker & Taylor Publisher Services